Tropical Medicine
from Romance to Reality

Anglo-American conferences:

1971: **Medical Care**

SBN 9501555 1 9

1973: **Drug Abuse**

ISBN 0 9501555 5 1

1974: **Continuing Medical Education**

ISBN 0 9501555 7 8

Reports of these conferences may be obtained
from The Publications Department, Royal Society
of Medicine, Chandos House, 2 Queen Anne Street, London,
W1M 0BR, or through any bookseller

1976: **Sexually Transmitted Diseases**

ISBN 0 12 164150 3

1977: **Care of the Elderly**

ISBN 0 12 244950

1977: **The Challenge of Child Abuse**

ISBN 0 12 265550 8

Published by Academic Press Inc (London) Ltd

Tropical Medicine
from Romance to Reality

Proceedings of a Conference 12–14 December 1977

sponsored jointly by the Royal Society of Medicine, London;
the Wellcome Trust, London;
the Royal Society of Medicine Foundation, Inc., New York;
the National Institute of Allergy and Infectious Diseases, Bethesda;
the John E. Fogarty International Center, Bethesda

Edited by
CLIVE WOOD

1978

ACADEMIC PRESS London
GRUNE & STRATTON New York

ACADEMIC PRESS INC. (LONDON) LTD
24/28 Oval Road
London NW1

U.S. Edition published by
GRUNE & STRATTON INC.
111 Fifth Avenue
New York
New York 10003

Library of Congress Catalog Card Number: 78-67901
ISBN (Academic Press): 0-12-763360-X
ISBN (Grune & Stratton) 0-8089-1141-4

Printed and bound in England by
Staples Printers Rochester Limited
at The Stanhope Press.

Contributors

Professor David J. Bradley *Ross Institute of Tropical Hygiene, London School of Hygiene and Tropical Medicine, Keppel Street, London WC1E 7HT, England*

Professor L. J. Bruce-Chwatt, CMG *21 Marchmont Road, Richmond, Surrey, England*

Dr A. E. Butterworth *The Seeley G. Mudd Building, 5th Floor, 250 Longwood Avenue, Boston, Mass. 02115, USA*

Professor Eli Chernin *Department of Tropical Public Health, Harvard University School of Public Health, 665 Huntington Avenue, Boston, Mass. 02115, USA*

Professor Sydney Cohen *Department of Chemical Pathology, Guy's Hospital Medical School, London SE1 9RT, England*

Sir John Dacie *President, The Royal Society of Medicine, London W1M 0BR, England*

Dr M. T. Gillies *University of Sussex, Biology Building, Falmer, Brighton, Sussex BN1 9QG, England*

Dr C. E. Gordon Smith *Dean, London School of Hygiene and Tropical Medicine, Keppel Street, London WC1E 7HT, England*

Dr George Hitchings *Burroughs Wellcome Co., 3030 Cornwallis Road, Research Triangle Park, North Carolina 27709, USA*

Dr Stephen C. Joseph *Deputy Assistant Administrator for Human Resources Development, Department of State, Agency for International Development, Washington D.C. 20523, USA*

Dr John H. Knowles *The Rockefeller Foundation, 1133 Avenue of the Americas, New York, NY 10036, USA*

v

Dr Richard M. Krause *National Institute of Allergy and Infectious Diseases, National Institutes of Health, Bethesda, Maryland 20014, USA*

Dr A. O. Lucas *Director, Special Programme for Research and Training in Tropical Diseases, World Health Organization, 1211 Geneva 27, Switzerland*

Dr Adel A. F. Mahmoud *Division of Geographic Medicine, Wearn Research Building, University Hospitals, Cleveland, Ohio 44106, USA*

Dr Louis H. Miller *Head, Malaria Section, Laboratory of Parasitic Diseases, National Institute of Allergy and Infectious Diseases, National Institutes of Health, Bethesda, Maryland 20014, USA*

Professor G. L. Monekosso *Centre Universitaire des Sciences de la Santé, Universite de Yaoundé, Yaoundé, Cameroon*

Dr S. R. Smithers *National Institute for Medical Research, The Ridgway, Mill Hill, London NW7 1AA, England*

Dr J. Stauffer Lehman *The Edna McConnell Clark Foundation, 250 Park Avenue, New York, NY 10017, USA*

Professor William Trager *Department of Parasitology, The Rockefeller University, New York, NY 10021, USA*

Dr Kenneth Warren *Director of Health Sciences, The Rockefeller Foundation, 1133 Avenue of the Americas, New York, NY 10036, USA*

Dr P. O. Williams *The Wellcome Trust, 1 Park Square West, London NW1 4LJ, England*

Professor A. W. Woodruff *Department of Clinical Tropical Medicine, London School of Hygiene and Tropical Medicine, Hospital for Tropical Diseases, 4 St. Pancras Way, London NW1, England*

Dr C. A. Wright *British Museum (Natural History), Cromwell Road, London SW7 5BD, England*

Contents

List of Participants   v

1   Introduction
Sir John Dacie   1

2   Introduction
Richard M. Krause   3

I. Scene Setting

3   The Real Face of Medicine in the Tropics
Stephen C. Joseph   7

4   The Scientific Neglect of Tropical Medicine
P. O. Williams   15

II. Malaria

5   The Challenge of Malaria: Crossroads or Impasse?
Leonard J. Bruce-Chwatt   27

Discussion   47

6   Cultivation of *Plasmodium falciparum*
William Trager   49

Discussion   62

7   Immunology and Malaria
S. Cohen   65

Discussion   76

8   The Metabolism of Plasmodia and the Chemotherapy
of Malarial Infections
George H. Hitchings   79

Discussion   98

9 New Methods of Vector Control: their Possible Role
in Malaria Campaigns
M. T. Gillies   99

   Discussion   111

III. Schistosomiasis

10 Bilharz's "Splendid Distomum"; Schistosomiasis, 1950–1977
Eli Chernin   115

   Discussion   134

11 Immunology and Schistosomiasis
S. R. Smithers   135

   Discussion   149

12 Cell Biology and Schistosomiasis
A. E. Butterworth   153

   Discussion   169

13 The Use of Chemotherapy in Schistosomiasis Control
A. F. Mahmoud   173

   Discussion   185

14 Possibilities of Intermediate Host Parasite
Relationship Studies
C. A. Wright   190

   Discussion   205

IV. Epidemiological and Environmental Approaches

15 New Epidemiological and Environmental Approaches
to Tropical Infections
David J. Bradley   209

16 New Environmental Approaches to Schistosomiasis
J. Stauffer Lehman   217

   Discussion   220

V. Strategies for the Future

17 The View from the Third World
    G. L. Monekosso   225

18 What the World Health Organization Plans to Do
    Adetokunbo O. Lucas   233

19 Science Knows no Country: the Contributions of the
    National Institutes of Health to Tropical Medicine
    Research
    Richard M. Krause   245

20 The Academic Potential
    C. E. Gordon Smith   255

21 The Role of the Foundations
    John H. Knowles   263

    Discussion: Who Can Do What—Gaps and Overlaps   273

22 Closing Remarks
    Richard M. Krause   281

    Index   285

1. Introduction

Sir John Dacie

This is the second Anglo-American meeting in a series of three organized jointly by the RSM, the RSM Foundation, Inc., of New York and the Fogarty International Center, Bethesda. The first such meeting was held in Bethesda in November 1976, and the title then was "Priorities for Use of Resources in Medicine". The third meeting of the series was also held there in March 1978, when the subject for discussion was "Issues in Research with Human Subjects".

In addition to the organizations I have just mentioned, this particular meeting has also been sponsored by The Wellcome Trust of London and by the National Institute of Allergy and Infectious Diseases, Bethesda. All these organizations have done much to help with the planning and, indeed, the financing of the meeting and we are grateful to them.

In addition, I should like to mention some individuals who have greatly assisted the organizers in the detailed planning of the meeting. First, there is Dr Krause who is a Director of the National Institute of Allergy and Infectious Diseases and who, in addition, I believe suggested the topic for the meeting.

Then, in alphabetical order, I should like to mention the following, to all of whom we are greatly indebted: Dr Alec Bearn, President of the Royal Society of Medicine Foundation, Dr Katherine Elliott from the Ciba Foundation, Professor Sidney Cohen of Guy's Hospital Medical School, Dr Warren from the Rockefeller Foundation, Dr Peter Williams from the Wellcome Trust, Sir Gordon Wolstenholme, Ciba Foundation, and Professor Woodruff of the London School of Hygiene and Tropical Medicine.

Finally, I should like to add that we are most grateful to the Ciba Foundation and to the Wellcome Trustees who arranged hospitality for the participants in the meeting.

2. Introduction

Richard M. Krause

This conference was conceived three years ago at the New York board meeting of the Royal Society of Medicine Foundation which endeavours to promote a special relationship between the medical profession in the United Kingdom and in the USA; these conferences are one of the mechanisms to achieve that objective. Considerable thought is given to the selection of the topics: we seek to examine critical issues of the day, issues which are common to both countries and yet, more often than not, we pursue solutions, understandably, from different points of view. At these conferences, then, there is opportunity to examine, to debate, to vitalize a common interest. In both countries tropical medicine is a specialty conceived out of the very specific needs of colonialism, here in the United Kingdom a legacy of Bruce-Chwatt, for the USA a legacy of Gorgas and Walter Reed. Now we seek the opportunity for a genuine partnership with all people to solve these intractable problems of tropical medicine, and so we welcome especially our World Health Organization colleagues to this conference. We applaud their leadership under Dr Lucas through the tropical diseases research programme which was initiated two years ago and in which we all participate.

Health in the developing countries will require the reapplication of old principles of public health on the one hand, and the generation of new knowledge through research on the other. The parasitic diseases in particular are the last of the known infections to be deciphered in biomedical and biochemical and biological terms. They represent intricate biological systems involving a multiplicity of hosts and a variety of biological life-styles, and we shall be on our mettle to decipher their mystery and their complexity, but I think that it can be done. It was Albert Einstein who said that Nature hides her secrets through her intrinsic grandeur but not through deceit, so I think that we can decipher the intrinsic grandeur.

We again owe a special word of thanks to the Royal Society of

Medicine for all they have done to help us in this conference, especially Sir John Dacie, the current President. I want to thank also past Presidents who have worked with us in thinking through the scope and nature of this conference, the immediate past President, Sir Gordon Wolstenholme, and before that Sir John Stallworthy. I should also like to thank especially Mr Richard Hewitt for all that he has done in the organization of the conference.

Finally, we at the National Institutes of Health welcome the opportunity to participate in this journey from romance to reality. The position has been embraced by President Carter in his message to the Thirtieth World Health Assembly last May in Geneva when he said: "These efforts will brings us closer to our goal, a world in which all people can live free from fear of crippling and debilitating diseases."

I. Scene Setting

3. The Real Face of Medicine in the Tropics

Stephen C. Joseph

Once upon a time there was a garden as full of weeds as of flowers. Three noted specialists were called in to recommend remedies for this situation. The first, a laboratory researcher, said "Until we know much more about the detailed distribution of weed and flower species, and unless we can develop more effective new herbicides and flower stimulants, we cannot do much." The second, a specialist in the organization and delivery of floral arrangements, demurred: "Unless we can make more efficient use of the rakes and shovels that we have, and train more and better gardeners and (especially) garden administrators, we cannot deal with the common weeds which are choking out our flowers." The third pundit, a flora-economist, disagreed with his colleagues. "Flowers and weeds are about equally good cattle fodder, and we probably have too many of both." The three specialists went their separate ways. The researcher turned his attention to the ultra-structure of rose-petals, a field in which much grant support was available. The administrator organized beautiful glass flower exhibits in the capital city. The economist persuaded the politicians to develop a herd of cattle that would require no forage at all. Meanwhile, the garden went on pretty much as before, at some seasons with more flowers and at others with more weeds. . . .

This fable is not without relevance to the focus of this Symposium. We do lack specific biomedical, epidemiological and social-science knowledge and technology with which to attack effectively many of the serious health problems of the developing countries, particularly those countries in which tropical ecologies are combined with rural poverty. The two major health problems which are the subject of this Symposium provide important examples of these gaps. Regarding malaria, increased knowledge is required both of the physiology and biochemistry of the parasite itself and of host-parasite relationships, to provide a basis for the immunological advances that will, it is hoped, lead eventually to an effective malaria vaccine, and to an improved therapeutic armamentarium for prophylaxis, suppression and clinical cure. These topics take on greater urgency in the face of the current resurgence of malaria in Asia and because of the increasing problems of insecticide resistance of the vector and of drug resistance of the parasite. The global incidence and prevalence of schistosomiasis is increasing, exacerbated by the pressure of rapid population growth on agricultural and sanitary resources, and by the association of the disease with large-scale water impoundment and irrigation programmes. Our available knowledge in the areas of case detection, molluscicide technology and human therapeutics has proved inadequate in most countries for the large-scale control of the disease, and the immunological knowledge necessary for vaccine development appears to be far over the horizon. In addition, our relatively feeble understanding of effective health education and behavioural change must be included in the list of constraints to health improvement requiring research advances for application to schistosomiasis as well as to other major health problems.

Similar gaps in knowledge and technology could be described for the other diseases which the World Health Organization has included in its Special Programme for Research and Training in Parasitic Disease—trypanosomiasis, filariasis, leishmaniasis and leprosy. To this list of major health problems requiring fundamental research advance may be added the problem of rapid population growth. Our biological and behavioural science understanding in such areas as the epidemiology of fertility, the behavioural modifications (both of the individual and society) necessary for control of excessive fertility, and the development of mass-applicable effective and safe contraceptive measures, is currently inadequate to the challenge at hand.

Returning to the fable, it is also true that unless we can improve our ability to apply the knowledge that we already have, and new knowledge that we may gain, maximal impact cannot be achieved on the health status of the majority of the population of the developing world. For example, suppose that we had, today, a reasonably effective malaria vaccine: to what proportion of the 425 million people of Africa could we deliver this vaccine, especially in those countries where villages are most isolated, roads least adequate, and trained personnel and petrol most scarce? Although the technical specifics of the problem are quite different from malaria, it is interesting to consider the situation of measles in much of West Africa. We have been in possession, since the 1960s, of a highly effective and increasingly inexpensive vaccine; vaccination programmes in the area in the late 1960s and early 1970s produced rapid local declines in measles incidence and mortality. But in virtually all West African countries these declines were not sustained, as national health ministries found themselves unable and/or unwilling to press on with mass campaigns at six-monthly intervals, as the problems of heat instability and cost of delivering the vaccine in rural areas were increasingly recognized, and as governments became unwilling to assume the costs of measles vaccination campaigns once foreign assistance was withdrawn. The result is that, in nearly all of West Africa, measles incidence appears to be about what it was before the campaigns began, and measles remains, especially in association with protein-energy malnutrition, among the greatest causes of early-childhood mortality. The proposed new WHO Programme in Expanded Immunization will have to grapple with all these problems: adapting bio-medical technology to developing country realities; strengthening health infrastructures so as to be accessible to the mass of the population and so as to sustain the hard-won gains of initial immunization campaigns; and doing all this within acceptable cost.

Beyond the issues of categorical disease control, the problem of organizing basic health services to reach dispersed rural (and also urban-poverty) populations remains a major constraint to the improvement of health in the developing world. It is now well established that prompt recognition and appropriate home and health-post treatment of early childhood diarrhoea with simple oral rehydration can have a major effect on lowering early-childhood mortality from this most common of disease entities. Yet how many developing countries currently possess a health system that reaches far enough into the rural periphery, with sustained contact with auxiliary personnel and village populations, to apply these or other simple promotive, preventive and therapeutic measures on a national basis?

Whether in the development of health systems which can provide basic medical services to dispersed rural populations, in bringing disease-preventive campaigns to bear, or in linking the availability of primary health care with secondary and tertiary levels of the system, it is clear that we have much to learn. Rhetoric, and innovative but limited demonstrations of new ways to train and support auxiliaries and village-based health workers should not obscure the fact that fundamental changes at all levels within existing health systems will be necessary if current and future biomedical knowledge is to be applied to the needs of mass populations. Changes in motivation and relevant competence of public-health administrators, clinicians and inter-mediate nursing personnel are probably even more difficult to achieve than the creation of the auxiliary and community health-worker cadres necessary to extend the reach of health services.

Along with the changes in, and extension of, health infrastructures outlined above, an important set of "application" issues resides in the development of appropriate technology within the health sector. Problems of cost, of technological relevance to the human and physical environment, and of cultural appropriateness to the populations to be served, frame guidelines for adapting existing biomedical technologies to the broader health-care needs of developing countries. This is not at all a question of the development of "second-class" technologies to fit within economic constraints, but rather of combined effectiveness, efficiency and acceptability within different ecological and cultural environments.

The third face of the fable, that of the dialogue between the health sector and economic and political decision-makers, poses the most difficult problem of all. It is of the first importance to recognize that unless or until the health community can be more persuasive about the social utility of investments in both knowledge-generation and efficacious application of health measures, our effectiveness on national and global scales will continue to be limited.

We have not, as yet, developed an adequate language of communication with either economists or politicians. Social, economic and political development decisions that have enormous impact on the health of populations are generally made without adequate consideration of their effects upon physical and mental health: examples abound in the history of schistosomiasis and malaria. Conversely, what is the role of health professionals in speaking to, and acting upon, the root causes of ill-health that lie embedded in social and economic structures? Without question, the amelioration of malnutrition in large parts of the world depends more upon changes in land ownership and land tenure, and upon global balances of power and wealth, than upon either the generation or the application of biomedical knowledge. What are our responsibilities in these areas? What are effective courses of action open to us within our own communities and as members of the global species?

At present, we are unable convincingly to calculate or demonstrate the economic benefits of investments intended to improve the health status of populations. Again, the case examples of schistosomiasis and malaria make this abundantly clear, but it is equally true of investments in basic health services. On another level of complexity, we cannot even assign, especially in economic terms, the relative proportion of contribution to improved health that has been, or can be, attributed to public health and medical activities, as opposed to broader economic and social change; the brilliant work of McKeown serves to illuminate serious questions concerning the impact of biomedical advances. As health workers, we are dependent upon political, economic and social contexts, and can no longer rely upon *a priori* arguments of scientific purity or professional humanitarianism to gain us a large share of scarce resources.

Virtually all of the arguments advanced so far in this paper refer not only to developing countries but to more affluent nations as well, my own among them. I am convinced that the "real face of medicine in the tropics" is only as different from the "real face of medicine in Boston" (or in London) as the physiognomic variation encountered in our species; the underlying structural elements remain basic and universal. Nevertheless, the assigned topic is the "real face of medicine in the tropics". It will be noted, however, that this paper refers to "health" rather than "medicine" and to "developing countries" rather than "the tropics". The reasons for this lie in the conviction that it is the improvement of the health of populations to which we are committed, that medicine (as narrowly defined) has only a limited role to play in this, and that climate and geography are less important determinants of health than are the social, economic and political factors outlined here.

So far I have sketched "the face" from the perspective of the health worker, whether involved in research or application. An outline of the major features of the profiles of the populations concerned may be useful as a context for the other papers of this Symposium: who are the people of developing countries, and in what transitions do they find themselves?

They are the majority of our species (70–75 % of the world's total population), they have demographic characteristics of high birth-rates and high death-rates, and thus have broadly-based triangular population pyramids weighted heavily towards the childhood age groups. They live a largely rural existence in subsistence agricultural patterns, but the massive global trend of urban migration is rapidly changing this picture in many parts of the developing world. This presents new magnitudes of health problems in the growing urban environments, narrowing the margin of existence supplied by the subsistence agricultural base, and eroding the patterns of extended family and village relationships that have provided the cement of survival in most traditional societies.

That the populations of developing countries are "poor", at least in modern economic terms, is part of the definition of their status, as is the statement that most of the developing countries of Asia and Africa are recent independent political entities with a legacy of colonial political and economic dependency. Of major importance is that, on a broad scale, individual and community poverty is increasing in many countries, with respect to the gaps between rich and poor countries, and between the elite and the masses within individual countries. The instances of newly controlled wealth in the oil-producing developing nations raise the possibility of rapid improvements of health status if the benefits of that wealth could be rapidly and broadly distributed across the population. As a contrasting theme, there is the example of the People's Republic of China, where extraordinary changes in health status have been accomplished without significant transfers of wealth from outside, but rather by internal social reorganization.

With few exceptions, the disease patterns of developing countries, especially of the poorest among them, remain fairly constant to the traditional pattern. Although it is clear that worldwide crude mortality rates have fallen significantly over the past century, there remains excessively high mortality largely clustered in children under five years of age, and largely due to the synergism of protein-energy malnutrition with infectious/parasitic diseases. Among the adult population, acute and chronic infectious diseases, and parasitic diseases such as those considered in this Symposium, provide an unmeasured, but probably severe, constraint to economic development.

Most populations of developing countries are poorly served by modern social and economic infrastructures such as education, marketing, transport and communications systems. This is exemplified by their health systems, which are largely based on Western biomedical models that are clearly inappropriate to the needs of the majority of the population, and which have only fragmentary contact with a fractional minority.

In analysing this profile for its implication for our tasks as health workers, where then shall we set priorities? I would like to make three points in this regard.

First, the emphasis must be on wide distribution and mass applicability of medical advances. The gap between sophisticated urban-centred technology and the majority of the world's population is simply too great to be allowed to persist, both for reasons of equity and because of calculations for the survival of our species. This is not an argument against "basic" research, but rather for a balanced consideration both of research priorities and the need to consider the broad application of technological advance. This poses a challenge to biomedical researchers, a new demand for a greater participation by society at large in decisions regarding priority-setting and funding—resisted in the past by many scientists as detrimental to scientific creativity. The balance also poses a challenge to those concerned with organization and delivery of health services, the challenge of developing a more systematic and intellectually rigorous—more scientific, if you will—approach to their activities.

Second, we need to develop an effective language and technology of integration—within the biomedical and health sector, and between this sector and others, particularly the economic and political. Within the health sector, it would seem that self-serving arguments between the "categorical disease" and the "basic health services" approaches are, in the end, sterile. What is required are methods for developing health infrastructures, delivery systems and technological advances in tandem, rather than competitively. Across sectors, we must learn to be persuasive in fostering health improvement as a factor in social and economic development, and we must be active in promoting those social and economic changes that will improve health.

Third, those of us who come from the Western affluent countries (whether we work in international or national agencies, academic institutions or foundations) need to adopt a more humble and collaborative posture *vis-à-vis* developing countries, learning to work with colleagues within their perspectives on their problems, rather than imposing our own preconceptions by the weight of our supposedly superior wealth or technology. There is no simple formula for achieving this, although it may be partly a matter of individual and institutional "style", and the need to think as much about changes to be made within our own societies as about changes desirable for others.

Returning once more to the fable, I suppose that all fables should end with a moral: if mine has one, it is this (with only slight injustice to Voltaire's "Candide"): "We can no longer, each one of us separately, afford to cultivate our own garden."

4. The Scientific Neglect of Tropical Medicine

P. O. Williams

The ink of Science is more precious than the blood of martyrs.

Arab Proverb

I have decided on an historical approach to my theme because I believe that we may be able to learn something from the way in which knowledge developed in the past that will help us to examine, with better perspective, proposals for the future. I limit coverage to the activities of the United Kingdom in relation to its former tropical colonies and their subsequent evolution because the message I wish to convey is well illustrated by this restriction of scope. Discussion may show whether the pattern I describe is mirrored in the USA and hence whether my conclusions can be substantiated by parallel evidence. My chapter falls into three parts, the colonial period, the post-colonial and the future.

The Colonial Period

During the colonial period, many citizens of the British Isles lived and worked in tropical countries either in the armed services, in government or in commercial civilian employment; they were exposed to tropical diseases and many died from them. Because these communities lived away from home, special medical services were developed to look after them, and as a consequence many British-trained doctors worked in the tropics. Their primary task was to care for the health of their fellow-citizens. During the early years of the Empire they were not charged with looking after the health of the local people except those who were employed by the government, the army or on major plantations. These doctors were, for the most part, in salaried appointments but were often allowed some private practice. In the course of their work they came to learn much about tropical diseases and gradually gained a better understanding of them. In India, particularly, from the late nineteenth century until independence, enormous advances were made in our knowledge of a wide variety of diseases: it is fascinating how the whole subject appeared to burst into flame between 1890 and 1910.

These advances at first came from individuals working in their spare time—Manson with his work on filariasis and Ross working on the transmission of malaria. Later, as different disease entities were identified, various organizational arrangements were made such as the Kala-Azar, Plague and Malaria Commissions and the Cholera Advisory Committee; in some cases, Institutes were established such as the Central Research Institute at Kasauli, the King Institute at Guindy and the Haffkine Institute in Bombay. The Medical Research Institute in Kuala Lumpur was also founded at an early stage in 1900. Important discoveries were made about the nature and causation of malaria, kala-azar, plague, cholera, rabies, etc. Men of great stature emerged, such as Sir Ronald Ross, Sir Leonard Rogers, Sir Rickard Christophers, W. G. Liston (who received the Karl F. Meyer Award in 1971 for his work on plague), Shortt, Leishman and Donovan. As a result of this work a great deal was done to control these diseases, usually by relatively simple public-health measures. A fascinating account of this period is being prepared by Colonel Hugh Mulligan and I have been privileged to see some of his manuscripts.

This interest in the elucidation of the nature of disease, leading to its control and treatment, extended to other parts of the world as the British Empire expanded. We all know of the important work undertaken by British doctors on malnutrition, trypanosomiasis, yellow fever, onchocerciasis, filariasis and schistosomiasis in Africa, the West Indies and the Far East. I could dwell at length on the history of tropical medicine during this period but it is an old story and what I wish to emphasize is that relatively few research workers (and they were nearly all medically qualified), mostly without formal research training, often using makeshift facilities, undertook an immense amount of important research. The work was done in the tropical countries and was relatively isolated from the university world of Britain. These doctors had two advantages, they were responsible for patients but were neither overwhelmed by having to care for an enormous number of sick people, nor were they likely to be much diverted by the financial opportunities of private practice.

When India became independent the British focus shifted to Africa, Malaya and the West Indies and there was a considerable build-up of activity there. By that stage the research institute pattern had developed so that the organization of research had shifted from the armed services and the Colonial or Indian Medical Service to the Colonial Research Service with its Institutes (four were established in East Africa alone in 1949), and also a few Medical Research Council Units. Thus, in the mid-1950s there were two British Medical Research Units in Malaya, three in Tanganyika, two in Kenya, three in Uganda, three in Nigeria, one on the Gold Coast, one in Gambia, two in Jamaica and individuals in a number of other places. The people who worked in these places were full-time research workers and nearly all came from Britain. This development of a full-time research service, separate from the medical departments, was a recognition that it is not possible to do much research if one is very busy looking after patients—the role that had by then developed for the members of the Colonial Medical Service. This separation of research carried with it the disadvantage that it became more removed from day-to-day problems and sometimes over-academic. The number of non-medical scientists entering research also began to increase at this stage, with the inevitable result that the work became less orientated towards the solution of specific medical problems.

Towards the end of the colonial period in Africa, universities began to develop in Uganda, Ibadan and Accra; the University of the West Indies was also established. These were at first very largely staffed by British graduates who themselves undertook research on such problems as cardiomyopathy, cancer and hypertension which had not previously been regarded as of significance for the tropics. The British research in the tropics was backed up by tropical schools in London and Liverpool, both founded in 1899 as a result of the efforts of Sir Patrick Manson and the influence of Joseph Chamberlain, the then Secretary of State for the Colonies. The overseas activities in tropical medical research were supervised by a Colonial Medical Research Committee in London and, after about 1960, by the Tropical Medicine Research Board which came under the Medical Research Council (MRC). The supervisory committees were responsible for overall budgets and general review but they did not direct the research of the overseas Institutes.

The pattern is as follows: individuals went to the tropics because jobs were available and through their own interest made important discoveries. The significance of their work was recognized and so gradually a more formalized structure for research was developed, at first through *ad hoc* commissions and later by the establishment of a central organization in London which supervised, but did not direct, the Research Institutes in the tropics. When the British left India they built up the research institute pattern in Africa. Only later were universities places of significance for medical research and their interest tended to be on diseases that would not strictly be called tropical. The universities and institutions in Britain trained these men before they went to the tropics and the Schools of Tropical Medicine acted as centres of knowledge for

those overseas; their staffs also undertook fundamental work. The research workers in the tropics were, however, for the most part, self-
propelled and not dependent for the day-to-day work on the academic
strength of Britain. This was not surprising since most of this development was before the days of air travel.

The Post-colonial Period

When independence came, British citizens who undertook research in
the tropics left and only a few islands of continuing British activity
remained, notably in the MRC Units in the Gambia, Jamaica and
East Africa. The other Institutes were taken over and gradually staffed
by local doctors and scientists. The withdrawal of these opportunities
for British graduates to work in the tropics meant that recruitment very
largely ceased; since British graduates could no longer make a career
in the tropics they diverted their interests in other directions. Over
comparatively few years we witnessed the disappearance from the
medical research scene of a whole generation of medical scientists and
the disappearance too of career opportunities, and hence recruitment
from the next generation. The Army, too, had gradually withdrawn to
Europe and so their research effort was also lost. Britain was effectively
out of medical research in the tropics except for a few individuals
supported by the MRC and the Overseas Development Ministry, the
Wellcome Trust, the Rockefeller Foundation and the Tropical Schools
in London and Liverpool.

After independence the new countries set about tackling their health
problems and naturally directed their primary attention to their sick
people. They therefore set up medical schools and the graduates were
faced with an enormous burden of untreated disease. It was not surprising, in this new milieu, that local doctors and research workers were
not available to take up the research task where it had been left by the
expatriates: the task was too great for the smaller economic units of the
new independent states. Research had, in any case, by this time come to
depend on more sophisticated technology which necessitated special
training. The priorities of the new states were different, their doctors
could not remain isolated from the pressing problems of sick people.

Coincidentally, around the period when Britain was withdrawing
from the tropics, major new medical weapons had become available for
tropical medicine; insecticides, antimalarials and antibiotics. It is
understandable that the tropical countries decided that they need not
put much emphasis on research; it was as much as they could afford to
apply the knowledge that was already available and the prospect looked
extremely bright. It was not understandable, however, that the World

Health Organization, which stood outside the local economic and social arena, and might have been regarded as the inheritor of the health responsibilities of the colonial powers, failed to take a longer-term view and failed to maintain a continuing impetus in medical research. It would be charitable to suppose that it saw greater good might come from the implementation of the measures already available and—being largely health administrators rather than medical scientists—its staff did not envisage the day when these would be inadequate. So research diminished, research workers interested in tropical diseases were no longer recruited or were frequently non-medical and often based in temperate climates where they studied animal models—making considerable fundamental scientific advances but, because they were not in the tropics, their work was not orientated to practical problems.

It had been the pious hope of many that research would be taken over by the activity of the new universities and the rebirth of the old research institutes under regional and national medical research councils. Unfortunately the leaders were, with few exceptions (Dr Lucas, Professor Monekosso and Sir Kenneth Stuart, for example) simply not available or too occupied with administrative responsibilities to be able to keep up their research activity.

All this can, of course, be simply considered an indictment of the method of government of the British Empire which failed to train local people for the tasks that were necessary. But I believe that research activity is directly related to the size of economic units: the British Empire was large enough to afford research, the tropical countries individually, are not. Now, at last, it has been realized by WHO that medical research on tropical diseases is essential, but it took so long to appreciate the effect of neglect that there is now only a sadly depleted group of research workers available to undertake the work required and to train the next generation.

Let us turn briefly to the source of the research activity leading to the discovery and development of the drugs, vaccines and insecticides that have been so significant in altering the medical scene in the tropics. These therapeutic measures did not have their birth in the tropics, they were a product of basic research in universities, institutes and pharmaceutical laboratories of the industrialized world. But even their discovery in these different types of institution would have been of no significance without the existence of the industrial organization willing to take up the new ideas and create suitable finished products for use in the tropics. Unfortunately many of these laboratories have also gradually turned away from tropical problems, partly because their involvement has diminished in the post-colonial phase and partly because the economics of drug development have changed enormously during the past twenty years. The ultra-cautious approach of the world to the toxicity reactions to drugs particularly militates against the needs of tropical countries (but there cannot be two standards).

The Future

This is a greatly abbreviated synopsis of the background to tropical medical research undertaken under the aegis of Great Britain during the period when it was a major colonial power, and of the situation of neglect that has since occurred. A question worth considering is whether knowledge of this pattern helps us to see what should be done to foster research now that there is a real chance that it will once more receive the attention that it deserves. In drawing my conclusions I would like also to draw on my experience, during the past 22 years, of administering medical research at the MRC and the Wellcome Trust and, especially, the tropical programmes of both agencies. I believe there are a number of rules that are just as true for the organization of tropical medical research today as they were in the colonial period, and that any plan for the future must take note of this experience so as to avoid costly mistakes.

First, some general points, not always appreciated by policy-makers.

(1) Research workers are much more interested in the particular topic on which they are working than the importance of their work for the health of man.
(2) It is very difficult to get research leaders of top quality to change their line of work, especially to some unfashionable area.
(3) Research workers must have time to pursue their research and therefore must not be overwhelmed by regular duties such as patient care, administration and committee work. They also require a reasonable degree of stability and security to achieve continuity of their work.
(4) New discoveries and ideas often emanate from university departments but such places are not equipped to develop, test and produce new drugs, vaccines, etc.
(5) It will not be the research workers who will implement the discoveries they make.
(6) A large and elaborate organization is required to develop, test and produce new drugs, etc., and this exists only in the pharmaceutical industry which almost invariably operates on a commercial basis.

A number of special points apply to the situation of tropical research.

(1) The staffs of universities in the tropics tend to see patients with international, not tropical, diseases because the latter are prevalent

in rural areas while the universities are sited in cities. They may also wish to belong to the international rather than to the local or tropical research scene.

(2) Tropical research undertaken in temperate climates tends to be academic and based on animal models.

(3) If research is to be relevant to the problems of medical practice then the research workers must work in close relation to the patients: short visits to collect samples are unlikely to produce deep understanding. The need to have medically qualified workers is therefore very significant.

(4) The research discoveries will only be used satisfactorily if the countries where they are needed have adequately developed health systems.

It may be noted that this list of points nowhere suggests that committees should decide what research needs to be done, followed by an attempt to try to get others to do it: research workers are independent people who pursue their own ideas.

To pull these various threads together and describe what I believe to be the logical way to promote future medical research in the tropics, I will concentrate on the two most important problems—the men who do the job, and the source of the pharmaceutical products which provide the most practical end-result of most research.

The requirements for research are threefold: men, facilities and running expenses, and of these three the men are absolutely paramount. The money available must therefore be used primarily for recruitment and training. The provision of facilities and running expenses is relatively easy. While it is necessary, in order to gather money, to show the opportunity open for tropical research by considering the state of progress in a variety of areas, this will not lead to any new research unless new posts are offered in these fields. But there is an additional qualification. The medical men required must be familiar with tropical disease and the conditions of life and this means that they must spend a part of their career in the tropics—therefore a suitable environment must be available. The major question is what is that environment? Logically it should be in the universities but, in fact, universities in the tropics are not as concerned with the major tropical health problems as might be expected. The alternative of special Institutes is not satisfactory either, as I believe was shown to be the case during the 1950s when this pattern was developed in Africa. The Institutes were in the right places but were too isolated from an intellectual environment as well as from the realities of life: special units in universities may be the solution.

Where should the men we require come from? My answer must be "anywhere they can be found". The opportunity must be made available to people of suitable calibre of any nationality: the object is to get the best men, not the nationals of particular countries where the problems exist. The really important discoveries in medicine have not necessarily been made by nationals working in their own countries: penicillin was discovered by a Scotsman working in London and developed by an Australian and a Russian working in Oxford; it was then produced on a large scale in the USA and was used, among other things, to eradicate yaws from the tropics.

So the first essential is to create an international cadre of research workers of the highest calibre who are interested in both the basic and the clinical aspects of tropical disease, selected simply on account of their quality, trained and offered a stable career. They must work both in the tropics and in the leading world centres, wherever these are. The places where they work should, as far as possible, be politically stable and should not all be in large cities. The recruits should be spared undue involvement in the day-to-day problems of patient care, university administration, etc.—but they should maintain contact with the realities of life. They must be given the requisite support to develop new ideas and to implement the good ones but, above all, they must be able to see a future before them. The precise detail of the framework in which they should be employed poses difficult questions but these must be resolved if we are to reverse the neglect that has been allowed to develop.

Since the pharmaceutical industry has to be the source of new drugs, a way must be found to see that it develops and tests those products that are needed. Clearly there must be some compromise possible between the necessity to work on the most profitable lines and the requirement of the poor people of the world. The most practical approach might be to create some form of contract with industry to develop and test the products required by the tropical countries.

If any use is to be made of the anticipated discoveries and the pharmaceutical developments, then a great deal of support has to go into improving the health service in the countries where the new products would be used. If this is not done, then we are likely to get into the same situation as is current, where valuable products such as measles vaccine are either not being used or are being used unsatisfactorily.

The role of the central organization for research needs to be carefully considered. In the colonial system research was decentralized with a very small administrative structure at the centre. The pattern now being developed by WHO is very heavily weighted centrally, with a large number of scientific and administrative meetings. While I recognize the need to substantiate the case for tropical research in order to obtain funds, it is my hope that once the programme has got under way, too much time and money will not be spent on writing reports and discussing them at a large number of meetings. Knowledge is not advanced by review committees but by research workers themselves.

The Annual Report for 1977 of the WHO Special Programme for Research and Training in Tropical Diseases arrived after this paper had been prepared. I admire the enormous effort that Dr Lucas and his colleagues have made during the past year and the clear way in which they have stated their plans. I am encouraged to see that WHO has already dealt with my points about the pharmaceutical industry, but disappointed that it has not yet been decided to create an international cadre of research workers: I hope that this meeting may recommend that such a step is taken. There still seems to me to be too much of an overlay of nationalism which cannot be the best way to obtain results.

I am apalled by the amount of paperwork being generated and the large cost of administration for the numerous meetings that it is proposed to hold. I fear that the governments of the world, in their anxiety to keep too close an eye on finance, are forcing WHO, I hope against its will, to create an administrators' organization for tropical research instead of the arrangement that would be most suitable for the advancement of knowledge.

The various organizations responsible for medical research in the tropics propose to tackle the novel problem of turning medical research workers back towards this grossly neglected area of medicine. The Wellcome Trust has used its relatively small funds for this purpose for many years during the era of the scientific neglect of tropical medicine. I am very glad that others are now giving this important field the strength of funding it requires.

II. Malaria

5. The Challenge of Malaria: Crossroads or Impasse?

Leonard J. Bruce-Chwatt

Introduction

So much has been said and written about all the ups and downs of the two decades of malaria eradication that any attempt to present once again the story of this rather controversial international endeavour is bound to evoke a "déjà vu, déjà entendu" response. And yet many complex issues of this particular case reflect and focus the unsolved dilemma of the socio-economic advance of the Third World.

From the early days of modern knowledge malaria had been the major endemic disease, though its true incidence and mortality was uncharted in tropical countries (Russell 1955). In the 1930s Sinton (1936) estimated that in the Indian peninsula alone there were about 100 million cases of malaria every year.

> "There is no aspect of life in that country which is not affected by this disease. It constitutes one of the most important causes of economic misfortune . . . hampering progress in every way."

Twenty years later Pampana and Russell (1955) stated that on a world scale the annual incidence of malaria was about 250 million cases with 2·5 million people dying of this disease year after year. There was no doubt that malaria not only killed more people than any other disease, but also interfered with the development of agriculture and growth of industry in the tropics. The intensive control methods of some western countries could not be easily applied in many tropical areas, even though a number of mining and plantation industries in India, Malaysia, Sri Lanka and elsewhere achieved a substantial degree of reduction of malaria using simple methods of prevention, mainly by destroying the Anopheles in its aquatic, larval stage, as advocated by Ross and his followers (Janssens, 1974).

Towards the end of the Second World War the advent of DDT

presented us with a new way of attacking the mosquito vector during its epidemiologically most important stage, when it feeds on man inside his home or near it. Spraying all inside wall surfaces of human dwellings and other domestic shelters with long-lasting insecticide such as DDT creates conditions in which a substantial proportion of Anopheles are killed before they can transmit malaria. DDT's long residual action bordered on the miraculous and it soon became obvious that a large-scale indoor spraying scheme, using this or other residual compounds, was the most practicable and economic method for the interruption of transmission (the attack phase), especially in the rural areas. In the next phase of the eradication programme (the consolidation phase) the remaining foci of infection could be detected by proper surveillance and eliminated by distribution of antimalaria drugs and focal application of insecticides.

The eradication of malaria did not require the total disappearance of all the vectors, and several early examples of successful campaigns (Italy, Cyprus, Greece, Guyana, Puerto Rico and Venezuela) were so impressive that the possibility of the global eradication of disease fired the imagination of many distinguished and experienced specialists. Not all of them realized the operational complexity of a country-wide programme and its utter dependence on meticulous planning, faultless administration, perfect execution, and reliable evaluation (Bruce-Chwatt, 1954). The ambitious worldwide enterprise was formally endorsed by the Eighth World Health Assembly in 1955 and the eradication programme was defined as

> "an operation aimed at stopping the transmission of malaria and eliminating the reservoir of infected cases in a campaign limited in time and carried to such a degree of perfection that, when it comes to an end, there is no resumption of transmission".

When in 1957 WHO took over the co-ordinating activities and the provision of technical assistance, many eradication programmes were initiated in all malarious countries in the Americas and Europe, and in the majority of countries in Asia and Oceania. But only pilot projects were attempted in Africa.

Over the next two decades an immense effort was deployed by some 60 countries, guided and co-ordinated by WHO and supported by multilateral or bilateral funds. Details of the progress of the first decade of this largest public health operation ever attempted have been published annually in the Official Reports of WHO (1961-69) and in a series of papers (Bruce-Chwatt, 1970; Brown *et al.*, 1976). The size of the global campaign can be gauged by the fact that at its peak in 1961 a total of 65 000 tons of DDT and 5000 tons of other insecticides (Dieldrin, HCH) were applied annually. Some 3000 microscopists throughout the world were fully employed by national eradication services. The initial successes in European countries, in the Middle East, in India, Sri Lanka, Taiwan and other countries of the Western Pacific, Mexico, the Caribbean islands and Venezuela were spectacular. It has been estimated (Brown *et al.*, 1976) that by 1968 the population living in endemic malarious areas of the world and virtually freed from the danger of transmission of the disease increased from 316 million to 997 million. Moreover, the direct mortality attributed to malaria decreased from an annual figure of some 2·5 million to less than 1 million. In India alone the annual malaria mortality was stated to have fallen from 750 000 in the 1950s to about 1500 fifteen years later. At the end of the first decade malaria eradication had been attained in 36 countries out of 140 where malaria was present. However

> "There is a tide in the affairs of men
> Which, taken at the flood, leads on to fortune—
> Omitted, all the voyage of their life
> Is bound in shallows and in miseries."

The same is true with some grandiose schemes, and the ebb of malaria eradication began in 1968, though the first signs of it appeared earlier.

The Uses of Adversity

The small cloud of resistance of Anopheles vectors to DDT which existed from the early days of the campaign grew steadily and soon extended to dieldrin, HCH and malathion in several countries. A second cloud, that of plasmodia not responding to prophylactic antifolic compounds and the failure of chloroquine to cure *P.falciparum* infection in two large areas of the tropics, cast an ominous shadow on the progress of malaria eradication. Moreover unsuspected exophilic habits of some anopheline vectors were an obstacle to attacking them by indoor spraying. At the same time a number of operational difficulties arose; some of them were related to the logistics of provision of supplies of insecticides according to precise time-schedules; others were due to the inaccessibility of outlying groups of houses and the primitive structure of dwellings; quite a few were caused by the lack of co-operation of householders who resented the periodic invasion of their privacy and objected, for various reasons, to the spraying routine. All this coincided with (or was perhaps caused by) a gradual decrease of financial support from international sources (such as UNICEF) and some bilateral agencies. Moreover an inflationary rise in the cost of insecticides and labour affected some of the largest eradication programmes of Afghanistan, India, Pakistan, Thailand, Sri Lanka and Indonesia. And yet in programmes at the periphery of the northern and southern boundaries of endemic malaria there was a steady improvement of the situation, and many remarkable achievements, especially in the USSR, Southern Europe and the Middle East.

Realistic assessment of the difficulties that have stopped the advance of malaria eradication in developing tropical countries recognized the paramount importance of administrative, socio-economic, financial and political factors, which affect the improvement of health in countries with inadequate basic health services and shortages of trained man-power (Bruce-Chwatt, 1974). Critical voices became more frequent, though not necessarily enlightening. One of the Presidents of the American Society of Tropical Medicine and Hygiene outlined recently the trends of malaria control in this century and castigated not only the conceptual flaws of the global eradication programme but also its doubtful results and over-optimistic evaluation by WHO (Jeffery, 1976). His main point was that the simplistic technology of eradication was applied mechanically, while our knowledge of the epidemiology of malaria was and still is less than adequate. He admitted that the eradica-tion programmes, though often forced on some countries, have stimu-lated a few public health efforts in the control of other vector-borne diseases, but felt that the overall benefits could have been obtained by less precipitate means and that the costs of the global programme were far too high in relation to its results.

Much of what Jeffery said was true and painfully obvious to many of us, when ten years ago some over-optimistic official reports on malaria as a disappearing disease were reflected in the headlines of the world's press. And yet Jeffery's stinging criticism, made with the benefit of hindsight, was not quite fair. One of the reasons for the early "take-off" of malaria eradication programmes in the 1950s was the realization that some species of Anopheles are becoming resistant to DDT; there was reasonable hope that a concerted, and relatively short universal campaign might eliminate the disease from very large areas before the insecticide resistance should spread all over the world. The second reason was the growing awareness of the damage caused by malaria to developing tropical countries, which elicited an honest attempt rapidly to improve the situation by a well-organized, vertical mass-campaign that would concentrate the effort of each country concerned. It was obvious that an alternative way of slow attrition of the widespread disease was unlikely to show any rapid results because of the time re-quired to build up the basic health services of tropical countries to a satisfactory quantitative and qualitative level. There simply was no inclination then, to indulge in more and more often abstruse research when the promise of the impact of the new tool was so bright. At the end of the halcyon decade of the 1960s a remarkable self-auditing study carried out by the WHO Secretariat was presented to the Twenty-second World Health Assembly (World Health Organization, 1969).

The main conclusions of this report stress that malaria eradication should remain the final goal—a long-term investment because of its overall impact on health and its socio-economic benefits. Wherever malaria-eradication programmes have good prospects they should be pursued with vigour towards their defined target. In countries where eradication does not appear to be feasible because of the inadequacy of financial resources, manpower requirements, or deficient basic health services, malaria-control operations may form a transitional stage towards the future launching of an eradication programme.

Experience has shown that in many tropical countries too little attention has been paid in the past to the availability of a network of elementary rural health services when the crucial consolidation phase of malaria eradication has been reached. It was soon obvious that the final success of any malaria-eradication programme depends not only on the availability of adequate technical tools but also on the community's will and means to use these tools to the best advantage. It comes down to the problems of good management; management and training of manpower, management of financial resources, stimulation of public co-operation—all this in relation to existing needs and conflicting priorities.

Where are we today, eight years after that "agonizing reappraisal" of the progress of the global campaign against the disease, the mastery of which seemed so near? A recent report (Noguer *et al.*, 1976) quotes that at the end of 1975, of the 2015 million people estimated to be living in the originally malarious areas of the world some 824 million (41%) were living in areas where malaria eradication has been achieved; 848 million (42%) were in areas where malaria-control measures are in progress. Comparative WHO data for 1960, 1965, 1970 and 1975 (see Table 1) indicate that in spite of difficulties antimalaria programmes are of benefit to an increasing number of people. However, at least 350 million people live in areas of highly endemic malaria with few if any measures of protection.

Naturally these figures are no more than estimates; it might still be argued that they are on the optimistic side, since the true beneficial effects of various antimalaria measures are difficult to assess. According to a recent report of the Audit Board of the United States Agency for International Development there are today over 480 million people with little or no protection from malaria.

On a geographical basis, judging from the latest WHO reports for 1975, malaria has been eliminated from the whole of Europe, including Cyprus, most of the Asian parts of the USSR, several countries of the Near East, much of North America including the whole of the USA,

Table 1

Population (in millions) covered by antimalaria activities

	1960	1965	1970	1975
Population freed from endemic malaria	298 (33·9%)	535 (45·7%)	727 (52·8%)	824 (49·3%)
Population protected by various antimalaria measures	581 (66·1%)	635 (54·3%)	650 (47·2%)	848 (50·7%)
Population in endemic areas without specific antimalaria measures	457 (34·2%)	405 (25·7%)	437 (24·1%)	343 (17·0%)
Total population living in former or present malarious areas	1336	1575	1814	2015

most of the Caribbean, large areas of the northern and southern portions of South America, Australia, Brunei, Hong Kong, Japan, Singapore, Macao and Taiwan. There is little information about China but it seems that endemic malaria has disappeared from most of that country.

In northern and southern Africa malaria is either absent or definitely on the retreat, while eradication has been accomplished in two islands: Mauritius and Reunion. However, in tropical Africa the situation has remained virtually unchanged over the past 20 years. The striking feature of the disease on that continent is its high endemicity with hardly any seasonal or annual changes; thus, the individual is infected at an early age and is subjected to repeated infections throughout his life. The toll of African malaria falls mainly on the very young, so that malaria is responsible for about 10% of annual deaths of infants and children. Those who survive gradually develop an increasing immunity. Some malaria-control activities, especially the distribution of drugs for prevention and treatment of the infection, are being carried out in urban centres, but the overall situation has not greatly improved in rural areas of tropical Africa, where malaria contributes in a large measure to the vicious circle of disease and poverty.

The numerical reports of WHO indicate that malaria eradication or various control operations cover today some 80% of the population of originally malarious areas. This optimistic statement is subject to caution if it is remembered that the remaining 20% of our unfinished task represents most of the developing tropical world. There is no doubt that what has still to be done will be much more difficult than anything so far achieved. But the most distressing problem of all is the resurgence of endemic malaria in areas where the disease has been kept in check until recently. Among these should be mentioned several countries of Central and South America (El Salvador, Guatemala, Guyana, Honduras, Nicaragua), and Costa Rica, Ecuador, Colombia, and others.

In Asia malaria has increased in Afghanistan, Pakistan, Sri Lanka, India, Burma, Thailand, Indonesia and the Philippines. It is estimated that in Pakistan alone there may be soon at least 5 million cases, and in India twice as many. The wave of endemic malaria that has swept over southern Asia may undo all the achievement of the past two decades.

It was the very complexity of the appraisal of the present situation that led the Director-General of WHO (World Health Organization, 1974) to formulate a set of questions for the attention of the 55th session of the Executive Board. Was malaria eradication a foolish enterprise to start with? Where, when and how did the programme go wrong? Could the technical setbacks have been foreseen by the scientists? Has the overall strategy been wrong? Have the governments and international bodies provided all the necessary support? Several of these questions are reflected and partly answered in the present paper.

As already mentioned, technical difficulties related to resistance of plasmodia or Anopheles to drugs or insecticides are only partly responsible for the present fiasco. The other factors are: inadequate case detection, premature move into the consolidation phase (since the health services were inadequate to deal with the sporadic outbreaks and continued transmission of malaria), shortage of experienced professional and field personnel and last, but far from least, the rising cost of anti-malaria activities as well as the inability, if not unwillingness, of many governments to make the requisite resources available for the control of a disease that was, or was supposed to be, close to eradication. It has become convenient, indeed fashionable, to put much of the blame for the present situation on WHO. The Director-General of the Organization pointed out that the formerly hallowed public health endeavour on a global scale is now being criticized because of setbacks, while the positive experience that it brought is easily forgotten (Mahler, 1976). But the fact is that not much change can be expected until the relevant governments demonstrate their own interest and concern through adequate economic and administrative decisions that will justify greater international support.

The present resurgence emphasizes the role of malaria as one of the many factors at the core of the great issue of socio-economic development of tropical countries. In spite of the great achievements of the global programme, a large reservoir of endemic malaria remains over most of the tropics. The problems as seen in tropical Africa and Asia explain why the eradication of malaria from the whole of these continents is now considered unlikely, as long as their basic health services are inadequate, and until they can muster the necessary human and material resources. One of the consequences is the increasing concern with malaria as one of the tropical diseases now frequently seen in Europe, the USA and other parts of the temperate world. The constantly rising speed and volume of international travel and the lure of exotic holidays at moderate cost have created new conditions for massive importation of communicable disease into countries where these infections were unknown or from which they had gradually disappeared with the advance of public health.

The Great Leap Sideways!

The metaphorical crossroads in the history of malaria eradication can be given the date of 1969; this was the year when for the first time the possibility of the global and rapid *eradication* of human malaria was officially questioned and the desirability of its *control* as an alternative target was endorsed by the World Health Assembly. Such a drastic change of orientation of the programme had not only a psychological impact. It confronted WHO and all the donor agencies with the need to replace the firm tenets of the strategy and tactics of eradication by the much more flexible, not time-limited and untried desiderata of malaria control (World Health Organization, Expert Committee on Malaria, 1974). The main issue was (and still is) how to adapt malaria-control operations to the new situation. A number of essential differences between malaria eradication and malaria control, which previously were only of academic interest, had to be taken into account in establishing operational criteria.

In the first instance, the malaria-control programmes had to be re-orientated to the reduction of the incidence of malaria to a tolerable level, but the degree of tolerance acceptable to the country concerned was left wide open, whether in terms of morbidity or mortality.

Secondly, and in relation to the previous point, malaria control operations would have to be concentrated in those parts of the country where endemicity of malaria is at the highest level and its impact on the health of the population greatest. The difficulty in delimiting such priority areas is obvious, not only for social, economic and political reasons, but also because beyond a certain degree of endemicity the adverse clinical and socio-economic effects of malaria are directed not at the whole indigenous community but primarily at its youngest age-groups.

Thirdly, a major difficulty in securing acceptance of the malaria-control concept stems from the fact that, in contradistinction to malaria eradication, malaria control held no promise of rapid, permanent effects but had to be planned in terms of long-term, continuous and unspectacular commitment, not likely to generate much enthusiasm, but demanding a great deal of steady devotion to a very distant goal.

The fourth important problem was the uncertainty whether malaria-control operations should be planned like malaria eradication, according to the principles of vertical target-orientated mass campaigns, or whether the responsibility for malaria control should be transferred to the basic health services. The latter choice might give to malaria control the broad basis that it requires, but could not provide the impetus of concerted mass campaigns.

The fifth factor is related to the availability of technically competent international and national staff, able to guide the complex national disease-control programmes whose very flexibility and dependence on local epidemiological conditions as well as economic, cultural and political constraints cannot be run "by the book" but require alert, inventive, bold and determined leaders. The shortage of such people is drastic and here a new training activity is of paramount importance and highest priority.

Finally, perhaps the most important question was whether the technical and financial assistance of international agencies and bilateral programmes, so generously provided during the past two decades, would continue to be available. It appears that the international funds allocated to antimalaria activities in 1976 represent only about 42% of those available ten years ago; if the monetary depreciation over that period is taken into account the present funds amount to less than 20% of the former financial assistance.

In 1976 the Executive Board of WHO reviewed, at its 57th session, the progress of the new strategy and recognized the potential gravity of the present situation. The Board took into the account the resolutions adopted by the WHO Regional Committees. The subsequent recommendations covered research, the integration of antimalaria campaigns into the basic health services, and the cost of malaria eradication or control (World Health Organization, 1976).

Some 60 years ago Ronald Ross (1911) stated a truth that should not have been forgotten:

> "The prevention of malaria on a large scale is a great economical as well as a great humanitarian undertaking. A genuine campaign does not consist merely in the formation of inexpert committees, the passing of ordinances . . .; and the issue of wise advice to the public . . . it must always be a permanent concern of the State, requiring careful measurements of the amount of sickness present, a nice appreciation of measures most suitable for the locality, exact estimates of their cost compared with the cost of the disease, a well-considered organization, and, above all, a fixed determination to succeed."

Search and Re-search

There is now a general consensus of opinion that our technical means of controlling, let alone eradicating, malaria from many endemic areas of the world are inadequate. A concentrated research effort may find new ways to attack the malaria parasite and its vector. Fields in which research is particularly important include immunological studies with the view to developing a malaria vaccine, improvement of serological surveillance methods, development and trials of new antimalaria drugs, search for better and more acceptable insecticides (Lepes, 1972, 1974).

Much has been said, written and done about the prospective malaria vaccine and during the past year the advance made by Trager and his group has been so striking that many of us admit the possibility of this achievement. Which of the three types of antigenic stimuli—viz. irradiated sporozoites, purified and lyophilized blood forms or emulsi-fied cultures of merozoites—is going to be the best, time only will show. In the meantime a number of difficulties will have to be solved and it may be premature to talk about the malaria vaccine as an ultimate technological solution of the problem of malaria control. Nevertheless research in this promising and expanding field of applied immunology must be stimulated and supported. The pioneering, imaginative, far-seeing and generous assistance of these studies provided over the past decade by the United States Agency for International Development deserves recognition and admiration.

The place of chemotherapy in malaria eradication depends on both the local epidemiology of the disease and operational facilities. The use of drugs for large-scale treatment is difficult since all those in use at present are rapidly excreted and have to be administered very fre-quently to be effective. Another handicap is the appearance of drug resistance due to the modified response of the parasite to the chemical compounds. Such instances of resistance have been reported in various parts of the world. The Walter Reed US Army Institute for Medical Research has carried out a tremendous scientific programme and dis-covered some 12 groups of new compounds (out of over 250 000 ex-amined) that represent potentially new and valuable antimalarials. This splendid effort should be further carried through by testing some of the new compounds in the field, providing that their toxicity has been fully investigated and that their use in humans presents no undue hazards.

When it comes to new residual insecticides the situation is grim. A systematic search for new compounds, at least as good as DDT, has been pursued by WHO for the past 15 years. During that time nearly 1500 compounds were tested in a series of stages and only a few that emerged were highly active and not unduly toxic to the human population or domestic animals. At the present time the supply of new candidate compounds for the WHO screening scheme has nearly ceased because of the stringent toxicity tests, poor yield of acceptable compounds and rising costs of research and production.

Between 1950 and 1975 the cost of development of pesticides rose by a factor of eight; the mean price of a discovery of a new compound suitable for field trials amounts today to 5 million dollars and takes not less than four years. Some hitherto commonly used compounds, such as malathion, have shown an unexpected degree of toxicity to man in new formulations. It should be added that the ambivalent attitude of several countries (including the USA) to the often imaginary environmental dangers of DDT has greatly hindered the provision of it for malaria control and its acceptance by some developing countries, suspicious of the real intentions of those who are unwilling to use the compound at home and yet foist it on others. The role of the United Nations Environment Programme was not helpful in this respect. For over 20 years DDT, the cheapest, highly effective and safe compound had been in use. With the rising tide of resistance to it, the alternative residual insecticides (HCH, dieldrin, malathion, propoxur) became available. However, many of these alternative insecticides, even if still active against some Anopheles, have a higher toxicity to man and require more frequent applications. Including the cost of transport and labour, residual spraying with malathion is five times more expensive than the application of DDT. Although residual insecticide spraying will remain the best method of attack on adult Anopheles the present trends are towards the older methods of source reduction, larvicides (when applicable), and such time-honoured but uncertain means of biological control as larvivorous fish. Genetic methods of Anopheles control have not fulfilled the early expectations.

There is much hope that the new programme of research on tropical diseases so actively promoted by the WHO will produce before long a few striking additions to the sadly depleted and blunted magic bullets on which we relied until now. The progress over the past year is a good augury for the future and the same can be said about the present concentration of WHO on the rationale of comprehensive malaria control and on training.

However, it would be equally pertinent to emphasize that we must not expect to conquer malaria, a disease rooted in the physical and socio-economic environment of tropical areas, by a miraculous vaccine, drug or insecticide. Each of such scientific tools will be of great value but their proper use will depend on other factors closely related to human ecology in its broadest sense.

Let me quote L. W. Hackett, one of those early pioneers whose lessons were so often ignored and forgotten:

"The mechanism of malaria transmission is so complicated and delicate that it has never been able to resist any long-continued sabotage. Persistence is more important than perfection and whether control is a partial failure or a partial success depends on the point of view. Above all, let us not allow ourselves to be discouraged by theorists . . . and

fight the disease now with weapons already proved useful, albeit im-
perfect, rather than to fold the hands while awaiting a problematical
therapia magna of the future." (Hackett, 1937.)

Vertical or Horizontal?

One of the mistakes of the past lay in failing to recognize that in the
consolidation phase of malaria eradication the surveillance mechanism
for detecting and dealing with the remaining foci of infection cannot be
vested entirely in the mass campaign. Its vertical uni-purpose organization is unsuitable and much too expensive for long-term deployment in
vast rural endemic areas of tropical countries. Sooner or later the surveillance activity will have to be taken over by the horizontally
orientated basic health services. And yet the well-known quantitative
and qualitative shortcomings of basic health services in many developing countries were such that this essential task of surveillance could not
be achieved. Therein lay the main flaw of the original strategy of malaria
eradication. In the present conversion from eradication of malaria to
its control, it has been recognized that satisfactory results can be better
achieved when at least some malaria control activities are the function
of the basic health services.

The WHO Expert Committee on Malaria attempted in the Sixteenth
Report (1974) to outline the relevant role of the basic health services
according to the traditional three-tier structure. But the experience of
the past few years showed the difficulty of determining any functional
pattern, mainly because the organization of basic health services varies
enormously from country to country. In the meantime, we have seen
examples of dismemberment of well-functioning antimalaria services
for the sake of the fashionable but often misunderstood concept of
"integration"—integration into a basic health infrastructure which is
defective, if it exists at all.

The answer to the question "vertical or horizontal" has been given
by Gonzalez (1968) ten years ago:

> "Unquestionably, in most developing countries the conduct of mass
> campaigns and the establishment of general health services must go hand
> in hand for many years towards the goal of a unified health programme.
> The progressive convergence and ultimate merging of the two ap-
> proaches will depend on a number of factors. The concept of integration
> is easily stated and understood but less easy to carry through and it
> cannot be reduced to any uniform pattern. It demands experience,
> imagination, caution and above all trained and abundant man-power."

There can be no doubt that the concept of malaria eradication was
born at the time when we believed that technological achievements

alone will be able to solve most of our health problems and certainly that of malaria. Admittedly the tactics of malaria eradication imply a degree of accurate planning and precise implementation that are the mark of a high degree of technological and executive maturity. But it would be wrong to believe that good malaria control is a simple matter. The present, however sound, philosophy of primary health care promoted by WHO cannot be expected to have a rapid impact on endemic malaria in tropical countries, though it may somewhat decrease its prevalence.

It may appear odd that the obvious difficulties of primary medical care, when it comes to control of some widespread tropical diseases, can be solved only by new therapeutic or other discoveries of the modern complex scientific technology—the very same achievements that are so often derided by Ivan Illich and his followers. True enough, any progress towards a significant decrease of malaria depends greatly on the motivation, co-operation, and determined action of the under-privileged rural societies in tropical areas (Djukanovic and Mach, 1975; Newell, 1975) but not without adequate tools for the job and not while millions of people live at the mere subsistence level. One wonders how their socio-economic conditions can improve in spite of the relentless demographic pressure. But this is a different story!

How Much?

Of all the human diseases malaria is the one that gave rise to the greatest number of attempts to quantify its direct and indirect adverse effects on socio-economic conditions. Sinton's (1936) study of India states that 40 years ago the annual cost of malaria to that country amounted to $400 million. A number of other workers tried to evaluate the burden of malaria on many countries but the results of their studies varied, even if they were not conflicting. A recent excellent study by Borelly (1974) and that by Conly (1975) concluded that the estimation of the true cost of malaria is extremely difficult to assess since a number of imponderables intervene in what appeared to be a simple equation. Abel-Smith (1976) points out that crude cost/benefit analysis, where the only benefits measured are economic, can have only limited application in health.

> "The economic and social appraisal of health programmes is difficult, especially according to a textbook concept of cost/benefit analysis. However, estimation of the probable consequences of a programme is essential for the determination of its priority within the health sector of the national budget. Analyses identifying the least costly option need

not be carried out in great detail; indeed, the uncertainties surrounding both costs and effects may be so great as to render precision specious. The determination of benefits presents overwhelming problems. The effects of a programme are diverse, and there is no method of summarizing the social consequences of changes in health. The common procedure of resorting to market prices is irrelevant because only a few effects have market counterparts and because the prices that are available (particularly wages) reflect existing distribution of incomes."
(World Health Organization, 1976.)

No one doubts that although the adverse effects of malaria vary, the ratio of "economic rentability" of eradication or substantial degree of control of this disease is fairly high, probably between 1:2 (in Italy) and 1:15, as in India (Pampana, 1969). An estimate of the cost of eradication of malaria from the world was made by WHO in 1959 and the average figures per capita per annum varied from US $0·11 for south-east Asia to US $0·80 for Africa. This estimate gave the total cost of eradicating malaria from the world over the subsequent 8–10 years as US $1691 million (Pampana, 1969). It may be of interest to compare this highly conjectural estimate with the actual expenditure on antimalaria programmes as known today.

Over the years 1957–67 WHO (including the Pan American Health Office) had spent on the malaria-eradication programme some US $87 million (including the funds available under the technical assistance component of the UN Development Programme). During the same period UNICEF provided supplies to the value of US $70 million. Assistance provided by the US Agency for International Development amounted during that decade to US $225 million in dollar grants, US $218 million in grants from US-owned local currency, and US $88 million in low-interest loans. The expenses of national governments (at four times the assistance of WHO/UNICEF) were estimated at US $650 million, though it is likely that they were higher. Thus the total cost of the first 11 years of malaria eradication would be of the order of US $1400 million of which not less than 35 % was contributed by the USA. During the period 1968–76 the estimated *annual* WHO/PAHO expenditure on malaria eradication and control was of the order of US $10 million, while the average assistance of AID in grants and loans probably doubled that figure. During the period 1968–76 the total estimated international assistance to antimalaria operations was not less than US $250 million while that of the countries concerned was probably not less than US $1000 million. Thus the cumulative expenditure on global malaria eradication over two decades since 1957 is not less than US $2650 million, a figure somewhat higher than that (US $2000 million) assumed by Jeffery (1976). It may be well to remember that nearly half of the larger sum is due to the generosity of the USA. It should perhaps be pointed out that the seemingly high amount of $2650 million represents about one-quarter of the present annual expenditure of the National Health Service in the UK and one-thirteenth of the sum spent every year on the "health industry" in the USA. Incidentally, the *annual* world expenditure on military hardware was, over the past ten years, of the order of US $300 000 million, or about 6% of the world's gross national product.

While this large amount of money spent on malaria eradication may appear to be excessive in relation to the results obtained in eliminating or curbing the effects of malaria throughout the world, it represents less than US $2·00 per person protected. This estimate may be reasonably accurate but it represents an average, with a range between US $0·70 for India and US $5·00 for the Americas.

We find ourselves on the horns of a dilemma when we consider the cost of malaria control in relation to the available means of the developing countries. It has been estimated (World Health Organization Expert Committee on Malaria, 1974) that in tropical Africa the minimal *annual* cost of anti-mosquito measures and treatment of infected cases is US $0·35 per person per year. However, the average expenditure on medical care and health protection in developing African countries is around US $1·00–1·20 per head per annum, but often very much less. It is this difficulty of the relatively high cost of malaria control, in conditions where there are so many other conflicting priorities, that constitutes the major obstacle to long-term plans for antimalaria campaigns in rural areas of the tropical world. Until the economic conditions of these societies rise to a certain level, commensurate with the present cost of various public health measures, it will be difficult to launch and to sustain a comprehensive and realistic malaria control programme, although small-scale project carried out by a community may improve the local situation.

One of the main lessons learned from malaria eradication is that too much emphasis must not be placed on health technologies alone, since our achievements depend largely on the economic involvement of the countries concerned (Lee, 1974). Many health administrators find themselves in a quandary; reducing malaria to the point where it would no longer be a major public health problem may require as much manpower and money as a time-limited malaria eradication, and it cannot be foreseen how long such support will be necessary. Freedom from malaria can be won, but as long as it remains endemic in large areas of the world the protection from the resurgent infection cannot be relaxed. Neither can it be obtained on the cheap. To the well-known saying: "The price of freedom is eternal vigilance" might be added "But what is the price of eternal vigilance?"

The Ghost in the Machine

Health services throughout the world are now confronted with challenges, resulting from rapid economic growth and technological advance, which manifest themselves in social stresses and pollution of the environment. In developing countries the paramount needs are still related to nutrition, communicable disease and poverty. A high rate of rural to urban migration exacerbates the disparity between the haves and have-nots, while the population pressure outpaces the capacity to provide even the minimal health services to people. The messianic call for "health for all by the year 2000", however emotionally satisfying, may be depressingly Utopian in the face of hard realities. Its mirage-like character, so well stressed by Dubos, becomes apparent when it is realized that 20 years from now the population of the world would reach 8000 million, at least two-thirds of them in the tropical developing countries.

When it comes to the population problem, the medical profession generally and the malariologists in particular have often been accused of being "sorcerer's apprentices" knowing how to do good but not how to undo evil, resulting from their actions. This charge should be seen in a proper perspective. It has been estimated that during the twenty years of the malaria eradication programme the mortality due to the direct effects of this disease fell by some 20 million; but over these two decades the population of the world increased by 1000 million, some two-thirds of it in the developing countries.

The standard of health and education both influences and is influenced by the economic conditions. Standards of health in developing countries cannot rise unless more wealth can be produced to provide for them; and as long as any increase of economic production must be divided by the growing common denominator of the population, higher standards of health and education cannot be attained. The role of health services in the developing countries must be extended to protect the social equilibrium of the community by incorporating the concept of family planning into each and every aspect of preventive medicine (Weller, 1974).

The pressure of populations on the diminishing resources of this planet and the insane way in which we are dissipating these irreplaceable assets form the core of the growing disparity of wealth between the developing and developed countries. Unrestrained population growth can bring development to frustration and can lead to the proliferation of human misery. Unrestrained utilization of natural resources and of geological capital is simply speeding up the day when everything will be gone. Deliberate family planning is alien to those societies where the mortality of infants and children is so high that only half of the new-born babies survive to adolescence. It is likely that the present high fertility of these populations will decrease when health improvements and socio-economic development will remove the instinctive stimulus for a better balance between life and death. But the time-lag between decreasing mortality and decreasing fertility must be counted in decades if not in generations, and no-one knows how the inevitable rise of the demographic pressure will affect the century that is closing upon us. The overriding priority is to stabilize the growth of the world's population at the present number of 4000 million or close to it. It is clear, however, that this is not possible in our time and one is left, like Sir Macfarlane Burnet (1971), with a gloomy certainty of a series of disasters of unimaginable dimensions, due to the development of nuclear weapons.

Two years ago, Lord Ashby compared the resistance of natural ecosystems, which have an astonishing capacity of recovering from disturbances to their equilibrium, with complex man-made systems that have evolved without a corresponding degree of inner stability. The latter systems when small and not too interdependent may preserve some degree of homeostasis. Their equilibrium may also be preserved for some time under a despotic rule that imposes draconian laws, similar to genetic coding in molecular biology. There is plenty of evidence of the lack of balance in the development of many of today's large technologically advanced societies.

The instability of advanced democracies is now acutely sensed. Their industrial base, economic security, moral stance and social systems are precarious. There is no obvious choice of action to preserve these societies from the results of their folly. But there is little evidence that developing countries will choose a different path as long as they are part of the present economic system, and a different system will demand sacrifices that no one is prepared to make.

Aid to developing countries by the advanced industrial nations has now become part of the new understanding of interdependence. However, it may be useful, though unfashionable, to remember, as Boulding (1973) says, that this relationship may create two traps: a "sacrifice trap" for the donor nations and a "dependency trap" for some recipients of aid. The defence against the "sacrifice trap" is an unsolved problem since up to a point it gives meaning to the solidarity of mankind. But it is easy to get locked into a situation that demands too much sacrifice from some and too little from others. The "dependency trap" opens when aids designed to meet a temporary need create such a successful adaptation to them that the need becomes permanent and a welfare mentality prevents an advance towards greater independence. Whether the lofty sentences about the transfer of technology within the "new economic order" will withstand the first cold winds of recession leading to still higher unemployment or a new turn of the screw of the price of oil, or that of essential commodities, is anybody's guess.

Much of what we see today is not really new: the evidence of it has been accumulating gradually. Man as a species has been expanding for half a million years in an even wider ecological niche—but the point has been reached when the prospect of the niche being filled is measured not in centuries but in decades. This has created a feeling of acute anxiety and is reflected in the present questioning of the value of science as a factor of "progress", when it is responsible for a chain of dislocations within societies and between them (Koestler, 1967). "This unease has resulted in equating the progress of science with the disasters of runaway technology, the vicissitudes of the business cycle, the decline of moral standards and the baffling complexities of human life"—these are the words of Dr Philip Handler, President of the United States Academy of Sciences, spoken last November in London at the Royal Society.

Science is no longer the good fairy, distributing her fruits to those who know how to ask her. It plays now a leading role in the drama of our hopes and fears; it has become open to social conflicts. In the process, everything that we owe to science and technology is fading from the memories of men and only the difficulties or perils of too much knowledge are being stressed. Medawar (1973) pointed out how often we wring our hands over the miscarriages of technology and take its benefactions for granted. There is, as he says, a sense in which science and technology can be arraigned for the deterioration of environment or for devising new instruments of warfare, but it is the height of folly to blame the weapon for the crime. As Medawar puts it: "In the management of our affairs we have too often been bad workmen, and like all bad workmen we blame our own tools."

Science and technology have a social dimension which calls not only for their better management in relevance to social needs but also for the maintenance of our civilization. The real problems are not created by the surfeit of human knowledge but by human behaviour and inept social systems. But the challenge presented by any or all these problems will not be met without the contribution of science as the factor of national and international responsibility and policy decisions. And yet, scientific and cultural aspects of social problems seem to be too complex to fit into the activities of social planners, swayed by this or that political credo.

The fundamental unity of human mind gives to knowledge its universal mark. But while the facts and laws of science are valid everywhere the application of science varies from one society to another (Dubos, 1970). Scientific knowledge is not sufficient to formulate values that govern human behaviour, nor can it impose them on the human society. However, it provides a basis for options and can indicate certain consequences that will result from technological or social practices. We have largely replaced the blind mechanism of natural selection by some forms of conscious interference and this is particularly obvious in the field of medicine and public health. Human societies must become aware of the consequences of their conduct and prevent the present drift of mankind to disaster by more deliberate tactics, with a view to a common goal.

Science cannot always provide the ultimate answers, but it can and does formulate pertinent questions. Knowledge, moral choice and a collective action on an unprecedented scale may yet save us but the time for decision is brief and getting shorter every day.

References

Abel-Smith, B. (1965). An international study of health expenditure. *WHO Public Health Papers*, no. 32, Geneva.

Abel-Smith, B. (1976). "Value for Money in Health Services". Heinemann, London.

Borelly, R. (1974). "L'économie du paludisme" (University of Grenoble thesis).

Boulding, K. E. (1973). "The Economy of Love and Fear". Wadsworth, Belmont (Colorado).

Brown, A. W., Haworth, J. and Zahar, A. (1976). Malaria eradication and control from a global standpoint. *Journal of Medical Entomology*, **13**, 1–25.

Bruce-Chwatt, L. J. (1954). Problems of malaria control in tropical Africa. *British Medical Journal*, **1**, 169–74.

Bruce-Chwatt, L. J. (1970). Global review of malaria control and eradication. *Miscellaneous Publications of the Entomological Society of America*, **7**, 7.

Bruce-Chwatt, L. J. (1974). Twenty years of malaria eradication. *British Journal of Hospital Medicine*, **2**, 381–88.

Burnet, Sir Macfarlane (1971). "Genes, Dreams and Realities". Medical and Technical Publishing Company, Aylesbury, Bucks.

Conly, G. N. (1975). The impact of malaria on economic development. *PAHO/WHO Scientific Publication*, no. 297, Washington, DC.

Djukanovic, V. and Mach, E. P. (1975). "Alternative Approaches to Meeting Basic Health Needs". World Health Organization, Geneva.

Dubos, R. (1970). "Reason Awake". Columbia University Press, New York.

Gonzalez, C. L. (1968). Mass campaigns and general health services. *WHO Public Health Papers*, no. 29, Geneva.

Hackett, G. W. (1937). "Malaria in Europe". Oxford University Press, London.

Janssens, P. G. (1974). Le procés du paludisme. *Journal of Tropical Medicine and Hygiene*, **77**, 39–47.

Jeffery, G. M. (1976). Malaria control in the 20th century. *American Journal of Tropical Medicine and Hygiene*, **25**, 361–6.

Koestler, A. (1967). "The Ghost in the Machine". Hutchinson, London.

Lee, J. A. (1974). Economic development in the Third World: Some implications for health. *Journal of Tropical Medicine and Hygiene*, **77**, 14–18.

Lepes, T. (1972). Research related to malaria. *American Journal of Tropical Medicine and Hygiene*, **21**, 640–7.

Lepes, T. (1974). Present status of the global malaria eradication programme and prospects for the future. *Journal of Tropical Medicine and Hygiene*, **77**, 47–53.

Mahler, H. (1976). Health strategies in a changing world. *WHO Chronicle*, **29**, 209–18.

Medawar, P. (1973). "The Hope of Progress". Anchor Books, New York.

Newell, K. (1975). "Health by the People". World Health Organization, Geneva.

Noguer, A., Wernsdorfer, W. and Kouznetsov, R. (1976). The malaria situation in 1975. *WHO Chronicle*, **30**, 486.

Pampana, E. J. (1969). "A Textbook of Malaria Eradication", 2nd edn. Oxford University Press, London.

Pampana, E. J. and Russell, P. E. (1955). Malaria—a world problem. *WHO Chronicle*, **9**, 31.

Ross, R. (1911). "The Prevention of Malaria". John Murray, London.

Russell, P. F. (1955). "Man's Mastery of Malaria". Oxford University Press, London.

Sinton, A. J. (1936). What malaria costs India? *Record of the Malaria Survey, India*, no. 6, Delhi.

Weller, T. H. (1974). World health in a changing world. *Journal of Tropical Medicine and Hygiene*, **77**, 59–61.

World Health Organization (1969). Re-examination of the global strategy of malaria eradication (Twenty-second World Health Assembly, Annex 13). *WHO Official Records*, no. 176, p. 106.

World Health Organization (1974). Twenty-seventh World Health Assembly. *WHO Chronicle*, **28**, 347–50.

World Health Organization, Expert Committee on Malaria (1974). Sixteenth Report. *WHO Technical Report Series*, no. 549.

World Health Organization (1976). Development of the antimalaria programme. (Report of Committee on Malaria to the Executive Board, 57th session, unpublished document EB 57/119.)

World Health Organization (1977). Thirtieth World Health Assembly. *WHO Chronicle*, **31**, 255–60.

Discussion

Professor Bruce-Chwatt thought it unlikely that malaria would be abolished in the near future, and although a malaria vaccine was desirable, control of the disease could not depend solely on possible technological advances. Health planning in tropical countries should incorporate malaria control into the development of basic health services.

Dr W. Ormerod (*London School of Hygiene and Tropical Medicine*) asked whether the consequences of eliminating malaria totally had been considered. It could lead to a rise in population, an increased food requirement, cutting down of forests, degradation of agriculture and starvation. Although he did not wish to belittle the achievements of malaria eradication which had been described, he felt it was necessary to consider the consequences of success as well as those of failure.

Professor Bruce-Chwatt said that Dr Ormerod had raised an important point, but that in his opinion, if malaria were eradicated from, say, South America it could lead to a reduction in infant mortality and general morbidity and an increase of agricultural and industrial production with probable benefits to the population concerned. Regarding malaria and population problems, he said that eradication of malaria had undoubtedly contributed to a certain amount of population pressure in some parts of the world, but not to the extent quoted by some authorities. Although malaria was an important element in morbidity and mortality, it was not the only element and the increase of the world population by some 1000 million during the past twenty years could not be attributed entirely to malaria control. He thought it quite likely that as population pressure increased, fertility would decrease; this had certainly happened in Europe and would probably happen elsewhere.

Dr Kenneth S. Warren (*Rockefeller Foundation, New York*) agreed with Professor Bruce-Chwatt on both points. He also felt it was very doubtful that any of the great tropical diseases in the world would be totally eradicated. He pointed out that a reduction in infant mortality, through a reduction in malaria and other infections, might well have a feedback effect in reducing population. Having recently arrived at the Rockefeller Foundation from a background in health, and being in charge of the population programme of the Foundation, he had become very interested in the entire issue. The same problem had to be faced in both areas, the lack of proper tools to control both disease and population.

Professor Bruce-Chwatt welcomed Dr Warren's remarks. At one time, research in tropical diseases had reached a very low level, with the Rockefeller Foundation contributing little; he was pleased that the Foundation was perhaps revising its philosophy.

Professor David J. Bradley (*Ross Institute of Tropical Hygiene, London*) asked Professor Bruce-Chwatt whether, if malaria control were turned over to the general health services, he saw any role for residual insecticides in, say, India or sub-Saharan Africa?

Professor Bruce-Chwatt doubted whether residual insecticides would play a major role after basic health services had taken over malaria control, which would then probably be limited to the diagnosis of malaria, treatment of acute cases, and the distribution of anti-malarial drugs. If there were residual insecticides still active against susceptible species of *Anopheles* vectors, they would be used only sporadically. He said that in the last year WHO had not received any single candidate insecticide when, in past years, up to 100 new candidate insecticides had been submitted for trial.

Dr Williams wondered whether, it it were not the tools that had failed in the past, but the socio-economic situation, it would make any difference if new tools were developed.

Professor Bruce-Chwatt said that it was not so much the immanent causes that produced the downfall of malaria eradication, as the absence of *new* tools. For instance, if there were an injectible drug available which would prevent malaria for six months without side effects he felt sure that many problems in malarial areas would be alleviated. This was a field where pharmaceutical companies could perhaps be urged to continue the work of Dr Thompson, (who had contributed so much to the development of amodiaquine) who had unfortunately died three years previously.

Dr Miller, introducing the next contribution, said that one of the best ways to start the search for future methods was with *in vitro* cultivation, and in this respect he believed this would prove a memorable decade in malariology. He referred particularly to the work of Professor Trager who had advanced research in trypanosomiasis and malaria, and whose recent findings had been most exciting.

6. Cultivation of *Plasmodium falciparum*

William Trager

The cultivation of parasitic organisms is only part science: it is also part art and part engineering. A recent article "The Mind's Eye: Non-verbal thought in technology", by Eugene S. Ferguson (1977), a professor of history and curator of technology, described the important role in design of the technologist's mental image of how a machine ought to look, as distinct from, and perhaps more important than, any mathematical calculations. In designing the apparatus that gave the first continuous *in vitro* growth of *Plasmodium falciparum* (Trager, 1976; Trager and Jensen, 1976), I imagined something that would permit the red blood cells (rbc) with their contained parasites to lie quietly, as they do through two-thirds of their 48-hour cycle in the human host, where the infected cells are sequestered in capillaries of the brain, heart and other tissues. At the same time a slow flow of medium and an appropriate gas phase had to be provided.

The so-called flow vial that was used is now, less than two years later, mainly of historical interest. It served to point out some of the essential conditions for continuous culture of *P. falciparum* in human erythrocytes: a thin settled layer of red cells, covered by a shallow layer (3–4 mm) of RPMI 1640 medium containing 25 mM HEPES (N'-hydroxyethylpiperazine-N'-2-ethanesulfonic acid) buffer and 10 % human serum, all with a gas phase with elevated CO_2 and reduced O_2, and provision of fresh erythrocytes as the parasite number increases. It soon led in two directions: (1) to a simple petri-dish method (Jensen and Trager, 1977) in which, however, frequent manual change of medium was essential; (2) to two partly automated methods, one based on continuous flow, the other on intermittent change of medium, and both capable of producing large amounts of parasite material.

Establishment of Additional Strains in Culture

In the spring of 1976 we had obtained growth in the flow vial of a
South-east Asian strain (FVO) of *P.falciparum* using infected *Aotus*
monkey blood as the starting inoculum, and we had subcultured this
to petri-dish cultures in a candle jar. It seemed of immediate importance to find out whether other strains of *P.falciparum* could be cultured
and whether cultures could be initiated directly from infected human
blood as well as from infected blood of *Aotus trivirgatus* monkeys. These
questions were soon answered in the affirmative (Jensen and Trager,
1978). At first the only strain available other than FVO was derived
from a patient in South America and had been passed twice in *Aotus*
monkeys, in which it produced only light infections. Nevertheless
we were able to get it going by the flow-vial method, but not in petri
dishes. Then Milton Friedman worked for two months at the Medical
Research Council Laboratory at Fajara, Gambia, through the courtesy
of Dr R. S. Bray. He sent us two infected human bloods and Jensen
started both of these directly in petri-dish cultures held in a candle
jar. We have now started a total of six culture lines: FCR-1, February
1976 from *Aotus* blood infected with FVO (South-east Asian); FCR-2,
April 1976 from *Aotus* blood infected with a South American falciparum;
FCR-3 August 1976 from infected human blood (designated FMG)
from the Gambia; FCR-4, November 1976 from another infected
human blood (patient 6252) from the Gambia; FCR-5 and FCR-6,
new isolates into petri-dish culture (R. Reese, unpublished data) from
Aotus monkeys infected with FCR-1 after a year in culture.

FCR-1 was maintained in continuous culture for about 14 months,
with infectivity to *Aotus* demonstrated after one year. It is now cryo-
preserved (Diggs *et al.*, 1975; Rowe *et al.*, 1968) and has on occasion
been reactivated. FCR-2 unfortunately was lost by contamination.
FCR-3 has now been in continuous culture for 16 months and is the
line we are working with mainly at present. This and FCR-4, 5 and 6
are also cryo-preserved. Other culture lines have been started in several
other laboratories (according to reports in abstract form and personal
communications). Hence there is every reason to believe that the
culture method is applicable essentially to all strains of *P.falciparum*.

The Culture Medium

This was RPMI 1640 (GIBCO) as first formulated by Moore *et al.*
(1967) plus 25 mM HEPES buffer plus human serum, originally at
15%. Small changes in the medium itself have given only discouraging
results: no effect or poor growth. By using the petri-dish method,

which lends itself to the rapid and economical testing of different culture conditions, we soon found that 10% human serum was as good as 15%, but 5% did not support good growth. It also became evident that human serum became unsuitable if stored for over a week at 4°C. It can, however, be stored at -20°C for long periods without losing its effectiveness.

From the outset we wondered whether human serum could be replaced by an animal serum, especially by foetal calf serum (FCS). Although some batches of FCS will support fairly good growth through two cycles (four days) it is never as good as in controls with human serum. Furthermore, the growth gets progressively worse on subculture (Jensen and Trager, 1977). Other animal sera (all inactivated at 56°C) were even less suitable than FCS.

Human serum is obtained from units of blood collected without anti-coagulant (through the co-operation of the New York Blood Center) that are allowed to clot and refrigerated overnight. The serum is drawn off, centrifuged and stored frozen. All manipulations are done aseptically. Serum of type AB+ is used for experiments where it is necessary to use different types of human erythrocytes or *Aotus* red cells, since it is compatible with all of them. Type A+ serum is used with type A+ cells for most work since this is the most common type and most readily available.

The Erythrocytes

Since human red cells are the natural host cell of *P. falciparum* and are also the easiest to obtain in quantity there seems little reason to use anything else. The blood is collected in ACD (acid-citrate-dextrose) or, more recently, in CPD (citrate-phosphate-dextrose) and stored at 4°C. Cells stored for a week have supported better growth than those freshly collected, and the cells are suitable for up to four weeks of storage (Jensen and Trager, 1977). This means that blood outdated for transfusion purposes can be used for the cultures.

Among numerous units of type AB+ and A+ blood used so far, only one has been observed that did not support growth. Type O cells from one individual have supported exceptionally good growth (J. B. Jensen, unpublished data).

Physical Conditions

A settled stationary thin layer of erythrocytes covered by a shallow layer (3–4 mm deep) of culture medium with an appropriate gas phase and with change of medium, either by slow continuous flow or intermittently at appropriate intervals, are essential.

The thickness of the erythrocyte layer is an interesting variable. At first a 25% red cell suspension was used in the flow vial and a 12% suspension in the petri dishes. It was soon found that a 6% suspension in petri dishes would permit the development of higher parasitaemias (J. B. Jensen, unpublished data). Of course a 20% parasitaemia in a 6% red cell suspension represents the same total number of parasites per ml as a 10% parasitaemia in a 12% cell suspension. This is a factor that is still under study and that will probably vary with other conditions of the cultures.

The proper gas phase seemed to present a problem. For the flow vials I used 7% CO_2 and 5% O_2 delivered through silicone tubing. This tank mixture had been arrived at empirically. When we found that the candle jars had an atmosphere of 3% CO_2 and 17% O_2 we took samples of the gas phase from flow vials of a new type (see below) and discovered that it contained 2–3% CO_2 and 10% O_2. Evidently the silicone tubing through which the gas was delivered was so permeable that CO_2 was lost and oxygen gained. M. Friedman (1978)g ood growth in atmospheres with 2% CO_2 and either 5% or 18% O_2. It seems likely that 2–5% CO_2 and 5–8% O_2 will ordinarily support good growth. I have obtained indications, however, that 5% CO_2 in air (21% O_2 at sea level) will not support continuous culture. It is most interesting that recent work with diploid human fibroblasts in culture has shown that they will not grow well in a semi-synthetic medium with reduced serum unless the O_2 tension is not more than 17% (McKeehan *et al.*, 1977). The air in Boulder, Colorado supported growth, but not that at sea-level.

In Vitro Screening of Antimalarials

The cultures obviously lend themselves to work on chemotherapy. Comparative studies of chloroquine-resistant and susceptible strains already show that these properties remain *in vitro* (Siddiqui *et al.*, 1972; Dinh and Trager, unpublished data). It should now be possible also to attempt to produce chloroquine resistance *in vitro* and to make comparative biochemical studies with resistant and susceptible strains (Nguyen Dinh and Trager, 1978).

Furthermore we can now screen for new antimalarials directly *in vitro* with *P.falciparum* developing in its natural host cell, the human erythrocyte. In studies of agents directed against the erythrocytic parasites there is no need for an animal screen. There is need, of course, for toxicity tests, especially in primates. But if an agent is effective against

P.falciparum in vitro, and if it has been shown safe at the effective levels, then clinical trial is the next logical step.

In collaboration with E. Lederer and his colleagues in France we have shown the antimalarial effect against *P.falciparum* in culture of a new type of compound: S.isobutyl adenosine (SIBA), an analogue of adenosyl homocysteine and an inhibitor of methyl transferase (Trager *et al.*, 1978).

Haemoglobin S and the Development of *P.falciparum*

Another obvious application of the cultures is for investigation of how it is that haemoglobin S (HbS) and also perhaps some other red-cell polymorphisms, confer relative resistance to falciparum malaria (Allison, 1961). The geographical distribution of these polymorphisms coincides with that of holoendemic malaria. Since falciparum malaria kills children, it seemed reasonable to suppose that the selective pressure of malaria would maintain a gene, such as that for HbS which is deleterious in the homozygous state, providing that the heterozygotes had a relative resistance to malaria. Since Allison first suggested this, considerable statistical evidence has accumulated in favour of this idea. But there has been no direct evidence and no understanding of how HbS might act to confer resistance to malaria. M. Friedman (1978) has compared cultures of *P.falciparum* in cells from sickle cell disease (S/S), from sickle trait carriers (S/A) and from normal people (A/A). In an atmosphere with 18% O_2 there is no sickling and the parasites develop equally well in all three types of cells. If, however, the O_2 tension is reduced to 5%, a level that occurs physiologically in certain blood vessels and tissues, the results are very different. In the S/S cells the parasites are destroyed within 24 hours. In the S/A cells young rings survive for a day but are unable to develop further. In the A/A cells development is normal, and the same as with 18% O_2. At 5% O_2 HbS becomes paracrystalline. It seems likely that this directly injures the parasites in S/S cells. In S/A cells, where 40% or less of the haemoglobin is HbS, the partial paracrystalline arrays probably interfere with the endocytic nutrition of the parasite.

Production of Gametocytes *in vitro*

Limited experience so far indicates that culture lines newly established from human material are most likely to produce gametocytes. To be fully mature and capable of exflagellation, gametocytes require about 10–11 days of incubation (Carter and Beach, 1977). Hence the conditions used for keeping a rapidly growing culture of asexual forms tend to dilute out gametocytes. Nevertheless an immature gametocyte was noted in line FCR-1 after a year of culture. With line FCR-3, placed after 13 months of continuous culture under conditions which would favour gametocyte formation, we have recently found several immature gametocytes and one fully mature-looking female gametocyte. Apparently, even after more than a year of rapid asexual growth, the parasites are still capable of gametocyte formation.

Large-scale Production of Parasite Material

All of us hope that the cultures may be of special importance as a source of antigens in attempts to develop a vaccine against malaria. Toward

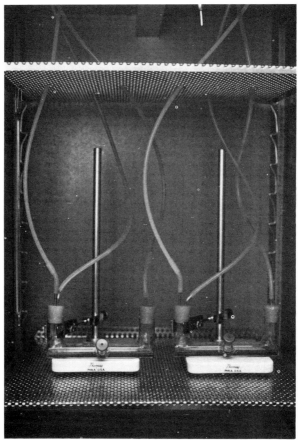

Fig. 1 Two flow vessels in an incubator. At left end of each are tubes for delivery of medium and gas; at right is tube for withdrawal of medium.

this end we have been especially concerned with scaling-up both the relative and absolute number of parasites.

We are now using a new type of flow vessel (Fig. 1) that will be described in detail in a separate paper (Trager, in press). It will suffice to say here that it consists of a horizontal, rectangular chamber 15 cm long by 2·5 cm wide and 2 cm high. It holds 12 ml of cell suspension, giving an area of settled red cells of 40 cm² and a depth of medium of 3 mm. At each end of the chamber is a vertical cylinder 6 cm high. The one on the left is equipped with a silicone-rubber stopper bearing a cotton-plugged delivery tube for gas and a delivery tube for the medium, which flows in at the left-hand end of the chamber. The vertical neck at the right end of the chamber bears a silicone-rubber stopper with the outlet tube for the medium. This is made of 4 mm glass

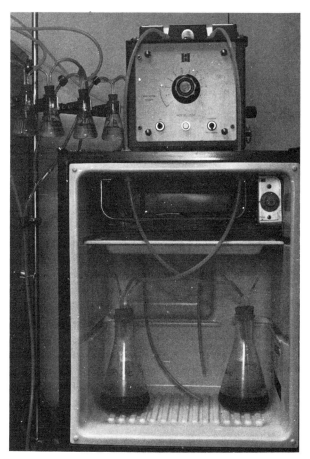

Fig. 2 Two reservoir flasks of medium in a refrigerator, with peristaltic pump above. Small flasks to left of pump are for bubbling of gas mixture.

tubing drawn to an opening of about 1–2 mm. It is passed through a hole in the stopper of larger bore and is held in place by a packing of non-absorbent cotton. This permits egress of the gas and also permits adjustment of the position of the tip of the tube, which controls the level of the medium in the chamber. At the centre of the front wall of the chamber is a short side-arm set at an angle and closed with a vaccine cap. This provides for removal of infected cell suspension and addition of fresh red cells by a syringe and needle.

Medium is delivered by means of a peristaltic pump from the reservoir flask held in a refrigerator (Fig. 2). The flask contains a week's supply of medium at a delivery-rate of 55 ml per day. Medium is drawn off from the surface by a separate pump set at a somewhat higher speed than the inflow, so that the position of the top of the withdrawal tube controls the depth of the medium. The spent medium is collected in sterile 250 ml flasks that are changed twice a week.

As already noted, the gas mixture from a tank containing 7% CO_2, 5% O_2, balance N_2 is delivered through silicone tubing and provides an atmosphere in the chamber of about 2% CO_2 and 10% O_2. Every Monday, Wednesday and Friday the contents of the vessel are gently mixed (with the flows shut off) and most (10 ml) of the suspension of infected erythrocytes is removed. Then 10 ml of fresh 10% erythrocyte suspension in complete medium are added and mixed with the small amount of suspension left in the vessel. Stained slides are prepared before and after dilution with fresh blood. Thus a 1:10 dilution is

Table 1

Growth of *P. falciparum* line FCR-1 (FVO) in two flow vessels after a year of continuous culture *in vitro* (Line begun 10 February 1976)

Date	Parasitaemia %		Remarks
	before addition of fresh rbc	*after addition of fresh rbc*	
17.1.77	8, 11	2, 1·5	Infectivity demonstrated in splenectomized *Aotus* (dose of 75×10^6 schizonts)
19.1.77	6, 7	1, 1	
21.1.77	7, 6	1, 1·5	
24.1.77	5, 5	1, 2	Rbc counts on material removed from vessels: $1·4, 1·1 \times 10^9$ ml^{-1}
26.1.77	8, 8	1·4, 1·6	Rbc counts: $1·8, 1·3 \times 10^9$ ml^{-1}
14.2.77	9, 7	1·3, 1·6	
16.2.77	5, 11	2, 0·9	
18.2.77	7, 6	2·5, 1·6	
21.2.77	10, 10		

typically effected three times weekly. The 48 hour cycle of reproduction of the parasites provides a 5–10-fold increase in parasitaemia by the time of the next dilution (Tables 1 and 2).

At each harvest one vessel of the size now used provides 1 ml of packed cells or 10_2 parasites if the parasitaemia is 10%. Since the

Table 2

Growth of *P. falciparum* line FCR-3 (FMG) in two flow vessels after over a year of continuous culture *in vitro*.

Date	Parasitaemia %		Fold increase between
	before addition of fresh rbc	after addition of fresh rbc	successive dates
7.10.77	8, 8[a]	0·5, 0·6	
10.10.77	10, 12	1, 0·9	20, 20
12.10.77	4, 8	2·7, 1·3	4, 9
14.10.77	6, 10	1, 1·2	2, 8
17.10.77	7, 8	1·5, 1·4	7, 7
19.10.77	5, 10	0·9, 1·6	3, 7
21.10.77	11, 12	0·8, 0·7	12, 8
24.10.77	8, 8	1·4, 1·5	10, 11
26.10.77	5, 6	1·7, 1	3, 4
28.10.77	7, 5	1·5, 1·9	4, 5
31.10.77	8, 10	1·4, 1·9	5, 5
2.11.77	6, 7[a]		4, 4

[a] Packed rbc volume in material removed was 10%.

average multiplication has been about 7-fold each time, the parasites increase each week 7^3 times or about 350-fold. The normal morphology of the parasites is illustrated in Fig. 3, as seen in stained slides and in Fig. 4 as seen in a fresh preparation by phase-contrast microscopy. Their fine structure as seen by electron microscopy is also entirely normal and has now been described in detail for all stages (Langreth, in press). Treatment of a 10% suspension with Physiogel (plasma extender) as recommended by Pasvol, *et al* (1977), provides for a high concentration of infected cells (60% parasitaemia or better) containing mostly large trophozoites and schizonts (Fig. 5). Furthermore, the cells which sediment include uninfected cells and those infected with young rings. This material, if put back into culture in petri dishes, yields a highly synchronous culture (for one cycle) from which large numbers of merozoites can be obtained about 30 hours later (Reese and Jensen, unpublished data).

A second semi-automated method for large-scale culture is being developed. This has been reported briefly by Jensen and Trager at the 1977 meeting of the American Society of Tropical Medicine and Hygiene and will be described fully later. It grew from a medium-

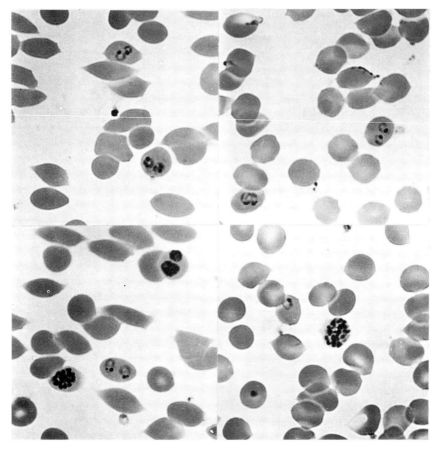

Fig. 3 Typical fields from a culture with 7% parasitaemia from a flow vessel with line FCR-3 after 14 months of continuous multiplication in vitro. Dried film fixed in methanol and Giemsa-stained (× 1200).

changing apparatus I had used (Trager and Jernberg, 1961) in work on extracellular survival and development *in vitro* of the bird malaria *Plasmodium lophurae*.

It depends on a culture vessel consisting of two chambers connected in such a way that when the vessel is tilted the medium flows out from the upper chamber, which contains the culture, into the lower. This spent medium is removed from the lower chamber while fresh medium is added to the upper culture chamber. Jensen supplied the important modification of a small glass shelf that traps the settled erythrocytes while permitting most of the medium to be decanted. In this apparatus conditions are much as in petri dishes except that the intermittent change of medium is done automatically rather than manually. The machine can thus readily make changes at short intervals as the parasit-

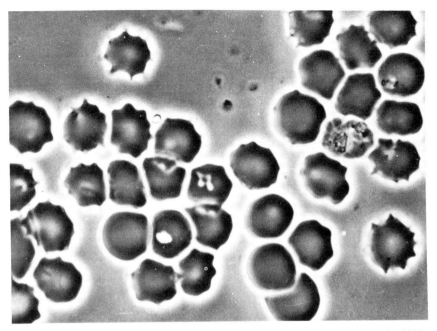

Fig. 4 Cells from the same culture as used for Fig. 3 as seen in a wet film with phase contrast (× 2000). Note the ameboid ring (moving when photographed), the bright trophozoite and the late schizont with forming merezoites.

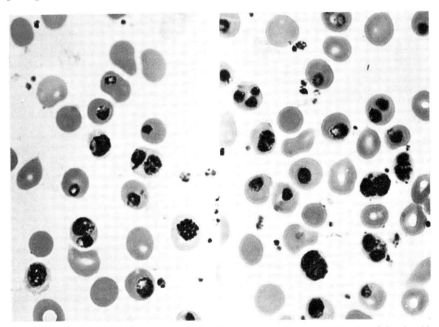

Fig. 5 Representative fields from a concentrate of the same preparation as used for Fig. 3 (made with Physiogel); fixed in methanol and Giemsa-stained (× 2000).

aemia gets high. With a 6% red cell suspension parasitaemias of between 20% and 30% have been obtained.

Although our experience with the tipping apparatus (as we call it) is still limited, the indications are that it will be especially useful for production of large amounts of parasite material. The continuous-flow vessels, on the other hand, already provide a convenient way for long-term maintenance of culture lines at levels of about 10% parasitaemia. The simple petri-dish method is ideal for short-term experiments involving drugs or multiple variables in the culture conditions. All of these methods together now make possible physiological and biochemical studies with the principal human malarial parasite *P.falciparum*. They also should lead to the large-scale production of appropriate antigens if vaccination against falciparum malaria is found to be practicable. Whether these methods will prove applicable to *P.vivax* or *P.malariae* remains to be seen.

Acknowledgements

It is a pleasure to acknowledge the superlative technical assistance of Ms Marika Tershakovec in the laboratory and of Mrs Diane Greene in the office. The work is supported in part by the United States Agency for International Development, Contract number Ta-C-1373.

References

Allison, A. C. (1961). Genetic factors in resistance to malaria, *Annals of the New York Academy of Sciences*, **91**, 710–29.

Carter, R. and Beach, R. F. (1977). Gametogenesis (exflagellation) by gametocytes of *Plasmodium falciparum* produced in culture. *Nature, London*, **270**, 240–1.

Diggs, C., Joseph, K., Flemmings, B., Snodgrass, R. and Hines, F. (1975). Protein synthesis *in vitro* by cryopreserved *Plasmodium falciparum*. *American Journal of Tropical Medicine and Hygiene*, **24**, 760–3.

Ferguson, E. S. (1977). The mind's eye: nonverbal thought in technology. *Science*, **197**, 827–36.

Friedman, M. J. (1978). Erythrocytic mechanism of sickle cell resistance to malaria. *Proc. Natl Acad. Sci.* **75**, 1994–97.

Jensen, J. B. and Trager, W. (1977). *Plasmodium falciparum* in culture: Use of outdated erythrocytes and description of the candle-jar method. *Journal of Parasitology*, **63**, 883–6.

Jensen, J. B. and Trager, W. (1978). *Plasmodium falciparum* in culture: establishment of additional strains. *American Journal of Tropical Medicine and Hygiene*, **27**, 743–6.

Langreth, S. G. Fine structure of *Plasmodium falciparum*. *Journal of Protozoology* (in press).

McKeehan, W. L., McKeehan, K. A., Hammond, S. L. and Ham, R. G. (1977). Improved medium for clonal growth of human diploid flagellates at low concentrations of serum protein. *In Vitro*, **13**, 399–416.

Moore, G. E., Gerner, R. E. and Franklin, H. A. (1977). Culture of normal human leukocytes, *Journal of the American Medical Association*, **199**, 519–24.

Nguyen-Dinh, P. and Trager, W. (1978). Chloroquine resistance produced in vitro in an African strain of human malaria. *Science*, **200**, 1397–8.

Pasvol, G., Weatherall, D. J. and Wilson, R. J. M. (1977). Effects of foetal hemoglobin on susceptibility of red cells to *Plasmodium falciparum*. *Nature, London*, **270**, 171–3.

Rowe, A. W., Eyster, E. and Kellner, A. (1968). Liquid nitrogen preservation of red blood cells for transfusion. *Cryobiology*, **5**, 119–28.

Siddiqui, W. A., Schnell, J. V. and Geiman, Q. M. (1972). A model *in vitro* system to test the susceptibility of human malarial parasites to anti-malarial drugs. *American Journal of Tropical Medicine and Hygiene*, **21**, 392–9.

Trager, W. (1976). Prolonged cultivation of malarial parasites (*Plasmodium coatneyi* and *P. falciparum*). *In* "Biochemistry of Parasites and Host-Parasite Relationships" (Ed. H. Van den Bossche), pp. 427–34. North Holland, Amsterdam.

Trager, W. and Jensen, J. B. (1976). Human malaria parasites in continuous culture. *Science*, **193**, 673–5.

Trager, W. and Jernberg, N. A. (1961). Apparatus for change of medium in extra-cellular maintenance *in vitro* of an intracellular parasite (malaria). *Proceedings of the Society for Experimental Biology and Medicine*, **108**, 175–8.

Trager, W., Robert-Gero, M. and Lederer, E. (1978). Antimalarial activity of S-isobutyl adenosine against *Plasmodium falciparum* in culture, *FEBS* Letters **85**, 246–6.

Discussion

Dr John H. Knowles (*President, Rockefeller Foundation, New York*) said that some eighteen months previously the Rockefeller Foundation had been one of the prime parties to the development of the International Laboratory for Research on Animal Diseases in Nairobi, and it was amazing to find a breakthrough in the culture of trypansomes within six or eight months of the laboratory being established. Clearly this was the first step in the development of a new technology. He asked Professor Trager when he had started the work, and how long it had taken.

Professor Trager said that Hirumi, who had carried out the work on the cultivation of *Trypanosoma brucei* had used the same medium—RPMI 1640 plus HEPES buffer; of the 90 different combinations of culture media and tissue-cell lines he had tried, only this single combination proved successful.

Regarding his interest in malaria cultivation, he said that this was of very long standing. He had considered a fundamental approach to the biochemical-physiological relationships between the malaria parasite and the host cell, and had thought that the red cell might provide a good starting point since it was not in itself a very actively metabolizing cell. Because of this, for many years he had not been concerned primarily with trying to grow malaria in a tissue culture system (that is, in its host erythrocyte) but rather in taking it out of its host erythrocyte to see what could be learnt when it was kept extracellularly *in vitro*. At a conference held several years ago by the Agency for International Development this matter was discussed, and it was clear that if a vaccine for malaria were to be a worthwhile goal, cultivation would be essential. A further important advance had been the success of Siddiqui, Schnell and Geiman in infecting *Aotus* monkeys with *P. falciparum*. Professor Trager said that the few preliminary experiments with *P. falciparum* which he had tried were on a limited scale, since only an occasional very lightly infected blood sample from a patient in the experimental malaria programme was available. These conditions had set the stage for his work. He began using *Plasmodium coatneyi*, a monkey malaria which is a good model for *P. falciparum*, and tried some of the newer tissue culture media which had become available, including RPMI 1640. A few trials showed that RPMI 1640 was an excellent medium for *Plasmodium coatneyi* and it was then applied to *P. falciparum*.

In reply to a question on why the parasitaemia reached a plateau at 12%, he said it was due partly to biological factors, but under the particular technical conditions in that culture system. With a flow rate in the medium of 55 ml per day, and a 10% erythrocyte suspension, if the culture were not diluted with fresh erythrocytes when it reached 10% it did rise, from 10% to 12 or even occasionally 15%, but then degenerating parasites are found. Therefore under those conditions there was some limiting factor which might simply be the glucose level. Glucose was measured in the effluent and, with this amount of culture, after two days the effluent contained only half the concentration of glucose originally present in the medium. Professor Trager thought that perhaps as the parasitaemia rose, the glucose level and the buffer should be simultaneously increased. In petri dishes, and in the tipping method, he had found up to 30% parasitaemia, but with very thin red-cell suspensions so that the total number of parasites was not great. Limiting factors seemed to be glucose acid, production and availability of cells. However, adjustment of the technical conditions could, in fact, raise the levels of parasitaemia.

Dr Miller said that the next speaker, Professor Cohen, had first entered this field with one of the outstanding workers in malaria today, Ian MacGregor; they had been the first to show the importance of antibody in the immune response to malaria. Since that time, papers from Professor Cohen's department had been a stimulus to everyone working towards vaccines, the biology, and many other aspects of malaria; in addition, his valued criticism and unending optimism had been a great help to all those in the field.

7. Immunology and Malaria

S. Cohen

Introduction

The developmental cycle of the malaria parasite exposes its vertebrate host to a succession of structurally distinct forms (Fig. 1) and at least some of these, e.g. sporozoites, tissue schizonts and blood parasites, appear to have individually distinct antigenic specificities. Studies of immunity have been mainly concerned with sporozoites, the naturally infective form derived from mosquitoes, and with the asexual erythrocytic stages of infection. The immune response to other stages, including exoerythrocytic (EE) schizonts (Foley and Vanderberg, 1977), EE merozoites (Holbrook *et al.*, 1974), gametocytes and gametes (Gwadz, 1976; Carter and Chen, 1976), have great potential interest, but have only recently come under immunological scrutiny and will not be considered here (see Cohen and Mitchell, 1977).

After several decades of endeavour the production of a vaccine against human malaria has become a realistic goal with the achievement by Trager and Jensen in 1976 of continuous culture of a human malaria parasite and the demonstrated immunogenicity of small amounts of merozoite antigen isolated in high yield and relative purity from cultured parasites (Cohen *et al.*, 1977). The production of a practical and effective human vaccine requires further improvement of culture techniques, and more detailed understanding of the mechanisms of induced immunity and their amplification through adjuvants acceptable for human use.

Malaria Life Cycle

Malaria infection is initiated through the bite of infected female anopheline mosquitoes which inoculate motile sporozoites into the bloodstream. In mammalian hosts these are cleared from the circulation within one and two hours and localize in hepatic parenchymal cells through mechanisms at present unknown. The EE forms become multi-nucleate, and after a variable period (usually about ten days) infected liver cells rupture and each discharge approximately 20 000 EE merozoites which invade erythrocytes. EE development does not appear to be cyclical in mammals, as is the case in avian malarias. Erythrocytic (E) schizonts rupture with a periodicity (24–72 hours) characteristic for individual species, and each liberates 10–20 E merozoites which attach to specific receptors on red cell membranes to initiate invasion. The erythrocytic cycle is associated with clinical manifestations of malaria. A proportion of blood parasites, influenced by mechanisms which remain obscure, develop into male and female gametocytes and these undergo sexual reproduction within the gut of the mosquito.

Immunity to the Tissue Stages of Malaria

Immunity to Infection
Human subjects living in hyperendemic areas and maintained on therapy to suppress erythrocytic stages of malaria are exposed to heavy and repeated natural sporozoite challenge and yet remain susceptible to infection when prophylaxis is suspended. The inference, that live unattenuated sporozoites are not immunogenic or else induce immunity of very brief duration is supported by observations in simian malaria (Garnham, 1966). On the other hand, rats maintained on chloroquine to suppress the erythrocytic stage of parasite development, and repeatedly inoculated with non-attenuated *Plasmodium berghei* sporozoites do develop resistance to this stage of the protozoon (Verhave, 1975; Beaudoin *et al.*, 1975).

Vaccination against Tissue Stages
Effective immunity against the exoerythrocytic stage has been induced in rodent but not in simian malarias by vaccination with sporozoites attenuated by irradiation. Induced protection is specific only for sporozoites, since immune animals remain susceptible to challenge with either blood parasites or hepatic schizonts which produce EE merozoites to initiate erythrocytic infection (Foley and Vanderberg, 1977). Immunity lasts for about three months in mice after intravenous administration of irradiated *P.berghei* sporozoites without the use of adjuvants. Protective sporozoite antigens are unstable and inactivated by high levels of irradiation, freezing and thawing, formol treatment or mechanical disruption (reviewed by Nussenzweig *et al.*, 1977).

A proportion of human subjects repeatedly inoculated with attenuated *P.falciparum* sporozoites through the bite of very large numbers of irradiated mosquitoes were resistant to challenge (Clyde, 1975). Despite this demonstration the practical implementation of human sporozoite vaccination confronts major difficulties (Table 1). The clinical manifestations of mammalian malaria are associated with the erythrocytic

Table 1

Current status of malaria vaccines in mammalian hosts

Characteristics of vaccine	Vaccine preparation		
	sporozoite	*parasitized rbc*	*merozoite*
Inactivation	Irradiation	[a]Formol	None
Route	[a]Intravenous	Intramuscular	Intramuscular
Adjuvant	None	[ac]FCA	[ac]FCA
Production	[a]Mosquitoes	Culture	Culture
Yield	[a]Low	[a]Low	High
Contaminating host antigen	Low	[a]High	Low
Storage	[a]Unstable	Stable	Stable
Immunity specificity[b]	[a]EE	E	E
duration	[a]3 months	> 1 year	> 1 year

[a] Unfavourable features of vaccines.

[b] EE exoerythrocytic forms   E erythrocytic stages.

[c] FCA Freund's complete adjuvant.

cycle of development. Effective vaccination against exoerythrocytic stages must therefore result consistently in the elimination of all viable-tissue parasites since any which mature would induce blood infection in a host fully susceptible to this stage of the parasite. Other constraints in regard to sporozoite vaccination concern the requirement for intravenous inoculation, the present inability to store the vaccine and the problem of producing sporozoites on a scale suitable for mass vaccination. Since neither sporogonic nor exoerythrocytic development is cyclical in human malaria spp., there is at present little prospect for successful serial cultivation of these stages.

Mechanisms of Immunity against Tissue Stages

The findings that intravenous administration is the optimum route of sporozoite vaccination, that attenuated organisms are more effective than killed, and that the use of adjuvant may reduce immunity, all suggest that sporozoites have to undergo some development in the mammalian host in order to induce protective immunity. The ability of irradiated parasites to enter the liver is suggested by the frequency of hepatic granuloma in vaccinated mice. Both humoral and cell-mediated effector mechanisms appear to play a part in acquired anti-sporozoite immunity, but the mechanisms involved have not been precisely defined. Antibodies directed against sporozoites have been detected by sporozoite-agglutination and by circum-sporozoite precipitation (CSP).

The latter reaction is independent of complement and involves the formation of a thread-like precipitate which appears within 10 minutes after incubation of parasites at 37°C with immune serum. The surface coat of fine fibrillar material is most prominent at the posterior end of the parasite, suggesting that the CSP reaction may result from posterior capping and shedding of surface immune complexes. Resistance to sporozoites may occur in the absence of detectable antibody and, conversely, anti-sporozoite antibodies are found in susceptible animals. Passive immunization has failed to establish a protective role for humoral antibody, but immune sera do increase the rate of sporozoite clearance while infectivity of sporozoites is reduced after incubation with immune serum (reviewed by Nussenzweig *et al.*, 1977; Cohen and Mitchell, 1977).

Acquired resistance to sporozoite infection is thymus-dependent. Thymectomized, irradiated, bone-marrow reconstituted mice or congenitally athymic (Nu/Nu) mice do not develop sporozoite-neutralizing antibody or clinical immunity after vaccination with irradiated sporozoites. Reconstitution with thymus cells restores the capacity of such animals to synthesize antibody and become immunized (Spitalny *et al.*, 1977). The possibility that cell-mediated effector mechanisms may act against sporozoites in the absence of antibody is suggested by the failure of passive serum-transfer studies and by the finding that mice treated with anti-μ-chain serum, which suppresses humoral immunity, may become clinically immune after vaccination with sporozoites (Chen, 1977—cited by Nussenzweig *et al.*, 1977). Adoptive transfer of sporozoite resistance with sensitized cells has proved unsuccessful (Spitalny *et al.*, 1976), but further evaluation of this system is needed.

Immunity to the Blood Stages of Malaria

Immunity to Infection
The pattern of acquired immunity to the erythrocytic stage of malaria varies widely in different host-parasite combinations. In some instances, involving infection of a non-natural host, no effective immune response occurs so that the disease is rapidly fatal, as is that produced by *P.knowlesi* in the rhesus monkey. Other experimental forms of malaria induce "sterilizing" immunity characterized by complete elimination of the parasite and lifelong resistance to challenge as *P.berghei* in the rat. Commonly, however, acquired immunity controls but does not eliminate blood infection which persists at low density over long periods—a sequence referred to as "premunition" (Sergent, 1963). This response is observed in the human malarias and, since

tissue forms do not develop cyclically, must be attributed to the periodic recrudescence of long-persisting blood infection (Cox, 1977).

Vaccination Against Erythrocytic Stages

Inactivated, parasitized red cells, fractions derived from these and, more recently, extracellular erythrocytic merozoites have been tested as vaccines in various forms of experimental malaria. The evaluation of different methods must take account of the divergent patterns of clinical immunity which characterize the experimental infections commonly studied.

Irradiated blood parasites proved effective in rat malaria, but gave weaker protection against more virulent infections of mice, rhesus and douroucouli monkeys. A parasite strain, attenuated by alternate *in vitro* culture and passage, effectively protected against rodent malaria, but the stability of such strains requires critical evaluation. Parasitized erythrocytes, killed by formol treatment or freezing and thawing, have been effective in rat malaria and partially successful in more virulent infections of mice and monkeys (reviewed by Cohen and Mitchell, 1977).

The elaboration of techniques for isolating blood-stage merozoites relatively free of host cell antigen has enabled this form of the parasite to be used for experimental vaccination. The cell-sieve culture chamber (Dennis *el al.*, 1975) provides an average yield of 6×10^{10} merozoites per ml parasitized red cells, equivalent to 60–600 vaccine doses in the rhesus. In conjunction with Freund's complete adjuvant (FCA) such vaccines have induced sterilizing immunity of broad serological specificity and long duration (more than one year) against normally lethal *P.knowlesi* malaria in the rhesus monkey (Table 2). In addition,

Table 2

Vaccination with various preparations of *P.knowlesi* merozoites (W1 variant)[a]

Merozoite	First challenge (strain, variant)			Total
preparation[b]	W1[c]	W3[c]	A[d]	survivors
Fresh	5/5	5/6	2/2	⎫ 17/18
Frozen	3/3	2/2		⎬
FD	10/14	4/4		14/18
Formol	0/1	1/1		⎫ 7/14
Formol, FD	2/4	1/4	3/4	⎬

[a] Figures refer to number of survivors in each group.
[b] FD = freeze-dried and stored 4°C for up to 20 weeks; Formol = 1 in 1000 formalin for 16 hours at 4°C.
[c] Challenge with 10^4 trophozoites by intravenous injection.
[d] Challenge with 10^3 sporozoites by intravenous injection.
Data from Mitchell *et al.*, 1975; Richards *et al.*, 1977; Voller and Mitchell (unpublished data); Richards and Mitchell (unpublished data).

merozoite vaccination has protected douroucouli monkeys against *P.falciparum*, the most virulent of the human malarias (Mitchell, *et al.*, 1977, Siddiqui, 1977). Merozoites require no inactivation since their infectivity for red cells is lost within an hour at room temperature.

Several problems remain in regard to the development of a blood-stage malaria vaccine suitable for human use (see Table 1). Apart from the exclusion of pathogens there will be a particular risk of contamination with blood-group substances if present techniques are used for cultivation of malaria parasites. In this connexion, vaccines prepared from extracellular merozoites are likely to prove more acceptable than those isolated from erythrocytes containing normal or attenuated parasites. A further problem concerns the requirement for the clinically unacceptable FCA in vaccines such as those which have proved effective against simian malaria (Table 3).

Table 3

P.knowlesi merozoite vaccination (W1-variant) of rhesus with various adjuvants[a]

Adjuvant	W1	W3	A	
FCA	8/8	7/8	2/2	17/18
FCA, FIA	1/1	0/1		⎫
FIA	1/3	0/1		⎬ 2/10
BCG, FIA[b]		0/1		⎭
FIA, MDP[c]	0/3			⎫
Adj.65[d]	0/4			⎬
Adj.65 + *M.butyricium*	1/3			⎬ 1/10
Adj.65 MDP	0/3			⎭

[a] Figures refer to number of survivors in each group.
[b] 2×10^6 BCG (Glaxo) 2 weeks before merozoites in FIA.
[c] MDP = muramyl dipeptide (Ciba).
[d] Adj.65 = adjuvant 65–4 (Mercke-Sharpe and Dohme).

Merozoite preparations were freshly prepared or frozen in liquid N. Data from Guy's Hospital, London, Nuffield Institute for Comparative Medicine, London (Dr A. Voller) and Wellcome Research Laboratories, Beckenham (Dr W. H. G. Richards).

The relevance to human populations of simian malarias studied in non-natural hosts is difficult to assess. Susceptibility to malaria is influenced by many factors including blood-group specificity, haemoglobin constitution and genetically determined differences in patterns of immune responsiveness. There is convincing evidence in human populations that malaria selects for genes controlling not only haemoglobin synthesis and blood-group specificity, but also HLA specificity. The immune response to malaria vaccination is likely to be strongly influenced by such antecedent selection as illustrated by the responses of natural (*Macaca fascicularis*) and non-natural (*Macaca mulatta*) simian hosts to *P.knowlesi* infection (Cohen *et al.*, 1977). The adjuvant require-ments in exposed human populations may, therefore, be less stringent than in experimental malaria which has concerned almost exclusively infections in non-natural hosts.

Mechanisms of Immunity against Blood Stages

The role of humoral antibody in immunity to the erythrocytic stage of malaria is established by the successful passive immunization of human subjects and experimental animals. In addition, antibody suppression using anti-μ-chain sera greatly increases susceptibility to infection. Anti-body appears to act by blocking the attachment of merozoites to red cells and preventing subsequent invasion of erythrocytes. Merozoite inhibitory antibody correlates with clinical immune status in repeatedly infected and most vaccinated rhesus monkeys, and the outcome of passive immunization is related to levels of merozoite inhibitory anti-body. The correlation between clinical immunity and inhibitory anti-body levels is not, however, invariable. Exceptions are observed in vaccinated animals (Butcher *et al.*, 1977) and in chronically infected rhesus (Miller *et al.*, 1977) indicating that cell-mediated effector mech-anisms have an important role in immunity to malaria.

Thymus-derived lymphocytes act as helper cells in the synthesis of malaria antibody, but efforts to demonstrate an effector role for im-mune lymphocytes have not been successful (reviewed by Brown, 1976). Damage to parasites within red cells, seen in malaria infections of mice previously given a large intravenous dose of BCG vaccine, has been attributed to specifically induced release of lymphocyte mediators having a non-specific cytotoxic action (Clark *et al.*, 1976). This effect is confined to certain inbred mouse strains and a similar phenomenon could not be demonstrated in simian malaria, while intracellular para-site damage is not a feature of immunity to human malarias. Specific antibody acts synergistically with macrophages to promote ingestion of parasites, but this phenomenon does not show consistent correlation with clinical immune status (Butcher *et al.*, 1977).

The survival of erythrocytic parasites in hosts manifesting specific cell-mediated and humoral responses could be promoted by several mechanisms (Cohen, 1975), and it is likely that the relative importance of these varies with different *Plasmodium* spp. Antigenic variation is associated with chronic *P.knowlesi* and *P.cynomolgi* infections in the rhesus, but its occurrence with other plasmodiids is uncertain. Immune suppression mediated predominantly by splenic cells may enhance parasitaemia (Wyler *et al.*, 1977). The fact that malaria infection is associated from the outset with production of circulating antigen, de-rived in part from the merozoite coat, may determine the outcome of immunization by infection or vaccination, respectively. In the former, antibody synthesis follows antigen release and this sequence could lead to formation of complexes in antigen excess able to block immune effector mechanisms and promote parasite survival. Vaccination with non-viable antigen, on the other hand, will induce inhibitory antibody in the absence of circulating malarial antigen. Subsequent challenge infections generate antigen and probably lead to formation of complexes in antibody excess; these could act synergistically with splenic cytotoxic cells, stimulated by FCA, to eliminate blood parasites (Cohen, 1977). If circulating antigen is involved in promoting parasite survival, then there is clearly a need to establish whether the outcome of vaccination is modified in subjects with an established malaria infection.

The above observations concerning mechanisms of acquired immunity to the erythrocytic stage of malaria indicate the need to identify the cellular components which may either act with antibody to mediate protection, or suppress immune effector mechanisms and favour parasite survival. In addition, it is necessary to analyse the role of FCA in promoting specific antibody formation or non-specifically stimulating immune effector cells. Such data would provide a basis for the rational choice of an adjuvant for use with a human malaria vaccine.

Clinical Trial of a Human Malaria Vaccine

At present blood-stage merozoites constitute the most promising form of vaccine for potential use in a human trial (see Table 1). This is so in terms of experimentally established immunogenicity of merozoites which induce immunity of broad variant specificity and long duration directed against the stage of the parasite causing clinical illness. In addition, E merozoites can be isolated from cultures in high yield and relatively uncontaminated with host antigens. Finally, merozoite antigens are stable and can be stored in the freeze-dried state. Purified merozoite fractions might prove to be effective, and their combination with vaccines active against tissue stages (Nussenzweig *et al.*, 1977) or gametes (Gwadz, 1976; Carter and Chen, 1976) would facilitate interruption of transmission.

Results in animal models cannot be extrapolated to man, and the evaluation of any vaccine will require controlled clinical trials in an exposed community. Before such a trial can be undertaken the vaccine and any adjuvant employed would have to comply strictly with the health and safety regulations of a responsible organization. A thorough prior knowledge of the endemicity of malaria in the population to be vaccinated will be essential. A trial would presumably be initiated some weeks before the onset of peak transmission. Immunized and control groups would be assessed on the basis of parasite prevalence and density during an extended period of observation. Monitoring would involve detailed clinical assessment with examination of blood films, haematological indices, body temperature and spleen size and therapeutic intervention, where necessary at the discretion of a clinician with full experience of local infectious diseases and with access to adequate hospital facilities. If the group selected comprised older children and young adults likely to have acquired partial immunity, the need for intervention with drug-therapy would be reduced, but the effects of vaccination might be less obvious.

It is evident that the organization of a malaria vaccine trial which could provide meaningful data under the circumstances which prevail in areas of continued transmission is a complex and difficult operation. Such a trial will require skilled personnel, close co-operation with the exposed population, detailed planning and careful supervision. Vaccination with relatively untested materials in poorly defined populations and with sub-optimum facilities for surveillance would involve serious risks without the prospect of conclusive results and should be most strenuously discouraged.

Acknowledgements

This work is supported by the Medical Research Council, London and the World Health Organization. Dr G. H. Mitchell, Dr W. H. G. Richards and Dr A. Voller kindly allowed me to record unpublished data.

References

Beaudoin, R. L., Strome, C. P. A., Palmer, T. T. and Bowden, M. (1975). Immunogenicity of sporozoites of the ANKA strain of *Plasmodium berghei* following different treatments. *American Society of Parasitology, Abstracts*, **231**, 98–9.

Brown, K. N. (1976). Resistance to malaria. *In* "Immunity to Parasitic Infections" (Eds. S. Cohen and E. H. Sadun), pp. 268–95. Blackwell, Oxford.

Butcher, G. A., Mitchell, G. H. and Cohen, S. (1977). Antibody mediated mechanisms of immunity to malaria induced by vaccination with *Plasmodium knowlesi* merozoites. *Immunology* (in press).

Carter, R. and Chen, D. H. (1976). Malaria transmission blocked by immunization with gametes of the malaria parasite. *Nature, London*, **263**, 57, 60.

Clark, I. A., Allison, A. C. and Cox, F. E. (1976). Protection of mice against Babesia and Plasmodium with BCG. *Lancet*, (i), 309–11.

Clyde, D. F. (1975). Immunisation against falciparum and vivax malaria by use of attenuated sporozoites. *American Journal of Tropical Medicine and Hygiene*, **24**, 397–401.

Cohen, S. (1975). Immunoprophylaxis of protozoal diseases. *In* "Clinical Aspects of Immunology" (Eds. P. C. C. Gell, R. R. A. Coombs and P. J. Lachman), pp. 1649–80. Blackwell, Oxford.

Cohen, S. (1977). Mechanisms of malarial immunity. *Transactions of the Royal Society for Tropical Medicine and Hygiene*, **71**, 283–6.

Cohen, S. and Mitchell, G. H. (1977). "Prospects for Immunization against Malaria. Current Topics in Immunology and Microbiology". Springer, Heidelberg **80,** 97–137.

Cohen, S., Butcher, G. A., Mitchell, G. H., Deans, J. A. and Langhorne, J. (1977). Acquired immunity and vaccination in malaria. *American Journal of Tropical Medicine and Hygiene,* **26,** 223–32.

Cox, F. E. G. (1977). Relapses in malaria. *Nature, London,* **266,** 408–9.

Dennis, E. D., Mitchell, G. H., Butcher, G. A. and Cohen, S. (1975). *In vitro* isolation of *Plasmodium knowlesi* merozoites using polycarbonate sieves. *Parasitology,* **71,** 475–81.

Foley, D. A. and Vanderberg, J. P. (1977). *Plasmodium berghei*; transmission by intra-peritoneal inoculation of immature exoerythrocytic schizonts. *Experimental Parasitology,* **63,** 69-81.

Garnham, P. C. C. (1966). Immunity against the different stages of malaria parasites. *Bulletin de la Societe de pathologie exotique,* **59,** 549–57.

Gwadz, R. W. (1976). Malaria: Successful immunization against the sexual stages of *Plasmodium gallinaceum. Science,* **17,** 1150–1.

Holbrook, T. W., Palczuk, N. C. and Strauber, L. A. (1974). Immunity to exoerythrocytic malaria: III Stage-specific immunization of turkeys against exoerythrocytic forms of *Plasmodium fallax. Journal of Parasitology,* **60,** 348–54.

Miller, L. H., Powers, K. G. and Shiroishi, T. (1977). *Plasmodium knowlesi*: functional immunity and antimerozoite antibodies in rhesus monkeys after repeated infection. *Experimental Parasitology,* **41,** 105–11.

Mitchell, G. H., Butcher, G. A. and Cohen, S. (1975). Merozoite vaccination against *Plasmodium knowlesi* malaria. *Immunology,* **29,** 397–407.

Mitchell, G. H., Richards, W. H. G., Butcher, G. A. and Cohen, S. (1977). Merozoite vaccination of douroucouli monkeys against falciparum malaria. *Lancet,* (i), 1335–8.

Nussenzweig, R. S., Cochrane, A. and Lustig, H. (1978). Immunology of murine malaria. *In* "Rodent Malaria" (Eds. W. Peters and R. Killick-Kendrick) (in press).

Richards, W. H. G., Mitchell, G. H., Butcher, G. A. and Cohen, S. (1977). Merozoite vaccination of rhesus monkeys against *Plasmodium knowlesi* malaria; immunity to sporozoite (mosquito-transmitted) challenge. *Parasitology,* **74,** 191–8.

Sergent, E. (1963). Latent infection and premunition. *In* "Symposium on Immunity to Protozoal Diseases" (Eds. P. C. C. Garnham, A. E. Pierce and I. Roitt), pp. 39–47. Blackwell, Oxford.

Siddiqui, W. A. (1977). An effective immunization of experimental monkeys against a human malaria parasite, *Plasmodium falciparum. Science,* **197,** 388–9.

Spitalny, G. L., Rivers-Ortiz, C. and Nussenzweig, R. S. (1976). *Plasmodium berghei*; the spleen in sporozoite-induced immunity to mouse malaria, *Experimental Parasitology,* **40,** 179–88.

Spitalny, G. L., Verhave, J. P., Meuwissen, J. H. E. and Nussenzweig, R. S. (1977). T-cell dependence of prozoite-induced immunity in rodent malaria. *Experimental Parasitology,* **42,** 73–81.

Trager, W. and Jensen, J. B. (1976). Human malaria parasites in continuous culture. *Science,* **193,** 673–5.

Verhave, J. P. (1975). Immunization with sporozoites. *Krips.Repro.B.V.Meppel.* p. 121. (Thesis.)

Wyler, D. J., Miller, L. H. and Schmidt, L. H. (1977). Spleen function in quartan malaria (due to *Plasmodium inui*); evidence for both protective and suppressive roles in host defence. *Journal of Infectious Diseases,* **135,** 86–93.

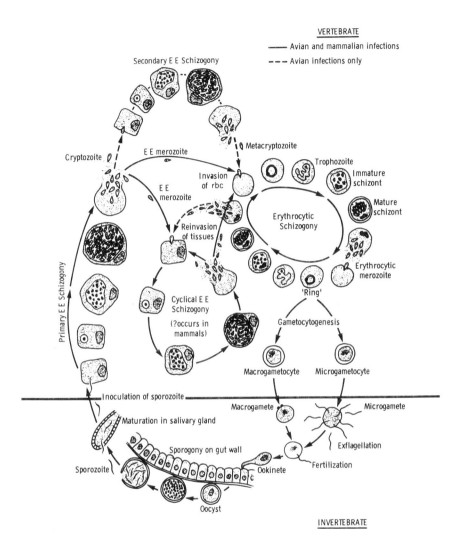

Fig. 1 Diagrammatic representation of the malaria life-cycle in the vertebrate host and the mosquito (Cohen and Mitchell, 1977).

Discussion

Professor Bruce-Chwatt said that it was not often a meeting was privileged to hear a presentation such as that of Professor Trager; it was a milestone in the history of malariology and would be in the textbooks for many years to come.

He agreed with Professor Cohen that Professor Trager's achievement had shown the right path, and wondered whether it would be possible to use his technique to assess the effect of protective antibody which was not always obtained by standard serological techniques.

Professor Cohen said that they had since 1970 made use of short-term cultures to assay antibody activity. There was no doubt that in some instances there was a dissociation between antibody activity and clinical immunity but he did not know whether this could be altered with continuous culture. Where continuous culture would be invaluable was in trying to assay the cellular components of immunity.

Dr J. R. David (*Harvard Medical School*) referred to the difficulties that Professor Cohen had experienced with some adjuvants. He said that a whole new range of adjuvants was being used, particularly in the cancer field, for instance *Nocardia rubra* which had been used clinically in Japan. He thought it might be interesting to see whether any of them could be applicable to malaria.

Professor Cohen felt that there were two aspects to this; firstly, they should examine the system already in use, with new adjuvants. He had already used muramyl dipeptide, which had given negative results, and would like to try others.

Secondly, he thought the question of the host-parasite relationship was fundamental. If they were dealing with a natural host-parasite system, then the host would have been exposed to selection over malaria and this influence on its immune responsiveness to the parasite could be of considerable significance in regard to adjuvant needs. For example, *Plasmodium knowlesi* is naturally infective for the kra monkey, *Macaca fascicularis*. When monkeys born in Britain, and therefore not exposed to malaria, were compared to the rhesus monkey with regard to their early immune responses to infection, the difference was astonishing. If infection in the rhesus monkeys were controlled so that they have an equal parasite load, after two weeks the rhesus had made no perceptible merozoite inhibitory antibody against the parasite. Meanwhile the kra monkey, which had no innate immunity, showed an increase of parasitaemia in the first week, as in the rhesus, after which it was controlled. There was antibody present in that monkey after about seven or eight days, in high titre, and with extremely broad variant specificity, which raised the question of whether a different antigen was involved. With the help of Dr. W. H. G. Richards, a trial of adjuvants in this natural host was being set up, which they hoped would give information more relevant to man.

Dr Miller said that one cause for concern in the use of dead antigens with adjuvants with erythrocytic infection, was the experience in the animal infections *Babesia* and *Anaplasma*. In both these cases killed antigen vaccines with adjuvants had been used, and on reinfection the animals had developed severe haemolytic anaemia. Dr Miller was concerned that when malaria immunization was begun, patients might develop autoimmune haemolytic anaemia, and asked Professor Cohen for his views.

Professor Cohen agreed that this was a danger, and said that so long as red blood cells were used for culture there was a risk of the inclusion of red-cell antigens in the vaccine. However, on the basis of evidence to date, red-cell destruction did not occur during vaccination, challenge or subsequent infections in monkeys; nothing in the *P.knowlesi* system or in the *P. falciparum* vaccinations carried out in the *Aotus* monkey, suggested that this would happen.

Dr Butterworth (*Harvard Medical School, Boston*) suggested that there were two components in the action of Freund's complete adjuvant. Firstly, a classical adjuvant effect in the induction of an antibody response, and secondly, a non-specific effect enhancing an effector cell which may be present in the spleen. If this was correct, it should be possible to dissect out the two different components; for example, by giving merozoites in one of the adjuvants which did not work, for instance BCG, and following it up some time later with FCA and observing whether there was a non-specific enhancement of an effector-cell response. If so, FCA was not working in a classical adjuvant fashion and it should be possible to look for different classes of material which would give the same enhancement of the non-specific effector-cell response.

Professor Cohen agreed with this suggestion, and said that it was something they had not investigated.

Dr Warren, referring to Dr Butterworth's remarks, said that at a recent meeting in France on the immunology of parasitic infections Cox and Allison appeared to be making rather sweeping claims, on the basis of studies in mice, that immunity to malaria was due largely to non-specific activation of immune-effector systems. He suggested that another approach would be to give BCG, or Freund's complete adjuvant without antigen, wait a while, then give a challenge and observe the results.

Professor Cohen said that the experiments Dr Warren referred to had been repeated unsuccessfully in the rhesus monkey with *Plasmodium knowlesi*. As he understood it, the effect was genuine in rodents, and seemed to be related to granuloma formation, but he did not think it had been observed in other species.

Dr Ruth Nussenzweig (*New York University Medical Center*) commented on the effect of non-specific immunity and its association with specific immune response. Using sporozoites, she had observed that giving *Corynebacterium parvum*, which was a simulant of the reticuloendothelial system, a certain amount of non-specific protection was obtained. If that was associated with a sub-optimal dose of sporozoites, namely, a single injection which protected only part of the animals, the effect was greatly enhanced. As had been suggested, the *C. parvum* was given separately about a week before the sporozoites were introduced.

Regarding sporozoite vaccine, she said that protection was of only short duration if the animals were not challenged, but that experiments in mice, and a few in man, had shown that challenge with a bite from an infected mosquito greatly boosted the immune response. Recent evidence, based on sera investigated in the Gambia, showed that even under natural conditions there was an immune response to sporozoites. Using sensitive antibody tests, such as immunofluorescence, it was possible to detect specific antisporozoite antibodies in these sera. They could be differentiated in relation to antibodies against red blood cells because, although sporozoites had both a sporozoite-specific and a common antigen, which was also present in blood forms, the former was on the surface of the sporozoites. Thus, by reacting with viable sporozoites, it could be shown that these were specific antisporozoite antibodies.

Dr Miller said that the discovery of pyrimethamine, and its synthesis by Dr Hitchings and his co-workers, had introduced a new, unique approach to antimalarial development. Dr Hitchings, who would be speaking next, had a rational approach to antimalarials which differed from most other work which used the empiric or drug-screening approach.

8. The Metabolism of Plasmodia and the Chemotherapy of Malarial Infections

George H. Hitchings

The metabolic capabilities of plasmodia are of interest not only to comparative biochemistry, but in providing leads for the discovery of new chemotherapeutic agents. Since plasmodia are intracellular phago-trophes (Rudzinska and Trager, 1957) it would be expected that their metabolic processes would differ from those of autotrophic micro-organisms through deletions of anabolic functions that are redundant because the products are readily available from the host tissues ingested. In the main, this is probably true, but documentation is sketchy. One possible exceptional persistence is the synthesis *de novo* by plasmodia of folates, in the face of high concentrations of (5-methyl) tetrahydro-folates in erythrocyte (see p. 89). The biochemical capabilities of plasmodia would be expected to differ from one another, since those of erythrocytes differ from species to species (for example, human erythrocytes are incapable of converting inosinate to other ribonucleo-tides (Lowy *et al.*, 1962) although those of species other than the hominidae can do so). Thus it appears probable that a dovetailing of host and parasite metabolic profiles may play a major role in the specificity of plasmodial infections.

Current knowledge of plasmodial metabolism is fragmentary. It is derived from several sources: (a) from observations and manipulations of infected hosts; (b) from observations on infected erythrocytes in culture; and (c) from direct observations on infected parasites and extracts prepared from them. The reliability of interpretations of the evidence derived from these types of experiment probably increases in the order listed.

For example, it was believed on the basis of experiments of types 1 and 2 that plasmodia require pantothenate. Pantothenic acid, however, did not support the growth of free *Plasmodium lophurae* parasites; they required co-enzyme A or a close relative (Trager 1957; Trager and

Brohn, 1975). Enzymes in the erythrocyte are necessary to convert the vitamin to the functional co-factor.

The main thrust of the present paper will be to explore plasmodial metabolism as it relates to nucleic acid biosynthesis and to the biosynthesis and utilizations of folate-containing co-factors. Antimetabolites such as sulphonamides and sulphones interfere with this biosynthesis, and inhibitors of dihydrofolate reductase (DHFR) block the formation of tetrahydrofolate-containing co-factors. These are the only antimalarial drugs of which mechanisms of action are known in detail. Many of the standard antimalarials such as quinine, quinacrine, chloroquine and primaquine apparently bind to double-stranded DNA. All except primaquine inhibit the incorporation of $^{32}PO_4$ into nucleic acids, probably by binding also to single-stranded DNA (Rollo, 1975). Most of them probably owe their selectivities to some as yet unexplored properties which engender a concentrative uptake into parasites and parasitized erythrocytes (Polet and Barr, 1968). The similarities in their *loci* of action are supported by studies of resistance and cross-resistance (Thompson, 1968).

Evidence for the biosynthesis *de novo* of folate in plasmodia began to accumulate along with the development of biochemical knowledge of the folate system. The starting point of both was observations on the activity of sulphanilamide, and its reversal by *p*-aminobenzoic acid (*p*-AB). Thus, at almost the same time that sulphanilamide had been identified as the active principle of prontosil, Coggeshall (1938) had found it effective against *Plasmodium knowlesi* infections in rhesus monkeys, although it was ineffective against other experimental malarias and *P.vivax*. Shortly afterwards, sulphadiazine, and a diaminodiphenyl sulphone derivative (Promin) were found active (with some failures) against both *P.vivax* and *P.falciparum* infections in human subjects (Coggeshall *et al.*, 1941). Maier and Riley (1942) quickly showed that the activity of sulphanilamide against *P.gallinaceum* was blocked by *p*-AB. Ball (1946) and Anfinsen *et al.* (1946) not only showed that *p*-AB could reverse the effects of sulphadiazine, but that this substance was a requirement of *P.knowlesi* in infected erythrocyte cultures. Hawking (1954) demonstrated that depletion of the host of *p*-AB (milk diet) inhibited plasmodial infections in mice and monkeys and that supplementation of the diet with *p*-AB resulted in a resurgence of the infection. Jacobs (1964) extended these observations by showing not only that *p*-AB was required for the growth and development of *P.berghei* in mice, but that the *p*-AB was used by the parasite to form a substance similar to, but not identical with folic acid (FA). Kretschmar and Voller (1973) added similar experiments with *P.falciparum* in *Aotus* monkeys; moreover, they reviewed the whole literature on *p*-AB as well as infant resistance to malaria, and concluded that *p*-AB deficiency can play a major role in determining susceptibility to malaria. Thus many of the earlier experiments in which diets were uncontrolled may have given somewhat misleading answers; the effects of sulphonamides observed are to be regarded as minimal limits.

Basic knowledge of plasmodial metabolism has advanced in fits and starts, reflecting the waxing and waning of interest in malarial therapy consequent upon military involvement of developed countries in tropical areas. Thus, the promising beginnings of the early 1940s were followed by a premature decline, and the apex of discoveries in the field of folate biochemistry coincided with a period of languishing interest in malarial research. As a result, centre stage was held by pigeons and *Escherichia coli* as the biosynthetic pathways of purines, thymine and methionine were elucidated, as the role of *p*-AB as a precursor and component of dihydrofolate became apparent, and the catalytic role of tetrahydrofolate was documented. It is pertinent to review briefly the present state of knowledge in the field (for reviews see Friedkin, 1963; Hitchings and Burchall, 1965) as a basis for the understanding of recent developments in the field of plasmodial biochemistry.

Most bacteria synthesize *p*-AB *de novo* ultimately from phosphoenol-pyruvate and erythrose-4-phosphate via chorismate. Nevertheless, most species are able to assimilate exogenous *p*-AB. The competitive relationship between sulphonamides and *p*-AB therefore prevails whether or not *p*-AB is produced *de novo*. The critical property for sulphonamide inhibition is the inability of the cell to concentrate and utilize exogenous folates. Synthesis of folates *de novo* follows as an obligate requirement for survival. On the basis of the studies cited above it is highly probable that plasmodia require *p*-AB from exogenous sources. It seems clear, too, that this is used in the synthesis *de novo* of dihydropteroate (DHP) (see p. 81). Information on other protozoa seems to be lacking and

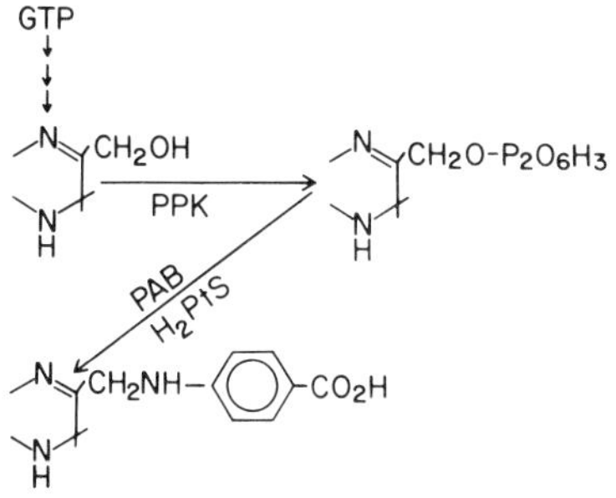

Fig. 1 Biosynthesis of dihydropteroic acid. Represented is the pyrazine portion of the pteridine molecule. Opening and excision of the 8-carbon atom of guanosine triphosphate (GTP) followed by reclosure and cleavage of the trihydroxypropyl side chain produces the hydroxymethylpteridine (partial structural formula). This is converted by the pteridine phosphokinase (PPK) to the pyrophosphate derivative which then condenses with p-aminobenzoate (PAB) in a reaction catalysed by dihydropteroate synthetase (H_2PtS) forming dihydropteroic acid (partial structural formula at bottom).

the inhibitions by sulphonamides of *Eimeria* (Joyner and Kendall, 1956) and *Toxoplasma* (Frenkel and Hitchings, 1957) point only to their synthesis of folates *de novo*.

The biochemical mechanism for folate biosynthesis was worked out with extracts of *Escherichia coli* (Brown, 1971). No inconsistencies with the scheme have appeared as other species have been investigated. It begins with opening of the imidazole rings of guanosine triphosphate (GTP) and proceeds in a multi-step sequence (Fig. 1) to the condensation of 2-amino-4-hydroxy-6-hydroxymethylpteridine pyrophosphate (AHMPP) with *p*-AB to form dihydropteroate. In bacteria, an additional enzyme that adds glutamate to DHP to form dihydrofolate (DHF) is widely distributed (Griffin and Brown, 1964). Plasmodia have been shown to contain DHP-synthetase (Walter and Königk, 1971; McCullough and Maren, 1974; Ferone, 1973), but DHF-synthetase has not been reported. It is true that the plasmodial enzyme will use *p*-aminobenzoylglutamate (*p*-ABG) which is a metabolite of folic acid in the rat (Murphy *et al.*, 1976) as substrate and thus produce DHF (Ferone, 1973) but the binding of *p*-ABG is much poorer than with *p*-AB, as is true with bacterial DHP-synthetases (Brown, 1971). Di- and triglutamates of *p*-AB seem not to have been investigated in any system. Ferone (1973), using *P.berghei* extracts, separated DHP synthesis into its two components, the pyrophosphokinase required for the activation of the pteridine, and the synthetase proper, although the two enzymes originally behaved as a complex with a molecular weight of between 200 000 and 250 000. Walter and Königk (1971), using extracts of *P.chabaudi*, were unable to effect a separation. McCullough and Maren (1974), also employing *P.berghei* extracts, used a system in which a preformed pyrophosphorylpteridine was required. Inhibition of pteroate synthesis by sulphonamides (Ferone, 1973; Walter and Königk, 1971) and sulphones (Ferone, 1973; McCullough and Maren, 1974) were reported. Ferone and Webb (1975) following an observation by Kisliuk *et al.* (1967) found dihydrohomopteroate to be a potent inhibitor of DHP-synthetase, 20 times as potent on the *P.berghei* enzyme as on the corresponding enzyme from *E.coli*.

The origins of the hydroxymethylpteridine used by plasmodia are unknown. It also is a product of cleavage of folates in the rat (Murphy *et al.*, 1976) and conceivably might be available to the parasite preformed. Either the pteridine, *p*-aminobenzoylglutamate or both may account for the stimulatory effects of exogenous folates (e.g. Trager, 1957). Antimetabolites to this portion of the folate molecule probably deserve attention.

A number of lines of investigation contributed to the current conception of tetrahydrofolate as a carrier of one-carbon units. Early work with secondary reversing agents of sulphonamides had implicated purines, thymine, methionine and serine in some system in which p-AB participated as a catalyst. Knowledge of the precursors of purine ring atoms and direct studies of enzymatic purine nucleotide synthesis led to the concept of an activated formate as a reactant and to tetrahydrofolate (THF) as the activator (for review see Buchanan, 1958–59). It is now known that THF-containing co-factors are formed by combining with one-carbon units at all levels of oxidation of carbon, and that these participate specifically in many biosynthetic reactions (Friedkin, 1963; Hitchings and Burchall, 1965). Those of particular pertinence for higher organisms are shown in the boxes in Fig. 2. In addition, co-factors participate in syntheses of many additional substances in autotrophic micro-organisms.

Only one of the co-factors, 5,10-methylene-tetrahydrofolate, is unequivocally important to plasmodia. This co-factor participates in the synthesis of thymidylate from deoxyuridylate, and the mechanism is unique. All other co-factor activities consist simply of a shuttle whereby THF alternately accepts and donates the one-carbon unit. When thymidylate is synthesized, the methylene unit is reduced to methyl and the hydrogen donor is the folate. Thus DHF is also a product of the reaction, and a second enzyme dihydrofolate reductase (DHFR) is required to keep the system running (see Fig. 2, upper left). The latter enzyme is of particular interest to malarial chemotherapy, as discussed below.

Synthesis *de novo* of thymidylate is an obligate requirement for growth and survival of plasmodia. Not only is the content of thymine nucleotides in the non-nucleated erythrocyte vanishingly small (Scholar *et al.*, 1973) but the thymidine content of body fluids is unsufficient to support cellular multiplication (Cleaver, 1967). Moreover, plasmodia have been found, in a variety of experiments, to be incapable of incorporating exogenous thymidine (Boden and Hull, 1973; Büngener and Nielsen, 1967; Davies and Howells, 1973; Gutteridge and Trigg, 1970, 1971;

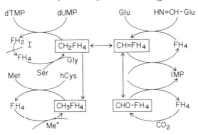

Fig. 2 Biosyntheses involving folate co-factors. The co-factors (shown in boxes) are derivatives of tetrahydrofolate (FH_4). Upper left, methylene FH_4, upper right, methenyl FH_4; lower left, 5-methyl FH_4; lower right, 10-formyl FH_4. Abbreviations used: dTMP, thymidylate; dUMP, deoxyuridylate; FH_2, dihydrofolate; Glu, glutamate, Gly, glycine; hCys, homocysteine; HN=CH–Glu, formiminoglutamate; I, inhibitor of dihydrofolate reductase; IMP, inosinate; Me, labile methyl groups; Met, methionine; Ser, serine. For enzymes see Hitchings and Burchall (1965), p. 425.

Jacobs *et al.*, 1974; Neame *et al.*, 1974; Omar *et al.*, 1975). This cannot be construed as demonstrating the absence of thymidine kinase, however, since most autotrophic bacteria also fail to incorporate exogenous thymidine although the enzyme is present and becomes expressed when synthesis is deleted (Singer *et al.*, 1966; Cleaver, 1967).

The enzymes needed for synthesis of thymidylate have been demonstrated to be endogenous products of plasmodial metabolism. These are serine hydroxymethyltransferase which synthesizes the co-factor, and thymidylate synthetase which transfers and reduces the methylene group. Serine hydroxymethyltransferase has been demonstrated by one author in one species (*lophurae*) of plasmodium (Platzer, 1970, 1972; Platzer and Campuzano, 1976) and indirectly by Smith *et al.* (1976) who found the hydroxymethyl group of serine to be incorporated into thymidylate by *P.knowlesi*. Further documentation in other species and human malarias in particular would be desirable. Thymidylate synthetase has been found present in *P.lophurae* (Walsh and Sherman, 1968), *P.chabaudi* (Walter and Königk, 1973) and *P.berghei* (Reid and Friedkin, 1973). The latter authors showed the enzyme to have a higher molecular weight and different responses to analogues than the host enzyme.

The most studied of the enzymes concerned with thymidylate synthesis is DHFR. This enzyme is necessary for two reasons. It is required in the first instance to convert the primary product of synthesis, DHF, to its active form, THF. The same reaction is needed to regenerate THF from the DHF which is formed in equimolar amounts with thymidylate. DHFR is the target of the agents, pyrimethamine, trimethoprim and cycloguanil (Hitchings, 1952; Rollo, 1955; Hitchings, 1960; Hitchings and Burchall, 1965; Ferone and Hitchings, 1966; Ferone *et al.*, 1969; Ferone, 1970; Walter and Königk, 1973; Platzer, 1970). The properties of the enzyme from *P.berghei* are strikingly different from those of the isofunctional enzyme of the host (Ferone *et al.*, 1969). The molecular weight was about 190 000 as compared with about 20 000 for bacterial and mammalian enzymes. A high molecular weight is a property shared by many other protozoal and helminth reductases (Jaffe, 1972). The plasmodial enzyme also exhibited tighter binding of substrates than those of the host enzyme and some differences in other properties. A striking feature, however, was the selective binding of pyrimethamine, giving IC_{50} values of 0·5 nM for the plasmodial enzyme as against 1 μM for the mouse-erythrocyte enzyme—a 2000-fold difference (Ferone *et al.*, 1969). In all, DHFR has been isolated from *P.berghei* (Ferone *et al.*, 1969), *P.vinckei* (Ferone *et al.*, 1970), *P.knowlesi* (Gutteridge and Trigg, 1971), *P.chabaudi* (Walter and Königk, 1973) and *P.lophurae* (Platzer, 1974) and, although extensions to other species are unlikely to provide any important surprises, further documentation would be desirable.

The substantive precursor of thymidylate, deoxyuridylate, and, in fact, all pyrmidines apparently are synthesized *de novo* by plasmodia. The original Harvard medium (Anfinsen *et al.*, 1946) for the cultivation of *P.knowlesi* in erythrocytes, contained both purines and pyrimidines. Trigg and Gutteridge (1971) apparently were the first to report that the pyrimidines were unnecessary. Meanwhile, and since, it has been reported by many authors that orotate is incorporated into the nucleic acids of plasmodia (Boden and Hull, 1973; Conklin *et al.*, 1973; Gutteridge and Trigg, 1970, 1971; McCormick and Canfield, 1972; and Polet and Barr, 1968). Two odd observations may be mentioned. Jacobs *et al.* (1974) found orotate not to be incorporated into developing sporozoites, and Ilan and Tokuyasu (1969) found it only in the 40s fraction of ribosomes.

Orotate phosphoribosyltransferase (OPRT) is an integral step in the synthesis *de novo* of pyrimidine nucleotides. Its presence would be inferred from the incorporation studies, but it remained for Walsh and Sherman (1968) to demonstrate it in extracts of *P.lophurae*. In the same paper the incorporation of $NaHCO_3$ was shown. This is important evidence showing that in this species, at least, pyrimidine biosynthesis follows the pathway that prevails in most organisms (Fig. 3) (Potter, 1960). Documentation is exceedingly skimpy. Of the many enzymes involved both before and after OPRT only aspartate transcarbamylase in *P.berghei* (Van Dyke *et al.*, 1970) and dihydro-orotate dehydrogenase in *P.gallinaceum*, *P.berghei* and *P.knowlesi* have been demonstrated (Davé *et al.*, 1976).

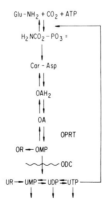

Fig. 3 *Biosynthetic pathway for pyrimidines. Abbreviations used: ATP, adenosine triphosphate; Car-Asp, carabamylaspartate; Glu–NH₂, glutamine; H₂N–CO₂–PO₃=, carbamylphosphate; OA, orotic acid; OAH₂, dihydro-orotate; ODC, orotate decarboxylase; OMP, orotate; OPRT, orotate phosphoribosyltransferase; OR, orotidine; UDP, uridine diphosphate; UMP, uridylate; UR, uridine; UTP, uridine triphosphate. Not indicated, dihydroorotate dehydrogenase (OAH₂OA) and formation of deoxyuridylate via reduction and dephosphorylation of UDP.*

Short-circuiting of pyrimidine biosynthesis by incorporation of uridine has been shown not to occur in a number of plasmodia: *P.lophurae* (Boden and Hull, 1973), *P.vinckei* (Büngener and Nielsen, 1967), *P.knowlesi* (Gutteridge and Trigg, 1970, 1971). Moreover, Schellenberg and Coatney (1961) found deoxyuridine as well as thymidine incapable of affecting the inhibition of DNA synthesis imposed by pyrimethamine. The only discordant note is the report by Conklin *et al.*, (1973) that uridine added to monkey blood infected with *P.knowlesi* appeared in the RNA but not the DNA of the parasites, whereas orotate appeared in both nucleic acids. These observations probably are explicable on the basis of details of host, rather than parasite, metabolism.

In contrast to the biosynthesis *de novo* of pyrimidines by plasmodia is their apparent dependence on preformed purines. The evidence consists of the requirement for exogenous purines in infected erythrocyte cultures, the demonstration of incorporation of exogenous purines by plasmodia—most significantly, in experiments with free parasites—and the apparent absence of all steps in the general biosynthetic pathway (see Fig. 2, right). It should be pointed out that the incorporation of pre-formed metabolites is not evidence for the absence of biosynthesis *de novo*. Most organisms possess the so-called "salvage pathways". The conversion of orotate to orotidylate is both salvage and an integral part of the biosynthetic sequence. Similarly, recycling of purine molecules is essential to metabolic balance. The incorporation of pre-formed purines suppresses synthesis *de novo* (e.g. Balis *et al.*, 1952) probably

Table 1
Incorporation of purines by parasites in infected erythrocytes

Plasmodial species	Substrates	Reference
lophurae	Ad	Boden and Hull, 1973
vinckei	Ad	Büngener and Nielsen, 1969
vinckei	AdR	Büngener and Nielsen, 1967
knowlesi	AdR	Concklin *et al.*, 1973
vinckei-chabaudi	AdR	Coombs and Gutteridge, 1975
knowlesi	Ad, Gu, H, AdR, GuR, dAdR	Gutteridge and Trigg, 1970
berghei	AdR, GuR	Neame *et al.*, 1974
knowlesi	Ad	Polet and Barr, 1968
lophurae	Ad, AdR, H, HR, Gu, GuR, XR	Tracey and Sherman, 1972
berghei	H, Ad, AdR	Van Dyke, 1975
berghei	AdR, dAdR, Ad, GuR	Van Dyke *et al.*, 1970
knowlesi	AdR	McCormick *et al.*, 1974

Infected erythrocytes were cultured in the presence of labelled precursors, the parasites were subsequently freed and extracted, and the DNA was purified and counted. The table lumps tritiated and ^{14}C purines.
Abbreviations used: Ad adenine; AdR adenosine; dAdR deoxyadenosine; Gu guanine; GuR guanosine; H hypoxanthine; HR inosine; XR xanthosine.

through feedback inhibition. The stimulatory effect of allopurinol (Büngener, 1974; Van Dyke, 1975) probably reflects its enhancement of recycling of purines (Hitchings, 1966).

The original Harvard medium (Anfinsen *et al.*, 1964) contained a purine supplement. Subsequent work has confirmed its necessity (e.g. Trigg and Gutteridge, 1971) and the incorporation of exogenous purines has been demonstrated repeatedly. The bulk of the incorporation data are derived from experiments with infected erythrocytes, as shown in Table 1. Such experiments leave undetermined the role of the erythrocyte. In view of the demonstration by Büngener and Nielsen (1969) that when erythrocytes were pre-labelled with ³H-adenine the label appeared in the parasite's purines, they perhaps show no more than that erythrocytic purine is available to the parasite. Feeding of tritiated adenosine and thymidine to mosquitoes bearing *P.cynomolgi* permitted tracing of the purine to the DNA of both oöcysts and sporozoites (Omar *et al.*, 1975). Thymidine was taken up by the mosquito tissues but not by the parasites.

More definitively, a limited number of observations show that free parasites can incorporate exogenous purines (Manandhar and Van Dyke, 1975; Tracey and Sherman, 1972). Moreover, two of the enzymes requisite to the incorporation of exogenous purines, hypoxanthine-guanine-phosphoribosyltransferase, and adenine phosphoribosyltransferase (Fig. 4, E1 and E2 respectively) have been purified several hundred-fold and characterized from *P.chabaudi* (Walter and Königk, 1974).

Investigations aimed at showing synthesis *de novo* from small molecule precursors have had the effect of bringing out the differences between erythrocytes of different species. Boden and Hull (1973) and Walsh and Sherman (1968) using *P.lophurae* found proffered formate in the purines of parasites liberated from infected erythrocytes, although the latter authors reported that free parasites incorporated few or none of the precursors. Formate was not incorporated in a monkey-erythrocyte

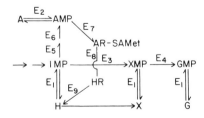

Fig. 4 Transformation and salvage pathways for purines. Abbreviations used: A, adenine; AMP, adenylate; AR, adenosine; E_1, hypoxanthine-guanine-phosphoribosyltransferase; E_2, adenine phosphoribosyltransferase; E_7, adenosine kinase; E_8, adenosine deaminase; G, guanine; GMP, guanylate; H, hypoxanthine; HR, hypoxanthine; IMP, inosinate; SAMet, S-adenosylmethionine; X, xanthine, XMP, xanthylate.

P.knowlesi preparation (Trigg and Gutteridge, 1971). Thus any indications of purine synthesis *de novo* in infected erythrocyte preparations can be attributed to the erythrocyte rather than the parasite. Consistent with this view is the absence of 10-formyl tetrahydrofolate synthetase, and 5,10-methylene tetrahydrofolate dehydrogenase from *P.lophurae* preparations although both enzymes were abundantly present in the duckling erythrocytes from which the parasites were derived (Platzer, 1972). Both these enzymes are required for the formation of the cofactors involved in purine biosynthesis *de novo* (see Fig. 2).

Very little is known about the interconversions of purines (see Fig. 4), E3–E6) by plasmodia. In the incorporation experiments of Table 1 the adenine and guanine of the nucleic acids were not separated, nor would there have been any way to distinguish between reactions of the erythrocyte and those of the parasite. Adenosine kinase (see Fig. 4, E7) as well as adenosine deaminase (Fig. 4, E8) were present (and difficult to separate) in extracts of *P.chabaudi*. The competition between these two enzymes can produce misleading results. At low (physiological) substrate concentrations kinase activity predominates almost exclusively (Miyazaki *et al.*, 1975). At higher concentrations the substrate is bound by the deaminase, and substrate inhibition of the kinase sets in. Thus, in experiments with both erythrocytes (Lowy *et al.*, 1962) and plasmodia (Van Dyke *et al.*, 1977) which report extensive deamination of adenosine are suspect. Since the human erythrocyte cannot convert hypoxanthine derivatives to either adenylates or guanylates (Lowy *et al.*, 1962) and the overwhelmingly predominant nucleotide in the erythrocyte is adenosine triphosphate (ATP) with almost negligible inosine triphosphate (ITP) (Table 2) it is clear that kinase activity prevails in

Table 2
Nucleotides of human erythrocytes[a]

Nucleotide	Concentration (mM)
NAD	0·075
NADP	0·028
AMP	0·003
ADP	0·061
ATP	0·970
ITP	0·001
GDP	0·010
GTP	0·052
UDP-G	0·193
UTP	0·003

[a] Nelson, D. J., unpublished data, 1977.
Abbreviations used: ADP adenosine diphosphate; AMP adenylate; ATP adenosine triphosphate; GDP guanosine diphosphate; GTP guanosine triphosphate; ITP inosine triphosphate; NAD nicotinamide-adenine dinucleotide; NADP NAD-phosphate; UDP-G uridine diphosphate-glucose; UTP uridine triphosphate.

this cell, probably utilizing adenosine released by the liver (Pritchard *et al.*, 1975). Although the A:G ratio of the human erythrocyte is about 20:1 while in the DNA of *P.knowlesi* the ratio is about 4:1 (Gutteridge *et al.*, 1971) there is no obvious reason why the parasite could not take both its adenine and guanine from the erythrocyte. It is to be hoped that the cultivation system of Trager and Jensen (1976) will be utilized to expand knowledge of the capabilities of plasmodia for purine transformation reactions. Human erythrocytes could easily be preloaded with labelled hypoxanthine derivatives (Nelson *et al.*, 1977) and any conversions to adenine and guanine taking place after infection would necessarily be reactions of the parasite.

Synthesis of methionine *de novo* also involves THF (see Fig. 2, lower left). The methylene group of 5,10-methylene tetrahydrofolate is reduced to 5-methyl group in a reaction requiring reduced nicotinamide adenine dinucleotide (NADH) and reduced flavin adenine dinucleotide ($FADH_2$). The methyl group is then transferred to homocysteine (h-Cys) and THF is regenerated. The transfer can involve either a cobalamine (vitamin B_{12}) co-factor, or catalysis by S-adenosyl methionine. Methionine was a constituent of the original Harvard medium (Anfinsen *et al.*, 1946). Its necessity was documented by McKee *et al.* (1947) and McKee and Geiman (1948) and many workers since have confirmed a requirement for this amino acid, and its incorporation into parasites, both free and in infected erythrocytes (see, e.g., McCormick *et al.*, 1974; Polet and Conrad, 1969; Sherman, 1977). Primate haemoglobins are somewhat deficient in methionine; they lack isoleucine entirely in contrast to those of lower mammals and fowl, and isoleucine must also, and possibly more critically, be supplied exogenously (Sherman, 1977) to primate plasmodia. Plasma, as well as haemoglobin, is a potential source of amino acids since they appear to enter cells by diffusion even where concentrative uptake is lacking. The methionine and isoleucine contents of human plasma are significant if not impressively high. Krebs' (1950) review places methionine at 0·06 μM and isoleucine at 0·12 μM, while Stein and Moore (1954) found somewhat lower values for methionine (about 0·03 μM).

If one accepts an absolute requirement for methionine, a consistent picture of folate biosynthesis and utilization appears. The relatively high THF content of the human erythrocyte (50–400 mμg per ml) and the adequate concentrations in plasma 5–10 mμg per ml) (Blakley, 1969) are not available to the parasite because they are present as 5-methyl derivatives and the parasite lacks the methyl group synthetic and transfer functions (see Fig. 2, lower left) as well as the whole purine biosynthetic cycles (see Fig. 2, right).

An inconsistency arises, however, with the finding of Smith *et al.* (1976) that *P.knowlesi*, in infected red cells, incorporated the hydroxymethyl group of serine into methionine-methyl to a much greater extent than did the uninfected erythrocyte. The methyl group of 5-methyltetrahydrofolate was not incorporated, however. A number of explanations exist alternative to the acceptance of this report as evidence for the existence in plasmodia of the 5-methyltetrahydrofolate cycle. This reluctance is amplified by the report (Platzer, 1972) that the vital enzyme, 5,10-methylene tetrahydrofolate dehydrogenase, is absent from *P.lophurae* though active in the duck erythrocytes. The prevailing evidence, therefore, is almost entirely consistent with the view that plasmodia retain only those portions of the complete pathways of folate synthesis and utilization which deal with the synthesis of dihydrofolate (see Fig. 2, upper left). Dihydrofolate reductase (DHFR, tetrahydrofolate dehydrogenase, E.C.1.5.1.3) is thus a critical enzyme for the growth and multiplication of the parasite.

The *locus* of action of pyrimethamine was identified as preventing the conversion of folic to folinic acid (Hitchings, 1952) before the isolation and characterization of DHFR. This was confirmed by the isolation of the enzyme from *P.berghei* and the demonstration of its selective binding to the plasmodial as compared with the host enzyme (Ferone *et al.*, 1969). Furthermore, the inhibitory concentrations for plasmodia *in vitro* are close to the concentrations required to inhibit the enzyme (Ferone *et al.*, 1969; McCormick *et al.*, 1971; Gutteridge and Trigg, 1971). The ultimate effect of inhibition of DHFR would be inhibition of thymidylate synthesis and subsequently DNA synthesis. Inhibition of DNA synthesis in *P.gallinaceum* and *P.berghei* by therapeutic concentrations of pyrimethamine was demonstrated by Schellenberg and Coatney (1961) using $^{32}PO_4$ incorporation as a measure of synthesis. They employed a 24-hour incubation of a suspension of erythrocytes. Moreover, a similar experiment with *P.gallinaceum in vivo* gave similar results.

Gutteridge and Trigg (1971, 1972), employing a shorter incubation period and a different species, *P. knowlesi*, agree that there is a close correlation between the enzyme and parasite-inhibitory concentrations of pyrimethamine. They find disconcerting, however, the differences in the time-course of incorporations of adenosine and orotate, that of adenosine alone paralleling the synthesis of DNA measured directly. They are also puzzled that the effects of pyrimethamine are apparent only at schizogony and not during the growth phase. They postulate that "either thymidylate is synthesized by a pathway not involving dihydrofolate reductase or that pyrimethamine penetrates to the malarial parasite only during schizogony" (Gutteridge and Trigg, 1972). A third alternative is more consistent with their facts. Pyrimethamine is known to be slow in its action (Goodwin, 1952). This and the data of Gutteridge and Trigg suggest that significant pools of thymidylate and/or 5,10-methylene tetrahydrofolate exist in the parasite. Synthesis of DNA during the early stages of growth would occur at the expense of these pools. In order to correlate incorporation and synthesis it would be necessary to determine the pool sizes of metabolites in both erythrocytes and parasite or, at least, to determine the relative specific activity (*vis-à-vis* orotate) of the thymine of the parasite DNA. Walter and Königk (1973), using synchronous cultures of *P.chabaudi*, found thymidylate synthetase and DHFR to wax and wane in synchrony, being minimal in rings and reaching a maximum accumulation just at cell division. Blockade of DHFR by pyrimethamine did not affect the synthesis of thymidylate synthetase.

Knowledge of the *loci* of action of sulphonamides and sulphones on the one hand and DHFR inhibitors on the other provides the basis for rational combination chemotherapy (Fig. 5). Sulphonamides and sulphones inhibit the biosynthesis of DHF through competition with *p*-aminobenzoate (*p*-AB). This inhibition manifests itself by slowing and ultimate cessation of multiplication as the pools of THF and products of its reactions are depleted through degradation and cell division. Inhibitors of DHFR (pyrimethamine, cycloguanil, etc.) block the reduction of DHF, both that newly formed and that generated as the result of the turnover of thymidylate synthetase.

This turnover accelerates the depletion of the THF pool, which is therefore more rapid with a reductase inhibitor than with a sulphonamide. Inhibitors of DHFR, however, are competitive inhibitors (Burchall and Hitchings, 1965) and their effectiveness depends on the inhibitor: substrate ratio, and unimpeded synthesis *de novo* of DHF tends to reduce the effectiveness of the block. It is advantageous, therefore,

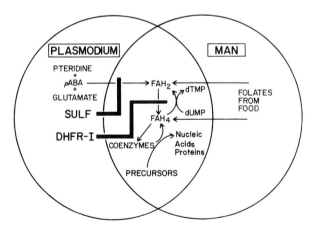

Fig. 5 Sites of action of sulphonamides and inhibitors of dihydrofolate reductase. Abbreviations used: DHFR-I, inhibitors of dihydrofolate reductase, SULF, sulphonamides and sulphones; for other abbreviations see legend to Fig. 2.

to combine the reductase inhibitor with an antagonist of p-AB. Potentiation in combinations of this type was observed early (Greenberg and Richeson, 1950) and has been confirmed repeatedly (e.g. Rollo, 1955; Hitchings, 1960; Hitchings and Burchall, 1965; McCormick and Canfield, 1972). Moreover, such combinations spread the range of sensitivities and reduce the likelihood of resistance (Richards, 1966).

The application of these findings to human malarias has been limited, although documentation has been adequate to demonstrate that potentiation does occur. Thus, Hurley (1959) and McGregor *et al.* (1963) showed the effectiveness of combinations of pyrimethamine and sulphadiazine (SD) while Basu *et al.* (1962) used combinations of pyrimethamine with diaminodiphenyl sulphone (DDS). One of the problems with such combinations is to match the two components with respect to pharmacokinetics. Pyrimethamine has a half-life of the order of four days in the human, while half-lives of DDS and SD are of the order of a half day. Better harmony is found in trimethoprim-sulphamethoxazole where both components are relatively short-acting, but the regimens employed have not always been designed to take this brevity into account. Pyrimethamine-sulphamethoxine and pyrimethamine-sulphalene are better matched. Both components in these have long duration of body levels and action. Trimethoprim-sulphalene also is a mismatch with a short-lived reductase inhibitor and a long-lived p-AB antagonist.

Some 95 references to the clinical use of combinations of this sort have been found. As prophylactics they have been successful even in areas where multiple drug-resistance has emerged (e.g. Chin *et al.*, 1966; Chin *et al.*, 1973; Shafei, 1975). Failures and recrudescences have occurred where these drugs were used therapeutically (Canfield *et al.*, 1971; Laing, 1974). Nevertheless, officialdom prefers to reserve them for therapeutic use, and to continue to use the best available therapeutic drug for prophylaxis (Laing, 1974; for comment, see Hitchings, 1968); thus, resistance to chloroquine continues to be disseminated (Peters, 1975; Tiggertt and Clyde, 1976). Fortunately, a sizeable group of new antimalarials, some with novel modes of action, awaits application (Canfield and Rozman, 1974). When, and if, further new antimalarials are needed, the prospects for success of a rational biochemical approach appear to be unusually high. The majority of plasmodial metabolic activities that have been examined have exhibited differences from host processes. Thus, in addition to the differences in isofunctional enzymes already mentioned, Schmidt *et al.* (1974) noted differences between the adenosine kinases of *P.chabaudi* and mouse erythrocyte. Reid and Friedkin (1973) commented on the difference in molecular weight between the thymidylate synthetases of *P.berghei* and mouse erythrocytes. Tsukamoto (1974) examined a battery of diverse enzymes of *P.berghei* and found them generally to have lower electrophoretic mobilities than the corresponding host enzymes; Carter and Voller (1973a) report similar findings with another group of enzymes, Büngener (1965) found an adenosine deaminase in *P.berghei*-infected erythrocytes that was not present in normal rat erythrocytes.

The possible requirements of plasmodia for vitamins and co-factors have been reviewed recently by Trager (1977). Apparent parasite requirements for ascorbic acid, riboflavin, thiamin (Rao and Sirsi, 1954) and vitamin E (Eaton *et al.*, 1976) have not been distinguished from similar host requirements. *P.lophurae* clearly requires co-enzyme A and is dependent on the host erythrocytes for its synthesis (Trager, 1977). The requirements of plasmodia for methionine and especially that for isoleucine (Sherman, 1977) are potentially exploitable—analogues with host: parasite selectivity would not be improbable. The co-enzyme Q metabolism of plasmodia seems distinguishable from that of the host, and antimetabolites based on this finding have significant selective action on malarial parasites (Porter and Folkers, 1974; Schnell *et al.*, 1971). It is possible that menoctone acts on this principle. This co-factor participates in parasite dihydro-orotate dehydrogenase activity (Davé *et al.*, 1976).

The carbohydrate metabolism of plasmodia has many possible points of difference from that of erythrocytes, but these have been difficult to demonstrate unequivocally (Homewood, 1977). The overlap with erythrocyte metabolism is only part of the problem; in malarial infections reticulocytosis and leucocytosis make inappropriate controls that are based primarily on a population of mature erythrocytes. However, several points of interest emerge. Oelshlegel, jr and co-workers (1975) have reported that in infections both of *P.berghei* in mice and *P.knowlesi* in monkeys, the infected erythrocyte shows an increase in ATP and a decrease in 2,3-diphosphoglycerate (DPG). This results from the introduction by the parasite of a new pyruvate kinase which alters the erythrocyte metabolism. By increasing the formation of phosphoenol-pyruvate, the formation of ATP is increased at the expense of phospho-glycerates. This is consistent with the high glycolytic activity and absence of the citric-acid cycle in plasmodia (Homewood, 1977).

A finding of particular interest is the apparent absence from plasmodia of glucose-6-phosphate dehydrogenase. This enzyme could not be found by Tsukamoto (1974) in extracts of *P.berghei*, and Theakston *et al.* (1976) found it only in food vacuoles of *P.falciparum*. The latter found, however, that phosphogluconate from the host could be carried through to pentose by the parasite; and the requisite parasite enzymes have been demonstrated by Carter and Voller (1973b). The implication is that host glucose-6-phosphate dehydrogenase is necessary for parasite growth and multiplication. This has an important bearing on the protective effect toward *P.falciparum* of a host deficiency in the enzyme, the selective infection of the normal erythrocytes when mosaicism occurs in heterozygotes (Luzatto *et al.*, 1969), and possibly the greater sensitivity of *Aotus* as against rhesus monkeys to infection with this parasite (Schnell *et al.*, 1969).

This paper presents only a sampling of the enzymatic and metabolic differences that have been observed between plasmodia and hosts, and one feels confident that deeper probing will uncover many more. To varying degrees all are grist to the mill of the drug designer.

Acknowledgement

I am greatly indebted to Robert Ferone for literature references and criticisms.

References

Anfinsen, C. B., Geiman, Q. M., McKee, R. Q., Ormsbee, R. A. and Ball, E.G. (1946). *Journal of Experimental Medicine*, **84,** 606–21.

Balis, M. E., Levin, D. H., Brown, G. B., Elion, G. B., Vanderwerff, H. and Hitchings, G. H. (1952). *Journal of Biological Chemistry*, **196,** 729–47.

Ball, E. G. (1946). *Federation Proceedings*, **5,** 397–9.

Basu, P. C., Mondal, M. M., and Chakrabarti, S. C. (1962). *Indian Journal of Malariology*, **16,** 157–75.

Bennett, T. P. and Trager, W. (1967). *Journal of Protozoology*, **14,** 214–6.

Blakley, R. L. (1969). "The Biochemistry of Folid Acid and Related Compounds", pp. 35–40. North-Holland, Amsterdam.

Boden, T. and Hull, R. W. (1973). *Experimental Parasitology*, **34,** 220–8.

Brohn, F. H. and Trager, W. (1975). *Proceedings of the National Academy of Sciences, USA*, **72,** 2456–8.

Brown, G. M. (1971). *Advances in Enzymology*, **35,** 35–77.

Buchanan, J. M. (1958–9). *Harvey Lectures*, **54,** 104–30.

Büngener, W. (1965). *Zeitschrift fur Tropenmedizin und Parasitologie*, **16,** 365–76.

Büngener, W. (1974). *Zeitschrift fur Tropenmedizin und Parasitologie*, **25,** 464–8.

Büngener, W. and Nielson, G. (1967). *Zeitschrift fur Tropenmedizin und Parasitologie*, **18,** 456–62.

Büngener, W. and Nielsen, G. (1969). *Zeitschrift fur Tropenmedizin und Parasitologie*, **20,** 67–73.

Burchall, J. J. and Hitchings, G. H. (1965). *Malarial pharmacology*, **I,** 126–36.

Canfield, C. J. and Rozman, R. S. (1974). *Bulletin of the World Health Organization*, **50,** 203–12.

Canfield, C. J., Whiting, E. G., Hall, W. H. and Macdonald, B. S. (1971). *American Journal of Tropical Medicine*, **20,** 524–6.

Carter, R. and Voller, A. (1973a). *British Medical Journal*, **1,** 149–50.

Carter, R. and Voller, A. (1973b). *Transactions of the Royal Society of Tropical Medicine and Hygiene*, **67,** 14–15.

Chin, W., Contacos, P. G., Coatney, G. R. and King, H. K. (1966). *American Journal of Tropical Medicine and Hygiene*, **15,** 823–9.

Chin, W., Bear, D. M., Colwell, E. J. and Kosakal, S. (1973). *American Journal of Tropical Medicine and Hygiene*, **22**, 308–12.

Cleaver, J. E. (1967). "Thymidine and Cell Kinetics", pp. 53, 84. American Elsevier, New York.

Coggeshall, L. T. (1938). *American Journal of Tropical Medicine and Hygiene*, **18**, 715–21.

Coggeshall, L. T., Maier, J. and Best, C. A. (1941). *Journal of American Medical Association*, **117**, 1077–81.

Conklin, K. A., Chou, S. C., Siddiqui, W. A. and Schnell, J. V. (1973). *Journal of Protozoology*, **20**, 683–8.

Coombs, G. H. and Gutteridge, W. E. (1975). *Journal of Protozoology*, **22**, 555–60.

Dave, D., Gutteridge, W. E., and Richards, W. H. G. (1976). *Parasitology (Proceedings)*, **73**, xvii.

Davies, E. E. and Howells, R. E. (1973). *Transactions of the Royal Society of Tropical Medicine and Hygiene*, **67**, 20.

Eaton, J. W., Eckman, J. R., Berger, E. and Jacob, H. S. (1976). *Nature, London*, **264**, 758–60.

Ferone, R. (1970). *Journal of Biological Chemistry*, **245**, 850–4.

Ferone, R. (1973). *Journal of Parasitology*, **20**, 459–64.

Ferone, R. and Hitchings, G. H. (1966). *Journal of Protozoology*, **13**, 504–6.

Ferone, R. and Webb, S. R. (1975). *In* "Chemistry and Biology of Pteridines", pp. 61–71, de Gruyter, Berlin.

Ferone, R., Burchall, J. J. and Hitchings, G. H. (1969). *Molecular Pharmacology*, **5**, 49–59.

Ferone, R., O'Shea, M. and Yoeli, M. (1970). *Science*, **167**, 1263–4.

Frenkel, J. K. and Hitchings, G. H. (1957). *Antibiotics and Chemotherapy*, **7**, 630–8.

Friedkin, M. (1963). *Annual Reviews of Biochemistry*, **32**, 185–214.

Goodwin, L. G. (1952). *British Medical Journal*, **1**, 732–4.

Greenberg, G. and Richeson, E. M. (1950). *Journal of Pharmacology and Experimental Therapeutics*, **99**, 444–9.

Griffin, M. J. and Brown G. M. (1964). *Journal of Biological Chemistry*, **239**, 310–16.

Gutteridge, W. E. and Trigg, P. I. (1970). *Journal of Protozoology*, **17**, 89–96.

Gutteridge, W. E. and Trigg, P. I. (1971). *Parasitology*, **62**, 431–44.

Gutteridge, W. E. and Trigg, P. I. (1972). *In* "Comparative Biochemistry of Parasites", pp. 199–218. Academic Press, New York.

Gutteridge, W. E., Trigg, P. I. and Williamson, D. H. (1971). *Parasitology*, **62**, 209–19.

Hawking, F. (1954). British Medical Journal, **1**, 425–9.

Hitchings, G. H. (1952). *Transactions of the Royal Society of Tropical Medicine and Hygiene*, **46**, 467–73.

Hitchings, G. H. (1960). *Clinical Pharmacology and Therapeutics*, **1**, 570–89.

Hitchings, G. H. (1966). *Annals of Rheumatic Diseases*, **25**, 601–7.

Hitchings, G. H. (1968). "Mode of Action of Anti-Parasitic Drugs", p. 76. Pergamon Press, New York.

Hitchings, G. H. (1971). *Annals of the New York Academy of Sciences*, **186**, 444–51.

Hitchings, G. H. and Burchall, J. J. (1965). *Advances in Enzymology*, **27**, 417–68.

Homewood, C. A. (1977). USAID/WHO Workshop on the Biology of Malaria Parasites (in press).

Hurley, M. G. D. (1959). *Transactions of the Royal Society of Tropical Medicine and Hygiene*, **53**, 412–13.

Ilan, J., Ilan, J. and Tokuyasu, K. (1969). *Military Medicine*, **134**, 1026–38.

Jacobs, R. L. (1964). *Experimental Parasitology*, **15**, 213–25.

Jacobs, R. L., Miller, L. H. and Koontz, L. C. (1974). *Journal of Parasitology*, **60**, 340–3.

Jaffe, J. J. (1972). "Comparative Biochemistry of Parasites", pp. 219–33. Academic Press, New York.

Joyner, L. P. and Kendall, S. B. (1956). *British Journal of Pharmacology*, **11**, 454–7.

Kisliuk, R. K., Friedkin, M., Schmidt, L. H. and Rossan, R. N. (1967). *Science*, **156**, 1616–17.

Krebs, H. A. (1950). *Annual Review of Biochemistry*, **19**, 409–30.

Kretschmar, W. and Voller, A. (1973). *Zeitschrift fur Tropenmedizin und Parasitologie*, **24**, 51–9.

Laing, A. B. G. (1974). *Bulletin of the World Health Organization*, **50**, 231–4.

Lowy, B. A., Williams, M. K. and London, I. M. (1962). *Journal of Biological Chemistry*, **237**, 1622–5.

Luzatlo, L., Usango, E. A. and Reddy, S. (1969). *Science*, **164**, 839–42.

McCormick, G. J. and Canfield, C. J. (1972). *Proceedings, Helminthological Society of Washington*, **30**, 292–7.

McCormick, G. J., Canfield, C. J. and Willet, G. P. (1971). *Experimental Parasitology*, **30**, 89–93.

McCormick, G. J., Canfield, C. J. and Willet, G. P. (1974). *Antimicrobial Agents and Chemotherapy*, **6**, 16–23.

McCullough, J. L. and Maren, T. H. (1974). *Molecular Pharmacology*, **10**, 140–5.

McGregor, I. A., Williams, K. and Goodwin, L. G. (1963). *British Medical Journal*, **2**, 239, 728–9.

McKee, R. W. and Geiman, Q. M. (1948). *Federation Proceedings*, **7**, 192.

McKee, R. W., Geiman, Q. M. and Cobbey, jr. T. S. (1974). *Federation Proceedings*, **6**, 276–7.

Maier, J. and Riley, E. (1942). *Proceedings of the Society of Experimental Biology and Medicine*, **50**, 152–4.

Manandhar, M. S. P. and Van Dyke, K. (1975). *Experimental Parasitology*, **37**, 138–46.

Miyazaki, H., Nanibu, K. and Hashimoto, M. (1975). *Journal of Biochemistry*, **78**, 1075–8.

Murphy, M., Keatin, M., Boyle, P., Weir, D. G. and Scott, J. M. (1976). *Biochemistry-Biophysics Research Committee*, **71**, 1017–24.

Neame, K. D., Brownhill, P. A. and Homewood, C. A. (1974). *Parasitology*, **69**, 329–35.

Nelson, D. J., Bugge, C. D. and Krasney, H. (1977). "Purine Metabolism in Man: II. Regulation of Pathways and Enzyme Defects", pp. 121–8. Plenum Press, New York.

Oelshlegel, jr. F. J., Sander, B. J. and Brewer, G. J. (1975). *Nature, London*, **255**, 345–7.

Omar, M. S., Gwadz, R. W. and Miller, L. H. (1975). *Zeitschrift fur Tropenmedizin und Parasitologei*, **26**, 303–6

Peters, W. (1975). *Journal of Tropical Medicine and Hygiene*, **78**, 167–70

Platzer, E. G. (1970). *Journal of Parasitology, Proceedings*, **56**, 267–8.

Platzer, E. G. (1972). *Transactions of the New York Academy of Sciences*, **34**, 200–7.

Platzer, E. G. (1974). *Journal of Protozoology*, **21**, 400–5.

Platzer, E. G. (1976). *Journal of Protozoology*, **23**, 282–6.

Platzer, E. G. and Campuzano, H. C. (1976). *Journal of Protozoology*, **23**, 282–6.

Polet, H. and Barr, C. F. (1968). *Journal of Pharmacology and Experimental Therapeutics*, **164**, 380–6.

Polet, H. and Conrad, M. C. (1969). *Military Medicine*, **134**, 939–44.

Porter, T. H. and Folkers, K. (1974). *Angewandte Chemie*, **13**, 559–619.

Potter, V. R. (1960). "Nucleic Acid Outlines: I. Structure and Metabolism", p. 292. Burgess Publishing Company, Minneapolis.

Pritchard, J. B., O'Connor, N., Oliver, J. M. and Berlin, R. D. (1975). *American Journal of Physiology*, **229**, 967–72.

Rao, R. R. and Sirsi, M. (1954). *Journal of the Indian Institute of Science*, **38**, 108–14.

Reid, V. E. and Friedkin, M. (1973). *Molecular Pharmacology*, **9**, 74–80.

Richards, W. H. G. (1966). *Nature, London*, **212**, 1494–5.

Rollo, I. M. (1955). *British Journal of Pharmacology*, **10**, 208–14.

Rollo, I. M. (1975). "The Pharmacological Basis of Therapeutics", pp. 1045–68. Macmillan, New York.

Rudzinska, M. A. and Trager, W. (1957). *Journal of Protozoology*, **4**, 190–9.

Schellenberg, K. A. and Coatney, G. R. (1961). *Biochemical Pharmacology*, **6**, 143–52.

Schmidt, G., Walter, R. D. and Konigk, E. (1974). *Zietschrift fur Tropenmedizin und Parasitologie*, **25**, 301–8.

Schnell, J. V., Siddiqui, W. A. and Geiman, O. M. (1969). *Military Medicine*, **134**, 1068–73.

Schnell, J. V., Siddiqui, W. A., Geiman, Q. M., Skelton, F. S., Luman, K. D. and Folkers, K. (1971). *Journal of Medicinal Chemistry*, **14**, 1026–9.

Scholar, E. M., Brown, P. R., Parks, jr. R. E. and Calabresi, P. (1973). *Blood*, **41**, 927–36.

Shafei, A. Z. (1975). *Journal of Tropical Medicine and Hygiene*, **78**, 190–2.

Sherman, I. W. (1977). USAID/WHO Workshop on the Biology of Malaria Parasites (in press).

Singer, S., Elion, G. B. and Hitchings, G. H. (1966). *Journal of General Microbiology*, **42**, 185–96.

Smith, C. G., McCormick, G. J. and Canfield, C. J. (1976). *Experimental Parasitology*, **40**, 432–7.

Stein, W. H. and Moore, S. (1954). *Journal of Biological Chemistry*, **211**, 915–26.

Theakston, R. D. G., Fletcher, K. A. and Moore, G. A. (1976). *Annals of Tropical Medicine and Parasitology*, **70**, 125–7.

Thompson, P. E. (1968). "Mode of Action of Antiparasitic Drugs", pp. 69–75. Pergamon Press, New York.

Tigertt, W. D. and Clyde, D. F. (1976). *Antibiotics and Chemotherapy*, **20**, 246–72.

Tracy, S. M. and Sherman, I. W. (1972). *Journal of Protozoology*, **19**, 541–94.

Trager, W. (1957). *Acta Tropica*, **14**, 289–301.

Trager, W. (1977). USAID/WHO Workshop on the Biology of Malaria Parasites (in press).

Trager, W. and Brohn, F. H. (1975). *Proceedings of the National Academy of Sciences*, **72**, 1834–7.

Trager, W. and Jensen, J. B. (1976). *Science*, **193**, 673–5.

Trigg, P. I. and Gutteridge, W. E. (1971). *Parasitology*, **62**, 113–23.

Tsukamoto, M. (1974). *Nettai Igaku*, **16**, 55–69.

Van Dyke, K. (1975). *Tropical Medicine and Parasitology*, **26**, 232–8.

Van Dyke, K., Trembly, G. C., Lantz., C. H. and Szustkiewicz, C. (1970). *American Journal of Tropical Medicine and Hygiene*, **19**, 202–8.

Van Dyke, K., Trush, M. A., Wilson, M. E. and Stealey, P. K. (1977). USAID/WHO Workshop on the Biology of Malaria Parasites (in press).

Walsh, C. J. and Sherman, I. W. (1968). *Journal of Protozoology*, **15**, 763–70.

Walter, R. D. and Königk, E. (1971). *Zeitschrift fur Tropenmedizin und Parasitologie*, **22**, 256–9.

Walter, R. D. and Königk, E. (1973). *Zeitschrift fur Tropenmedizin und Parasitologie*, **24**, 250–55.

Walter, R. D. and Königk, E. (1974). *Zeitschrift fur Tropenmedizin und Parasitologie*, **25**, 227–35.

Discussion

Dr Miller pointed out that the Walter Reed Programme had screened between 200 000 and 300 000 drugs; from that screening programme there had been little or no success in developing new antimalarials. The success of the programme had been obtained by going back to Second World War drugs and synthesizing their various analogues. It seemed that the general screening approach had reached the end of its useful life, and more work was needed to develop new groups of antimalarials.

Dr Krause said that Dr Hitchings had given an excellent review of what was known about plasmodial metabolism, although there were many gaps in our knowledge. He asked if it was correct that little was known about the electron transport, and Dr Hitchings replied that the whole citric acid cycle was missing. Dr Krause added that the reason for cytochrome oxidase being present was also still unknown.

9. New Methods of Vector Control: their Possible Role in Malaria Campaigns

M. T. Gillies

I should like to start by posing a very elementary question, namely, that if malaria transmission can be broken by intervention at any point in the cycle, either in man, or against the parasite or the mosquito, why has most malaria control been directed against the mosquito? And this leads on to the second question—should this continue to be the case in the future?

Robert Koch, on the basis of his studies on malaria in what was then German East Africa said "Treat the patient, not the mosquito" (Jaramillo-Arango, 1950). However, his advice was seldom followed, probably because of the truism that prevention is better than cure. If you eliminate the vector, or at least that section of the vector population responsible for transmission, namely the older age-groups of females, you eliminate the disease. The second reason for the predominance of anti-mosquito measures was that they worked. Wherever it was possible to implement this strategy, the reduction of vectors at source by larval control, or the elimination of infective females by house-spraying, amply fulfilled expectations. And the advent of residual insecticides enormously increased the possibilities of effective control, almost—it seemed—as to embrace the malarious regions of the whole world. Other speakers have described the fading of this dream. In the light of the situation that now confronts us, we must enquire whether mosquito control will still play a leading part in malaria campaigns or whether the development of resistance to insecticides and the problems of economic development are forcing us to a radical change in policy. In other words, are the present setbacks merely a hiccough in the long history of successful vector control, or are they a turning-point in our whole approach to the problem of malaria? The outstanding feature of residual house-spraying was that, for the first time, it permitted the mounting of mass campaigns in rural areas on a country-wide scale. If we are driven to abandon house-spraying, is there any new form of mosquito control, at present under development, that in the foreseeable future can replace it? That is the question I shall attempt to answer today.

It now seems clear that the progressive development of resistance in vectors may very well outstrip the capacity of the chemical industry to produce new insecticides. This, as much as anything else, is why eradication has dropped out of the malariologist's vocabulary. Before going on to look at other methods, I should like to mention one or two new types of chemical control that are currently under development.

Synthetic Pyrethroids

One such group comprises the synthetic pyrethroids. The first advance was the synthesis of knock-down agents with greatly increased toxicity to insects when compared with natural pyrethrins. These included S-bioallethrin and biomesrethrin. The latter has been shown to be 55 times more toxic to flies than the pyrethrins (Potter, 1973), and field trials against salt-marsh *Aedes* have been very encouraging (Brooke *et al.*, 1974). But of greater interest to malariologists has been the development of the first long-acting pyrethroids, notably permethrin, NRDC-161 and NRDC-167. Panels treated with the last-named compound gave good kills of *A.quadrimaculatus* for over two months (Reed *et al.*, 1977). Here, for the first time, we have residual insecticides of great potency and of extremely low toxicity to vertebrates. At the present time the cost of these compounds and the duration of their residual effect does not make them suitable for mass campaigns; future developments, however, may very well change the picture. We must expect that resistance may arise in time if they are widely used against mosquitoes. But the risk would be diminished if this group of compounds were not suitable for use against agricultural pests. Unhappily, this may be too much to ask.

Monolayers

One new type of agent has been tested in recent years that acts through its physical rather than its chemical properties. These agents are the monolayers, phospholipids or high alcohols that form a monomolecular film on water surfaces and thus interfere with the respiration of larvae and pupae (McMullen *et al.*, 1977). Their action is primarily against pupae, which respire entirely through the surface, while the effect on larvae is less marked (Reiter, 1978). Little has been published so far on field trials of monolayers, but early results suggest that the film is rather rapidly destroyed in natural breeding-sites, so that its effectiveness in killing pupae may be reduced to a few days or even, in the case of natural lecithins, to a matter of hours. In oxygenated water the larvae can survive without access to the surface purely by cutaneous respiration; but at low oxygen-saturation levels they are killed in the course of a few hours (Reiter, 1977). In natural waters with abundant plant life, oxygen tensions are known to fall to low levels at night, and it has been suggested that under these conditions monolayers may be fatal to larvae as well as pupae. Certain preparations have been found to be effective against *Anopheles* larvae under semi-field conditions (Garrett and White, 1977). These agents have virtually no environmental impact, but their usefulness remains to be established.

Insect Growth-regulators

One entirely new group of agents to have entered the field in recent years are the insect hormones, which may be growth-regulators, developmental inhibitors or hormone mimics (Chamberlain, 1975). For convenience they are known collectively as insect growth-regulators or IGRs. When applied to larval breeding-sites, they cause death or greatly retarded development with consequent suppression of adult emergence. As control agents they have two disadvantages, namely, their rapid breakdown in natural waters and the restricted period in the life of the larvae in which their effect is maximal. These shortcomings can be overcome by formulating the agents in such a way as to release them slowly into the water (Majori *et al.*, 1977). In this way the duration of effectiveness can be increased to two weeks. Certain IGRs have been shown to be very effective against *Anopheles* (Lowe *et al.*, 1975). Although expensive, they are showing great promise in the control of floodwater-pest mosquitoes. Their value for the control of malaria vectors remains to be determined. But it may be noted that cross-resistance to an IGR of a dieldrin-resistant strain of *A. gambiae* has already been recorded (Kadri, 1975).

Genetic Control

If chemical control is ruled out, what alternative ideas and methods are available? Perhaps the most convincing of the new concepts is that of genetic control. Two main approaches have been advocated: population suppression by the sterile male technique and population replacement by the introduction of chromosomal rearrangements into wild populations. The principle underlying the latter approach is to use radiation to induce chromosomal aberrations, which may be either translocations or inversions. It has been proposed that these could be employed in a number of ways (Rai, 1973). The simplest would be to release a strain homozygous for a particular translocation. The translocation heterozygotes resulting from hybridization with wild-type mosquitoes would be sterile. By releasing strains with multiple translocations a high degree of sterility in the wild population should result. Another use of translocations would be to introduce genetic characters favourable to disease control, such as insecticide susceptibility, low infectivity to malaria parasites or perhaps even with altered feeding preferences (Curtis, 1968). A third and even more esoteric idea has been proposed, that envisages the isolation of conditional lethal genes, such as temperature sensitivity. These would not be expressed under rearing conditions in the insectary, but at certain seasons would be lethal in the wild (Davidson, 1974).

Development of the sterile male technique is much more advanced, and a number of pilot projects have been carried out. The principle here is to inundate a local population with males that have been sterilized by irradiation or by chemical sterilants. Since females normally mate once only in their lives and, other things being equal, do not discriminate between fertile and sterile males, a high proportion of sterile eggs are produced and the population declines. If sequential releases of sterile males are maintained, this decline should progress to the point of total elimination of a vector population. The most successful trial of this new technique was carried out by American workers against *A.albimanus* in El Salvador (Lofgren *et al.*, 1974). Releases of over four million sterilized males into an area of 15 km^2 over a five-month period resulted in a 99 % reduction of the vector population. Thus the validity of the technique in malaria control was amply demonstrated. Additional importance should be attached to this experiment since the suppressed population of *albimanus* was an isolated focus of the vector. Because of this, permanent eradication of such foci of transmission appears to be feasible.

A further method of inducing sterility operates by producing hybrids of certain species complexes; *A.gambiae* is one of these. Hybrid males resulting from crosses between sibling species are sterile. A field trial in West Africa using hybrids of two species to suppress a population of a third species was not successful, probably because of insufficient mating competitiveness (Davidson *et al.*, 1970). It has been shown in laboratory cages, however, that it is possible to produce stocks with the sex chromosomes of one species and the autosomes of another which it is aimed to control. Since mating behaviour is likely to be controlled by autosomal genes, the released hybrids should be fully competitive with the wild population. Hybrids of a cross between females of this stock and males of the target species yield sterile males which are then used for releases (Curtis, 1978).

The best known and most successful application of the sterile male technique is, of course, the campaign against the screw-worm in the USA. Yet even here, although dramatic reduction of fly was achieved and the economic benefits were enormous, eradication of the species over the whole area has not been achieved. One reason for this is thought to be inadvertent selection for loss of competitive ability in nature resulting from factory conditions of rearing (Davidson, 1974). This points up an inherent weakness in any technique involving mass releases, namely, the difficulty of producing genotypes with optimal fitness for the local environment. There are other major objections to the technique that I will return to after discussing other new tools now being forged or on the drawing-board.

Biological Control

The idea of biological control probably has an instinctive appeal for all of us. It fits in, too, with the contemporary mood that sees nature as something to be manipulated in a way favourable to our interests rather than confronted and overpowered. Medical entomologists are not immune to its appeal either, and at present a wide range of biological agents is being studied (Chapman, 1974; Arata and Briggs, 1976). These include both predators and pathogens. Few new predators have been tested, and larvivorous fish are still quite widely used in mosquito control. Good control of *A. freeborni* in rice-fields in the USA has been achieved by stocking with 300 mature *Gambusia* per acre (Hoy *et al.*, 1971), and in some areas of that country routine stocking of rice-fields is carried out. Trials using laboratory-reared *Hydra* for the control of *Culex* in natural ponds have been reported (Yu and Legner, 1973). Planarians have been used in the same way (Legner, 1977). On the other hand, a great deal of research is going on into potential pathogens belonging to a variety of different groups.

Microsporida

Numerous microsporidans are known to occur as natural infections both in the wild and, accidentally, in mosquito colonies, particularly *Anopheles*. This has suggested their possible value as biological agents against malaria vectors. Their use has the additional attraction that, in *A. albimanus*, reduced longevity of infected females has been reported, and it has been suggested that this effect alone could cause an important reduction in the survival-rate of vectors (Anthony *et al.*, 1972). A further point in their favour is that microsporidans are transmitted through the eggs so that their chances of dissemination in nature are enhanced. However, I know of no published accounts of field trials with these agents.

Bacteria

The success of *Bacillus thuringiensis* in the control of forest insect-pests has suggested its use against mosquitoes. A related species, *B. sphaericus*, has been found to have considerable pathogenicity for mosquitoes, including certain *Anopheles*. A lot of groundwork has been done on the mass dissemination of *thuringiensis* in pest control, which provides a valuable background for developing studies on *sphaericus*. One major advantage is that the mass production of bacterial spores does not require sophisticated technology, a major consideration in developing countries.

Viruses

No useful viral agents against *Anopheles* have been isolated yet.

Fungi

Coelomomyces is probably the best known of mosquito parasites and has been recorded from many species of *Anopheles*. The discovery that the Copepod *Cyclops* is the intermediate host of this fungus (Whisler *et al.*, 1974), has made possible the cultivation of the parasite in the laboratory, an essential first step towards mass production. On the other hand, the complexity of the life-cycle, involving two obligate hosts, makes it clear that successful control involves more than simple dissemination of infective spores. Infected larvae usually die before pupation so that the frequency of infection in adult mosquitoes is very low. Natural spread of the fungus from one body of water to another is therefore rather slow. On the other hand, long-term persistence of the infection in particular breeding-sites has been shown in *A.gambiae* (Muspratt, 1963).

A more recently isolated fungus, *Metarrhizium*, has been found to show considerable promise as a pathogen of *Anopheles*, even though no natural infections in mosquitoes have been reported. In the laboratory, *A.gambiae* has been shown to be highly susceptible to it (Arata and

Briggs, 1976). In the case of this fungus specific toxins have been isolated, the destruxins, and one wonders whether these might form the basis for new types of insecticides.

Nematodes

Considerable progress has been made in the study of the preparasitic Mermithids, which have been found, usually at low frequencies, in many species of mosquitoes. The problems of culturing the worms in the laboratory have been solved, and the cultures can be applied to natural breeding-sites in much the same way as chemical larvicides (Levy *et al.*, 1976). Spraying from the air is also feasible (Petersen and Willis, 1974). Field trials have shown that a high degree of parasitization of *A.crucians* can be achieved by spraying 1000–2000 preparasitic nematodes per square yard. The adults are free-living and the eggs can survive in damp soil. This, coupled with the relative ease of mass production, suggests that this form of control could be of considerable value in controlling local sources of pest mosquitoes. Its value in malaria control remains to be determined. It is perhaps significant that the susceptibility of a laboratory strain of *A.quadrimaculatus* to infection with Mermithids dropped to a half of the original level after four years' use for culturing the parasite (Woodward and Fukuda, 1977). The mechanism of resistance appeared to be behavioural, the mosquito larvae becoming more active on contact with nematodes.

This is a formidable list of potential biological agents for controlling mosquitoes. But what does it add up to at the present time in practical terms? Commenting a year ago, a leading authority on the development of biological control observed that, of all the predators and pathogens under study in mosquito control "only a few fishes can be called operational" (Chapman, 1976). This is not to discount the possibility that we may discover new and potent pathogens that will establish themselves in natural populations of vectors, and research towards this end is highly desirable. But it does mean that this method of control is still something for the future.

Other Methods

I should now like to ask the question, what other forms of entomological interference might be useful in malaria control? The most direct approach is to attempt to break contact between man and the mosquito by some form of physical protection. The screening of houses and the use of bed-nets are long-established examples of this. The former demands a standard of housing seldom attained in rural areas of the tropics. But interestingly enough, there is an experiment in self-help along these lines being tried out in Ujama villages in Tanzania (N. Kolstrup, personal communication). Using funds from international aid, bedrooms are being converted by the householders into mosquito-proof rooms by installing ceilings, blocking-in the eaves with mud, and screening the windows and door. This is being done as part of an experiment to control bancroftian filariasis, transmission of which requires much more intense man/mosquito contact than does malaria. Nevertheless, it is a novel idea and one that, in conjunction with other methods, might help to relieve the burden of malaria in developing countries.

The use of some form of bed-net is widespread. It is true that their state of repair and the way in which they are used often turns them into mosquito-traps rather than a form of protection. However, it has been suggested that the mass distribution of nets and propaganda on the importance of using them properly might help to diminish the level of transmission. It is hard to be dogmatic about this. There is the obvious fact that some transmission occurs in the early part of the night before people go to bed and that on festive occasions people may stay up until all hours, especially in Africa. More importantly, no precise information is available on the proportion of people normally sleeping under nets in any particular region, nor do we know in any quantitative way the degree of protection afforded by nets when used normally. Interest in this subject has been raised by the suggestion that insecticides could be more economically used if bed-nets were sprayed rather than the walls of houses. Preliminary trials with organophosphorus compounds have been encouraging (Brun and Sales, 1976). It would presumably be necessary to supply bed-nets to the whole population, which would add to the cost. On the other hand, when the insecticidal effect waned, the inhabitants would still be enjoying some protection from attack. Again, this would be no answer to the ultimate development of resistance.

Space repellents should also be mentioned. These have been used experimentally either on wide-mesh cotton netting or, more effectively, sprayed on to the mud walls of houses (Sholdt *et al.*, 1976); it seems unlikely, however, that they could ever be used on a large scale. Other possibilities are suggested by the control of agricultural pests, for example, the possible place of chemical attractants in mosquito control. The answer is not encouraging. Sex attractants, so successful against an increasing number of crop-pests, are unsuitable, since with rare exceptions they play no part in the mating behaviour of mosquitoes. On the other hand, host attractants are of major importance for blood-sucking insects: could these be used, one might ask, as lures to divert mosquitoes from human hosts? Again, the answer must be no, for a number of reasons. The first is that a warm-blooded host is superior in its power of attraction to any specific factor that has been isolated from human sections; the chances of developing a "super-attractant" therefore seem remote. CO_2 is indeed a useful attractant, but its range of effect is limited and if used at high rates major problems arise in trapping or killing mosquitoes attracted to it. Secondly, the analogy with crop pests is misleading. Sex attractants are used where the pests are most concentrated, i.e. within standing crops. Vector mosquitoes are most concentrated in and around human settlements. This means that an artificial attractant, even if one were discovered, would merely serve to draw extra insects into the village where it would have to compete with the superior power of attraction of human bodies.

Conclusions

In evaluating the future of vector control it is essential to make the distinction between mass campaigns and localized projects. The most striking feature of residual house-spraying was that it permitted the mounting of country-wide campaigns. This is the yardstick by which one must measure the new tools being developed now and in the future; and it is by this that they will stand or fall. In my view, none of the methods that entomologists are working on can foreseeably take the place of house-spraying in major malaria control operations. To be fair, it is probably true that none of them is intended to. They could provide local solutions to particular malaria problems such as occur in densely populated areas and special communities. Before the DDT era, larval control in the tropics was limited to these types of situation; the new methods, should they prove to be practicable, will be as limited in their application. The tools may be new, but the strategy is an old one.

It is still too early to assess the potential of the new pyrethroids, although some of them are of great potency. The same is true of the IGRs. They may become valuable in dealing with localized pest-mosquito problems, but their short biological life and high cost militates against their widespread use in malaria control. Of the other new tools listed, only the sterile-male technique has been proved capable of suppressing a vector population in the field. The population of *A.albimanus* was an isolated one. Given the wide and continuous distribution of most vectors and their high reproductive-rate, it would seem that population suppression can only be achieved in special situations. As regards the more sophisticated methods of genetic control by population replacement, I would quote the words of one experienced reviewer of the subject: ". . . passing from small-scale projects to large-scale application is largely wandering into the unknown. . . . To many people, the extension of such techniques to the control of insects with a known high rate of reproduction is inconceivable" (Davidson, 1974).

The role of biological controlling agents is likely to be as restricted as the other new methods.

Despite the limitations on their use there are, nevertheless, a number of potential situations where the new tools could play a useful part. One such is the malaria generated by irrigated rice-growing schemes in Africa. These are frequently in areas of moderate rainfall, and transmission, which was formerly seasonal, now occurs all the year round. The limits of the breeding-areas are well defined and their distribution is strictly focal. Similarly, the malaria of urban and periurban areas and of islands and oases might be susceptible to more sophisticated methods. One could envisage, for example, population suppression by genetic methods, releases being made on a regular basis at seasons appropriate to the type of control. Population replacement and the use of pathogens and predators could also be important here.

To return to the question of whether vector control should still play the dominant part in malaria control—we are talking here about mass campaigns in rural areas for which none of the new entomological tools would seem adequate at present. Only two methods of control can be regarded as practicable on this scale, house-spraying and the administration of antimalarial drugs. In general, the organophosphorus insecticides are likely to be of most value until high resistance becomes an overriding obstacle to their application. The high cost of some of these compounds might demand economical use; for instance, spraying might be restricted to certain areas or carried out at longer than optimal intervals, making sure, however, that effective control was maintained during the main transmission season. It might be wise to restrict their use to areas where crops do not require heavy inputs of insecticide, which would mean, for example, abandoning mosquito control in cotton-growing areas.

Vector control measures could usefully be supplemented with drug administration; the relative amount of effort put into the two methods might vary according to the local situation. This would be integrated control at its simplest. It might be supplemented in time with improvements in personal protection from mosquito attack and in housing, and when an effective vaccine becomes operational this would allow much greater flexibility in the choice of other methods. It seems improbable that integrated control using a wide range of sophisticated techniques could ever be practised on a wide scale: apart from the cost, the amount of expert assessment that would be continuously required would be beyond both national and international resources. In the mass control of malaria, anti-mosquito measures will remain dominant only as long as effective insecticides are available; should we be deprived of them in the future, the responsibility for the large-scale control of malaria could pass into other hands.

References

Anthony, D. W., Savage, K. E. and Weidhaas, D. E. (1972) Nosematosis: its effect on *Anopheles albimanus* Wiedemann, and a population model of its relation to malaria transmission. *Proceedings of the Helminthological Society Washington* (Special Issue), **39**, 428–33.

Arata, A. A. and Briggs, J. D. (1976). Biological control of vectors. (WHO) unpublished working document, TDR/WP/76.22.

Brooke, J. P., Giglioli, M. E. C. and Invest, J. (1974). Control of *Aedes taeniorhynchus* Wied. on Grand Cayman with ULV Biomesrethrin. *Mosquito News*, **34**, 104–11.

Brun, L.-O. and Sales, S. (1976). Stage IV evaluation of four organophosphorus insecticides: OMS-43, OMS-1155, OMS-1197 and OMS-1424 applied at 0.2 g/m^2 to cotton mosquito nets. (WHO unpublished working document. WHO/VBC/76.630.)

Chamberlain, W. F. (1975). Insect-growth regulating agents for control of arthropods of medical and veterinary importance. *Journal of Medical Entmology*, **12**, 395–400.

Chapman, H. C. (1974). Biological control of mosquito larvae. *Annual Review of Entomology*, **19**, 33–59.

Chapman, H C. (1976). Biological control agents of mosquitoes. *Mosquito News*, **36**, 395–7.

Curtis, C. F. (1978). Possible use of translocations to fix desirable genes in insect populations. *Nature, London*, **218**, 368–9.

Curtis, C. F. (1968). Hybrid sterility in the *Anopheles gambiae* complex: mechanism and possible means of using it for genetic control. *Transactions of the Royal Society for Tropical Medicine and Hygiene* (in press).

Davidson, G. (1974). "Genetic Control of Insect Pests". Academic Press, London and New York.

Davidson, G., Odetoyinbo, J. A., Colussa, B. and Coz, J. (1970). A field attempt to assess the mating competitiveness of sterile males produced by crossing two member species of the *Anopheles gambiae* complex. *Bulletin of the World Health Organization*, **42**, 55–67.

Garrett, W. D. and White, S. A. (1977). Mosquito control with monomolecular organic surface films: II. Larvicidal effect on selected *Anopheles* and *Aedes* species. *Mosquito News*, **37**, 350–3.

Hoy, J. B., O'Berg, A. G. and Kauffman, E. E. (1971). The mosquito-fish as a biological control agent against *Culex tarsalis* and *Anopheles freeborni* in Sacramento Valley rice-fields. *Mosquito News*, **31**, 146–52.

Jaramillo-Arango, J. (1950). "The Conquest of Malaria". Heinemann, London.

Kadri, A. Bin Haji. (1975). Cross-resistance to an insect hormone analogue in a species of the *Anopheles gambiae* complex resistant to insecticides. *Journal of Medical Entomology*, **12**, 10–12.

Legner, E. F. (1977). Response of *Culex* spp. larvae and their natural insect predators to two inoculation rates with *Dugesia dorotocephala* (Woodworth) in shallow ponds. *Mosquito News*, **37**, 435–40.

Levy, R., Murphy, L. J. and Miller, T. W. (1976). Effects of a simulated aerial spray system on a Mermithid parasite of mosquitoes. *Mosquito News*, **36**, 498–501.

Lofgren, C. S., Dame, D. A., Breeland, S. G., Weidhaas, D. E., Jeffery, G. M., Kaiser, R., Ford, H. R., Boston, M. D. and Baldwin, K. F. (1974). Release of chemosterilized males for the control of *Anopheles albimanus* in El Salvador: III. Field methods and population control. *American Journal of Tropical Medicine and Hygiene*, **23**, 288–97.

Lowe, R. E., Schwarz, M., Cameron, A. L. and Dame, D. A. (1975). Evaluation of newly synthesized insect growth-regulators against *Anopheles quadrimaculatus*, *Anopheles albimanus*, and *Aedes taeniorhynchus*. *Mosquito News*, **35**, 561–3.

McMullen, A. I., Reiter, P. and Phillips, M. C. (1977). Mode of action of insoluble monolayers on mosquito pupal respiration. *Nature (London)*, **267**, 244–5.

Majori, G., Bettini, S. and Pierdominici, G. (1977). Methoprene or Altosid for the control of *Aedes detritus* and its effects on some non-targets. *Mosquito News*, **37**, 57–62.

Muspratt, J. (1963). Destruction of the larvae of *Anopheles gambiae* Giles by a *Coelomomyces* fungus. *Bulletin of the World Health Organization*, **29**, 81–6.

Petersen, J. J. and Willis, O. R. (1974). Experimental release of a mermithid nematode to control *Anopheles* mosquitoes in Louisiana. *Mosquito News*, **34**, 316–9.

Potter, C. (1973). Environmental outlines: I. Safe clean insecticides: the pyrethroids. *Developmental Forum* 1 (1), United Nations Centre for Economic and Social Information. (Cited in Brooke, J. P., 1976. *Mosquito News*, **36**, 402–11)

Rai, K. S. (1973). Genetic control of biting flies: progress and prospects. *In* "Symposium on biting-fly control and environmental quality", pp. 79–88. University of Alberta.

Reed, J. T., McWorthy, L. A., Eulberg, J., Sullivan, W. N. and Grothaus, R. H. (1977). Longevity of two new pyrethroids and pyrethro-organophosphate combination against two species of mosquitoes and against house-flies. *Mosquito News*, **37**, 135–6.

Reiter, P. (1977). The influence of dissolved oxygen content on the survival of submerged mosquito larvae. *Mosquito News* (in press).

Reiter, P. (1978). The action of lecithin monolayers on mosquitoes: II. Action on the respiratory structures of larvae and pupae. *Annals of Tropical Medicine and Parasitology*, **72**, 169–176.

Sholdt, L. L., Holloway, M. L., Grothaus, R. H. and Schreck, C. E. (1976). Dwelling-space repellents: effect upon behavioural responses of mosquitoes in Ethiopia. *Mosquito News*, **36**, 327–31.

Whisler, H. C., Zebold, S. L. and Shemanchuk, J. A. (1974). Alternate host for mosquito parasite *Coelomomyces*. *Nature (London)*, **251**, 715–6.

Woodard, D. B. and Fukuda, T. (1977). Laboratory resistance of the mosquito *Anopheles quadrimaculatus* to the Mermithid nematode *Diximermis peterseni*. *Mosquito News*, **37**, 192–5.

Yu, H. S. and Legner, E. F. (1973). Inoculation of *Hydra* (Coelenterata) and predation effectiveness in experimental mosquito (*Culex*) breeding-habitats. *Proceedings of the 41st Annual Conference of the Californian Mosquito Control Association*, 131–6.

Discussion

Dr Miller said that much of the work on malaria control had arisen from the one major discovery, made in 1898, that the mosquito was the vector of malaria. Another discovery of that magnitude was now needed so that once again malaria could be controlled.

Dr J. E. Scanlon (*University of Texas*) referred to diethyl toleramide (DEET) which had been mentioned by Dr Gillies. At the recent meeting of the Advisory Committee on Entomology to the Army Surgeon-General in the USA, DEET had been discussed; it had proved to be a potent teratogen and would soon be withdrawn from the market. Another subject discussed at the same meeting was a fungus which was showing tremendous promise; a small trial carried out in California showed a complete absence of mosquitoes in highly potential breeding sites more than one year after application of the fungus: neither larvae nor pupae could be found. The man responsible for the work had been urged to go to field trials for at least three years, but so far had not done so.

Dr Scanlon said that a panel of the National Academy of Science which had met in 1975 had reached the same conclusions as Dr Gillies, that for the foreseeable future nothing would replace the synthetic pesticides. He thought Professor Bruce-Chwatt might wish to mention a more recent study which had reached the same conclusions about malaria in Asia.

Dr Karl Maramorosch (*Rutgers University*) said that the reason why integrated control had not yet succeeded was that, for economic reasons, only the chemical and one other agent had been tested. He thought that not one or two, but three methods should be used; that is, the fungal with the biological and chemical control, and perhaps viral control. Although at present there were no effective viruses, this was a promising area which could be developed, and might lead to a reduction in the mosquito population.

Dr Gillies agreed that integrated control could be effective in localized situations. However, the point of his argument was that the expert assessment, programme handling, monitoring and the amount of detailed information required for a large-scale programme, would be beyond the resources available.

Professor Bruce-Chwatt said that Dr Scanlon had presented the current situation with regard to insecticide control, as far as malaria was concerned. Few suitable new insecticides had been found; not only was there the problem of growing resistance, but also the cost, toxicity and other factors. Traditional methods of control were again being used—source reduction, prevention of larval breeding, decrease of potential breeding places and intermittent irrigation—all the methods which had been mentioned by Dr Gillies. He said the tactics in malaria eradication strategy were simple—"Let us spray" —and hope to succeed.

Speaking of malaria control, as opposed to eradication, he said that sophisticated and knowledgeable malariologists and entomologists were needed, who were fully conversant with the bionomics of local malaria vectors, and able to adapt the methods of control to the prevailing conditions. Unfortunately such people were not available; they had been eradicated by residual insecticides! He said the current role of WHO was to retrain, train and create a new cadre who would be able to carry out field research, and to apply the kinds of cheap, economical and reasonably satisfactory methods of control which could be incorporated into active community participation. Therein lay the future of malaria control in urban and rural areas of developing countries.

He accepted the role of residual insecticides in malaria control, but in local conditions, strictly applicable to the needs of the area, and no longer on a very large scale. In limited areas all types of residual insecticides could be of considerable value, but the synthetic pyrethroids were impossibly expensive and he did not imagine that they would ever become cheaper.

III. Schistosomiasis

Kenneth S. Warren

At a symposium on the immunology of parasitic infections in June 1977 in Bethesda, one of the participants said that we should not only consider what immunology has done for schistosomiasis, but what schistotosmiasis has done for immunology, and I think that this holds for biomedical science in general. Briefly *Schistosoma mansoni* and *S. japonicum* cause a unique form of liver disease in which there is very little damage to the liver parenchymal cell, but marked changes in the liver circulation. All other major forms of liver disease do both simultaneously, so that we have biochemical changes due to sick parenchymal cells in the presence of marked circulatory changes. Studying schistosomiasis we can separate the symptoms and the physiological and biochemical changes that are due to alterations in circulation from those that are due to alterations in liver parenchymal cell function.

Another interesting distinction is that schistosomiasis causes liver fibrosis, not liver cirrhosis. A major factor in all forms of liver cirrhosis is fibrosis, but there are very few, if any, good animal models for this phenomenon. Recently, a group at the Albert Einstein Hospital has realized that murine schistosomiasis might make a good model for studying collagen formation and fibrosis, and they have been doing exciting work in that area. The first paper has been published in the *Journal of Clinical Investigation* and studies are now complete on liver fibrosis in patients with schistosomiasis in Egypt, not because of an interest in schistosomiasis but because of an interest in the biochemistry of liver fibrosis.

Schistosomiasis is a granulomatous disease, and one might be able to say that we know more about the mechanisms of granuloma formation for schistosomiasis than for any other disease, including tuberculosis: and what is learned of the mechanisms of granuloma formation in schistosomiasis is facilitating the understanding of this process in other fields where the models are actually more difficult to work with.

Another area of great interest is the mechanism for the natural immuno-suppression that occurs in schistosomiasis. All the work done on suppressor T-cells has usually involved antigens such as those found on sheep red-blood cells. Nevertheless, these suppressive phenomena are going on naturally in experimental animals with schistosomiasis, and now evidence is increasing that they are occurring in humans with schistosomiasis and maybe a major factor in preventing disease. This is of great importance because it appears that most chronic diseases that have significant immunological components have suppressor-cell or modulating immunological factors. This includes many different kinds of cancer.

Another area which schistosomiasis has pioneered is in our understanding of the eosinophil. It is possible at this moment to say that we may finally have found a function for the eosinophil; it appears to be the killer cell in antibody-dependent cellular cytotoxicity in schistosomiasis, and possibly in trichinosis; I think that if we look further we shall find it in many other common helminth infections.

Finally, I should like to mention the anti-schistosomal drug niridazole which appears to have potent immunosuppressive activity; this was discovered by people working on schistosomiasis. British investigators have recently shown that in cardiac transplants done in rats, niridazole in combination with other immunosuppressive drugs is a most powerful means of preventing cardiac graft rejection. Recently a group working in a pharmacology department in the USA have been able to isolate the active immunosuppressive metabolite of niridazole and it is an extremely powerful substance in suppressing cell-mediated immunity in tiny amounts. So it is possible that niridazole may become one of our major tools for suppressing graft rejection in the future.

Schistosomiasis has done at least as much, and perhaps more, for biomedical science than biomedical science has done for schistosomiasis, so there are good reasons on both sides why research should be fostered on this major problem for hundreds of millions of people, not only for their benefit but for those with many other diseases.

Professor Eli Chernin, author of the following paper, has been working on schistosomiasis for many years and has experience of many different aspects of the problem.

10. Bilharz's "Splendid Distomum": Schistosomiasis, 1950–1977

Eli Chernin

Introduction

One hundred and twenty-five years ago the young Bilharz stumbled onto his "splendid distomum", now *Schistosoma haematobium*. In the early 1900s Sambon validated the new *Schistosoma mansoni*. These two parasites, together with *Schistosoma japonicum*, several *japonicum*-like worms in Southern Asia and the Orient (Sasa, 1972; Wright, 1973; Yokogawa, 1974), some *haematobium*-like worms in small foci in India, and several zoonotic worms that infect man—these all represent our foes.

It would be presumptuous to sermonize on the past 25 years of work in schistosomiasis. We lack a true perspective against which to make confident assessments; the past is too close, and the future is too uncertain. I have, therefore, elected to mention only parts of the whole, leaving the rest to the articles that follow.

General

Our perceptions of schistosomiasis have changed against a background of astonishing geopolitical evolution and population growth. Africa, for example, has doubled its population since 1950, and since the Second World War the number of self-governing African states has risen from four to 48, their birth and existence accompanied by endless complications. They are young, poor, hungry, ill-educated, diseased, and anxious to move beyond their past into a future of their own making. This is the stuff of which crisis is made. A modern novelist addressing a different problem inadvertently spelled out the true malaise of developing countries. "The crisis", Grameci writes (see Holmes, 1977), "consists precisely in the fact that the old is dying and the new cannot be born; in this interregnum a great variety of morbid symptoms appear". I shall try to highlight some of these "morbid symptoms" by asking, "where are we?".

"Where are we?" can be measured in several ways, not all of them equally informative. The 93 schistosomiasis entries in the *Index Medicus* of 1950 rose to 365 in 1975, which says nothing, of course, about the quality of either group of papers, but such numbers do underlie bio-medicine, academic promotion, tenure, etc. (Chernin, 1975). Other numbers reveal the lopsided policy of the USA in disbursing its research funds: $800 million were allocated for cancer research in the USA last year, but only $40 million were expended by *all* nations for research on tropical diseases ". . . [although] the parasitic diseases are the 'cancers' of developing nations . . . the forgotten problems of forgotten people" (Schultz, 1977). Others estimate the outlays as $270 million and $30 million, respectively (Gordon Smith, 1976). Lepes of the World Health Organization (1976) referring now to the worldwide investment in WHO's new and exciting Special Programme, points out that its support represents about 12–15 % of the annual investment in research on cancer and cardiovascular disease in the USA alone. We must also acknowledge still other accountings rarely rendered in public. And so I stop here to recall the colleagues we all knew and loved and lost. It is only right that we remember those who made their mark and died in recent years: men such as Elvio Sadun and Don McMullen, R. T. Leiper and George Macdonald, who still live among us in their work; we owe to them and to others a conscious remembrance.

Prevalence of Infection and of People

Since schistosomiasis is worldwide, we would want, among other things, to know its supposed prevalence. In Stoll's famous paper on the prevalence of helminthiases (1947), his guess for schistosomiasis was 114 million infections; in the mid-1960s WHO's Expert Committee estimated 150–200 million cases; more recently WHO edged up to 180–200 million infections (of 0.5 billion at risk); one worker estimated 300 million cases (Jordan, 1975); another chose 117 million (Wright, 1968); while a schistosomiasis conference at Tulane (Miller, 1972) settled for 150 million. The only certainty is that we do not know the true figures; diagnoses are questionable, and reporting is incredibly bad. One example will suffice: Willard Wright (1968) discovered that during 1963–64 more than 10 times as many cases of schistosomiases were reported to the Pan American Health Organization from New York State than from all of Brazil.

But a closer look at available data gives us pause, for in the developing countries children under 5 years make up from 15% to 20% of the population as compared with 8% in developed countries (USA, Agency for International Development, 1972b). As Weller (1975) points out, most African countries are growing at 2–3% per year, doubling in about 27 years; however, urban areas will double in about 15 years and, according to Gratz (1974), the extensive peri-urban shantytowns will double in about 4–6 years. Urban and peri-urban schistosomiasis constitutes an obvious health threat as water accumulates in borrow-pits and stagnant drains. As Weller says, a growing, schistosome-infected, young population will excrete more eggs into a more finite environment, and thus intensity of infection and morbidity will likely increase henceforth.

Food, Power and Dams

Burgeoning populations demand food, and more food requires irrigation, the arable land having long since gone under the plough. The food shortage, and the need for hydro-electric power have caused people to change the face of the earth by building irrigation schemes and dams of unimaginable size and complexity without, as a rule, considering the ecological and disease problems they were courting. WHO warned member nations in 1950 of the unhealthy connection between irrigation and schistosomiasis, and of the equally unhealthy prospects inherent in shifting agriculture from basin to perennial irrigation. That this warning was ignored is testimony to the shortsightedness of those governments that stumbled ahead anyway, until the infection caused the abandonment of some costly irrigation schemes. In what must have been the understatement of 1953, the first WHO Expert Committee dealing with schistosomiasis wrote that the co-operation between health and irrigation authorities had not been achieved or been as close as necessary (World Health Organization, Expert Committee on Bilharziasis, 1953). Note that when perennial irrigation was first introduced into lower Egypt, schistosomiasis prevalence shot from 5% to 80% within a few years—so it is not surprising if fishermen now living on Lake Nasser, i.e., behind the High Dam, already "enjoy" a 60% prevalence of urinary schistosomiasis. But that is only part of the story, for Aswan's ecological impact is varied and incalculable: loss of fertile silt behind the dam; deltaic soil erosion by the sea; soil salinity; evaporation and seepage; and effects on fisheries near the Nile's Mediterranean outflow.

And Lake Nasser is "only" 5000 km² in area. The other three huge dams in Africa created Lake Kariba (Zambia–Rhodesia), 4300 km², Lake Kainja (Nigeria), 1280 km², and the largest, Lake Volta (Ghana), with its 8500 km² area (Obeng, 1975; Waddy, 1975). The size of Lake Volta can best be appreciated by comparing its shoreline (6400 km) with the sea-coastline of the entire African continent, about 30,000 km. The Akosomba dam on the Volta was completed in 1964. By 1966 *Bulinus truncatus rohlfsi* (intermediate host of *Schistosoma haematobium*) was established in the lake and *Biomphalaria pfeifferi* (intermediate host of *S.mansoni*) was moving in via the Dayi River, one of several streams feeding the lake. According to Paperna (1969, 1970) the prevalence of *S.haematobium* infection in and around the lake, in children under 16, increased sharply, sometimes to 100%, within a few years. The main bright spot of the last decade is the WHO research team, funded by the United Nations Development Programme (UNDP), studying schisto-somiasis and the lake. I am glad to have had a minor hand in WHO's Volta activity early in the planning stages. Let me mention, too, that lakes undergo ecological successions just as do woodlands; the point is that the Volta lake will be different in 10 years from now and certainly 50–100 years hence when it has reached "climax" conditions. New techniques will be needed to deal with evolving problems in the future.

Disease and irrigation aside, dams are also built for profit. The Akosombo Dam produces about 883 MW per year, 300 MW of which goes to the Volta Aluminium Co at Tema, on the coast, for its alu-minium smelter; the power costs over $5 million per year, and the pro-duction of aluminium (about 12 000 tons) brings in a profit of $15 million (Farid, 1975). Eighty thousand people had to be re-settled in building this dam, and according to Waddy (1975) Lake Nasser displaced 120 000 and Lake Kainja over 40 000 people. Between 1960 and 1967 the prevalence of schistosomiasis in some lakeside villages increased 20 times (Deom, 1975), and schistosomiasis is only *one* of several diseases whose epidemiology centres on or near impounded water. Although this discussion is confined to Africa, huge dams are going up in south Asia and in South America, each to the accompani-ment of its own set of health problems.

We cannot live without dams and we cannot live with them. Con-ventional control methods with molluscicides (World Health Organiza-tion, 1973; Webbe, 1972) and other means (McMullen, 1973) are less than satisfactory, and new control methodologies still lie over the hori-zon. But the past 25 years of dam building leaves us with the need some-how to cancel their noxious effects so that man can enjoy his measure of health. "Measure of health", one might say, is all the Pilgrims ex-pected given the rigours of their seventeenth-century New England environment. I'll wager that no economists can convert "measure of health" into dollars and cents, but they insist that we must do so.

Hygeia and Environmental Engineers

To turn to a related subject—it seems desirable to include sanitary engineers in anti-schistosomal planning, but the dearth of such people is disturbing. The few engineer-survivors such as Dr Kaz Kawata at Johns Hopkins complain that the American Society of Tropical Medicine and Hygiene does not seem to want or need them; either drop the "Hygiene", he says, or encourage that aspect of the Society's activity. He is right, of course, and we mean to revivify "Hygiene" and its implications. As if one needed further evidence supporting Kawata's position, along comes a letter (22 August 1977) from the American Board of Preventive Medicine, sent to the Deans of all schools of public health. The letter reads, in part, ". . . the MPH [Master of Public Health] programs at certain schools . . . do not contain courses in environmental health as a formal requirement for all students receiving the degree. The Board considers this subject to be one of the major areas of preventive medicine". The letter includes the instruction that after June 1978 no MPH student will be Board-certified if he cannot document having had a course in environmental health. The pendulum swings again. . . .

It seems well to close this section with the words of yet another engineer. Jerome Weisner (1977), president of the Massachusetts Institute of Technology, said in June 1977 that:

> "Today we face new kinds of risk . . . those associated with man-made technology. Unlike natural disasters, the probability of man-made disasters can usually be adjusted. Unfortunately, the cost of making the risks very small is apt to be very large, and finding an appropriate balance is not just a technical question or an analytical one, but a question of values—which risks are worth what costs?"

In 1953's Craig Lecture, Henry Meleney (1954) made what has become an oft-repeated remark: "We are now in the stage of the conquest of schistosomiasis," he said, "comparable to the stage in malaria control when we had only quinine for treatment, oil, paris green, and ditching for larvae control, and fly-swatters and screening for adult mosquitoes." How ironical! He could hardly have imagined that quinine and paris green would reappear as antimalarial measures, or that the anti-schistosomal tools would start improving as malaria eradication programmes disintegrated—a full turnabout in less than a quarter century.

The Literature of Schistosomiasis

Warmth, water, and poverty are the basic ingredients of tropical life: add a few snails and a dash of faeces or urine, and you have schistosomiasis; the recipe is simple and will serve any number. One of the by-products of the recipe is the scientific "literature" which all of us have suffered with and contributed to.* We can count ourselves lucky in that Warren and Newall (1967) took on the 10 000-plus references (1852–1962) and made of them a usable and unique bibliography. Warren followed it up with an annotated bibliography comprising a selected 4% of the papers, representing nearly 8000 pages of reading (Warren, 1973c). Recently published (co-authored with Hoffman, 1976) is a compendium of abstracts from the *Tropical Disease Bulletin*, *Helminthological Abstracts*, and Medlars (for 1963–74), and still to come is a selected and annotated treatment of that literature. The literature of no other biomedical field has been treated so as to serve well both the novice and the experienced worker. We are all in Warren's debt for his bibliographic and his other imaginative efforts on our behalf.

Additional Highlights—a Melange of Achievements and Under-Achievements

The following lists additional highlights, each reflecting a different facet of 1950–77.

(1) The Rockefeller Foundation altered its 1950 policy of withdrawal from international health and began its generous support of the St Lucia project. Finances aside, the psychological impact of the Foundation's move has been immeasurable. The Edna McConnell Clark Foundation has also entered this research field to everyone's benefit. The new Special Programme of WHO emphasizes schistosomiasis reduction among its several goals (Buck, 1976). Further support comes from the United Nations Development Programme (UNDP), from our National Science Foundation, from the National Institute of Health (NIH) extra-mural research programme (Narin and Shapiro, 1977), and from its support (with the State Department) of the Parasitic Disease Panel of the US–Japan Co-operative Medical Sciences Program. Aid in Britain comes from some of the sources mentioned and from the Medical Research Council and various private organizations, most notably the Wellcome Trust. To me, however, two of the most hopeful signs came when AID (USA Agency for International Development, 1972) and then the World Bank (International Bank for Reconstruction and Development, 1975) came to demand health-impact

---

* "Schisto Packet I" provides a novel, useful and aesthetically pleasant way to keep up with the literature. The packet is free and available through J. S. Lehman, jr, MD, Vice-President, The Edna McConnell Clark Foundation, 250 Park Ave., New York, N.Y. 10017. The first issue of the packet was made possible by grants from the Edna McConnel Clark Foundation, The Rockefeller Foundation, and Warner-Lambert Company.

reports before disbursing huge sums for development schemes in developing countries.

(2) The St Lucia project itself, now over 10 years old, is a marvel of planning and execution; in no way does it resemble the field schemes of recent years elsewhere in the world, the results of which are still being argued (Farooq *et al.*, 1966a, b; Gillies *et al.*, 1973; Jordan, 1974; Chu, 1976). For the first time we have equatable data on three methods of schistosomiasis control applied in three separate valleys simultaneously (Christie and Upatham, 1977; Unrau, 1975; Jordan *et al.*, 1975; Jordan *et al.*, 1976; Cook *et al.*, 1977a; Cook *et al.*, 1977b). During one two-year period, incidence was reduced from 19% to 4% with hycanthone chemotherapy (cost = $1·10 per capita), from 22% to 10% with snail control (cost = $3·70 per capita), and from 23% to 11% by providing domestic water supplies (cost = $4·00 per capita). While the results from St Lucia may not be fully reproducible everywhere, the methods of control that succeeded there merit consideration wherever an effective control scheme is required (Jordan, 1977). This may prove even truer if the new drug, praziquantel, now under field trial, lives up to its laboratory promise as a superior schistosomicide (Gönnert and Andrews, 1977; Pellegrino *et al.*, 1977; Webbe and James, 1977; James *et al.*, 1977).

(3) The People's Republic of China has broken its self-imposed silence *vis-à-vis* the world and schistosomiasis. US experts visited China in 1975 and learned that *Schistosomiasis japonicum*, once endemic in the Yangtze plains and delta, had engaged the labours of some 20 million people in control work. Control took many forms but none was more spectacular than the mass burial or drowning of oncomelanids by the shovels of millions of people, a control approach that could work only in China. The area's schistosomiasis prevalence, if a 20-year-old base figure is to be accepted, is said to have been reduced from about 10 to about 3 million infected people. The Chinese running the programme were pragmatists: use any method that works and do not bother with research. Hence, it was no surprise to learn from the Report (US Government, Schistosomiasis Delegation, 1977) that no research was in progress even at the Shanghai Institute of Parasitology. Recent political events in China may, however, redress the balance. Dr William Trager, and others from the Rockefeller University, visited China in May 1977, and found the Shanghai Institute humming with research; indeed, about one-half of the 300 professionals were working on schistosomiasis (Trager, personal communication, 1977). However, Harrison Salisbury (1977) reported in the *New York Times* that, "in August, officials [in Peking] began using the figure of 900 million for the total population [of China] after five years of using the figure of 800 million. The new figure indicates that, despite a birth control program, popula-

tion continues to rise more rapidly than food production." And so the inevitable: more irrigation, more schistosomiasis, more shovels—and more Chinese.

(4) Puerto Rico, Venezuela, and Japan have all but eradicated their schistosomes. Control techniques varied from molluscicides and drugs to biological means. To the best of my knowledge biological control has been used effectively only in Puerto Rico (with *Marisa cornuarietis*; Chernin *et al.*, 1956; Ferguson, 1977; Jobin *et al.*, 1977). Despite great efforts, other good control agents have not been found. The most interesting ones biologically (Lum and Heyneman, 1972) may or may not be effective in the field. But these otherwise disparate countries had one important thing in common, namely, their post-Second World War socio-economic improvement. Paved-over swamps are now shopping malls, water in each home obviates visits to the river, and even industrial pollution kills noxious snails. I recall seeing from a train window in Japan a wonderful spot for *Oncomelania*. The Japanese had, however, converted the area to a golf course, so presumably only the duffers who played into the water hazards were at risk. Just as malaria began to disappear from the southern USA long before DDT and "eradication" took hold, so, too, will schistosomiasis disappear as the socio-economics of lesser-developed nations improve; nevertheless the prospects for this improvement, wholesale, are less than good.

(5) Meanwhile we are learning, however slowly, to search out and quantify infections whether they be in faeces or urine; Scott (1938) first did such egg-counts. Finding eggs gives us some notion of prevalence. Counting eggs in a standard manner gives some insight into intensity of infection. It seems now, for example, that a low output of eggs may not necessarily reflect perceptible disease, at least in Puerto Rico (Cline *et al.*, 1977). Heavy egg burdens, as in Egypt, frequently are disease associated. But this is too simple, for in fact light infections may indeed produce disease (Woodruff, 1969; Weller, 1976). We have also learned in the near past to study infested areas longitudinally, rather than in cross-section (Forsyth, 1969; Forsyth and Bradley, 1966; Ongom and Bradley, 1972; Cline *et al.*, 1977; Cook *et al.*, 1977a; Lehman, jr *et al.*, 1976; Kloetzel, 1962). It has long since been shown, of course, that intensity of infection increases directly with prevalence (Jordan, 1972a), and this is now reconfirmed. A useful description of schistosomiasis as a disease is provided by Jordan (1977b).

This Symposium could well have included contributions on the pathology caused by the schistosomes, or on the quantitative data drawn from post-mortem counts of worms and of eggs in the tissues. Cheever (1968) pioneered this important work for *S.mansoni*, and Edington *et al.* (1970), Smith *et al.* (1974), Smith *et al.* (1975), and von Lichtenberg *et al.* (1971) for *S.haematobium*, and Cheever *et al.* (1977) for both parasites. Descriptive pathology is provided by von Lichtenberg *et al.* (1971), von Lichtenberg (1975), Warren (1973a), and by Marcial-Rojas (1971), Miyake (1971), and by Gazayerli *et al.* (1971). The reversibility of schistosomal lesions is reviewed by Farid *et al.* (1976), a line of study first developed by Lucas *et al.* (1966).

Lest we forget, man is also susceptible to certain of the schistosomes of his domestic cattle, *S.bovis*, and *S.mattheei*, for example. No definitive picture exists of the seriousness of disease these worms produce in man, but, along with *S.spindale* and *S.nasalis*, they produce epidemics of severe disease in cattle and sheep (Hussein, 1973; Islam, 1975; Bailey, personal communication, 1977; Reinecke, 1970; Lawrence and Condy, 1970), and *S.japonicum* decimates cows in the Tone River Basin in Japan (Yokogawa *et al.*, 1972). One cannot but suspect that the worldwide loss of domestic stock is larger and costlier than has been reported.

(6) Many of the complexities of schistosomiasis have come under study, but only in scattered ways. One such lies in measuring human contact with water, obviously an important element in transmission. I know of only a few such studies, two in Egypt (Farooq, 1963a; Farooq and Mallah, 1966), one in Rhodesia (Husting, 1970), one in St Lucia (Dalton, 1976), and one in Puerto Rico (Lipes and Hiatt, 1977), among others. More concerted efforts may yet yield up data useful in prevention. Surprisingly, we also know little about how schistosome eggs really do reach water, and we are only beginning to learn how the miracidia behave under laboratory (Chernin, 1974; Stibbs *et al.*, 1976) and under field conditions (Sturrock and Upatham, 1973). That miracidia can be decoyed from their proper host is of interest (Chernin, 1968).

Certain laboratory-based efforts have been surprisingly successful. The cultivation of worms *in vitro* (Senft and Weller, 1956; Cheever and Weller, 1958) has opened many investigative doors, including the continued effort to cultivate the worm's tissues *in vitro* (Weller and Wheeldon, 1970). And from the same laboratory came the discovery of antigen circulating in the blood of infected hamsters (Berggren and Weller, 1967), a finding which soon led to the discovery by others of circulating immune complexes, and of kidney disease in animals and man infected with *S.mansoni*. Through the support of the USA–Japan Programme a snail cell-line is now available (Hansen, 1976).

(7) But now follows a litany of under-achievement. First, little is known about the genetics of the intermediate-host snails (Richards, 1970; Richards and Merritt, 1972), and almost nothing about the worms' genetics. Second, as one colleague put it to me, we know volumes about the biochemistry of *Hymenolepis nana*, a perfectly innocuous tapeworm, but relatively little about the schistosomes' biochemistry. Third, we have had a series of mathematical models proposed and then mostly ignored because many of the assumptions on which they rested turned

out to be wrong or contradictory (Fine and Lehman, jr, 1977; J. E. Cohen, 1973). All these points need investigation and not derogation. Fourth, one cannot but wonder what has happened in the Philippines since the exhaustive and unique studies of Pesigan and his colleagues were published in 1958 (Pesigan *et al.*, 1958a, b, c). Fifth, vaccine: I would urge most guarded thinking about the chances of achieving an anti-schistosomal vaccine, a goal which Sadun felt was not even in sight in 1972, although he urged ". . . expanded fundamental research conducted in close collaboration with parasitologists and immunologists." And with this last I would agree wholeheartedly, *provided* that those who dispense research largesse maintain a reasonable sense of proportion *vis-à-vis* other research needs. The stimulatory antigen(s) are yet to be found, they must elicit *protective* responses, and we still do not know how many immunologically distinct variants the vaccine will be called upon to protect against. Sadun (1972) also cautioned against the possibility of renal disease produced by vaccine-antibody complexes, a matter worth remembering. Smithers (1976) discusses some of these problems in a recent publication, including the virtues and shortcomings of potential vaccines, live or dead, and the certain need for a non-toxic adjuvant. We will learn much from this work whether or not a vaccine eventuates. Sixth, there are unpublished and as yet unconfirmed hints to the disturbing effect that hepatic dysfunction may occur if women taking oral contraceptives are infected or became infected with schistosomes. If tropical countries may have schistosomiasis or oral contraceptives, but not both, which will they choose? These rumours may prove false, but what of the interaction between schistosomiasis and hundreds of other drugs available *ad lib.* to the tropical public? What of any interactions between schistosomiasis and other infections affecting the liver? Finally, field workers frequently report an unexplained reduction in egg output in children about 15–17 years old. The common explanations are that immunity or reduced contact with water account for the phenomenon (Clarke, 1966a, b; Warren, 1973b). I cannot help but wonder whether the post-pubertal endocrine, metabolic and growth changes also play some role in reducing egg output, at least under some circumstances.

It is only a slight exaggeration to say that among the first effects of the malaria eradication programme was the eradication of the classical malariologists. Years later, right now, we need them and they or their offspring are not to be had. Schistosomiasis is at least as complex as malaria and we can ill afford decisions that go unilaterally for vaccines or for some other single approach, while the needed talents of many scientists wither away.

(8) Decisions based on ambiguous data are difficult to reach or to rationalize. This applies especially in the case of the schistosomes which infect many but cause flagrant disease only in some. Olivier (1974),

Wright (1968, 1972), Farooq (1963b, 1964), Macdonald and Farooq (1973), and others, have written most trenchantly about analysing the economics of human parasitic infections; I will not repeat the extensive literature they cover. Oliver, however, pleads that prevalence and intensity data are badly needed because they ". . . are embarrassingly meagre, surprisingly fragmentary and unsuitable for quantitative analysis . . .". As the economist Cummins (1972) dryly observes, "It must be apparent that economic analysis in underdeveloped countries is itself underdeveloped."

More recently, economists at the University of Wisconsin looked at the world distribution of schistosomiasis and did some quantitative economic analyses and comparisons. Their first footnote reads: "These studies, self-admittedly, are constrained by inadequate prevalence and severity estimates." The second sentence of their summary reads: "We are naturally disappointed to find out that the only significant explanatory variable is income levels, after all the efforts to add in other socioeconomic variables thought to be important links in the schistosome transmission process" (Andreano *et al.*, 1974). I am sorry that the authors' self-expressed biases did not work out to their liking, and that when they say that the "factors governing the world distribution of schistosomiasis are infinitely complex . . . therefore, to view the transmission process on a worldwide ecological scale is probably of limited usefulness" they are stating the self-evident. Meanwhile, it remains unclear whether schistosomiasis affects work ability (Fenwick, 1972; Fenwick and Figenschou, 1972) or learning ability (Bell *et al.*, 1973).

In a discussion session of the conference from which emanated "The Careless Technology" (1972), Gunnar Myrdal, well-known Professor of International Economics at the University of Stockholm, participated. The discussion swirled about economics, social change, and disease. Myrdal remarked:

> "My friends, I am a displaced person who knows very little about the problems you are discussing. I thought I was a broadminded economist . . . but this conference is already giving me a new education in the historical narrowness of developmental economics. In my opinion we have a basic moral imperative to cure a man from illness and to try to prevent his death . . . When we change one factor in a society, we must take on the responsibility for all changes which result and try to deal with them intelligently."

Conclusion

Tropical medicine is coming into a new and vigorous era (Minner, 1977), or so all the signs suggest, and that is a good note on which to conclude. My favourite essayist, Lewis Thomas, of the Sloan Kettering

Cancer Center, provides some typically lucid thoughts. First, he makes it clear that "the major research effort . . . must be in the broad area of basic biological science . . . the highest yield for the future will come from whatever fields are generating the most interesting, exciting, and surprising sorts of information—most of all surprising" (Thomas, 1977b). Elsewhere he expands incisively on this thought: "[Surprise] is the element that distinguishes applied science from basic. Surprise is what makes the difference" (Thomas, 1974). Finally, in concluding one of his essays, he remarks that because of the new information garnered during the past quarter-century we can now begin to elucidate the mechanisms underlying certain major diseases, provided, as he says, "we do not set time schedules or offer dates of delivery" (Thomas, 1977a). The complexities of tropical diseases are no less formidable than those of the diseases Thomas referred to, and rigid time schedules (for which read Gannt Charts or similar documents) will do nothing but harass the researcher and foul up the research.

Acknowledgement

This work was supported in part by a Research Career Award from the National Institute of Allergy and Infectious Diseases, US Public Health Service.

I am indebted to many colleagues at Harvard and at other institutions for the stimulating discussions from which grew this paper.

References

Andreano, R. L., Helminiack, T. W. and Li, J.-Y. A. (1974). The world distribution of schistosomiasis: some quantitative economic comparisons. *Journal of Tropical Medicine and Hygiene*, **77,** 170–6.

Bell, R. M., Kanengoni, J. D. E. and Jones, J. J. (1973). The effect of endemic schistosomiasis and hycanthone on the mental ability of African schoolchildren. *Transactions of the Royal Society of Tropical Medicine and Hygiene*, **67,** 694–701.

Berggren, W. L. and Weller, T. H. (1967). Immunoelectrophoretic demonstration of specific circulating antigen in animals infected with *Schistosoma mansoni*. *American Journal of Tropical Medicine and Hygiene*, **16,** 606–12.

Boulding, K. (1972). Ballad of Ecological Awareness. *In* "The Careless Technology" (Ed. M. T. Farvar and J. P. Milton), p. 3. Natural History Press, Garden City, N.Y.

Buck, A. A. (1976). Epidemological research on tropical diseases. World Health Organization, unpublished working document, TDR/WP/76.18.

Cheever, A. W. (1968). A quantitative post-mortem study of schistosomiasis in man. *American Journal of Tropical Medicine and Hygiene*, **17,** 38–64.

Cheever, A. W., Kamel, I. A., Elswi, A. M., Mosimann, J. E. and Danner, R. (1977). *Schistosoma mansoni* and *S.haematobium* infections in Egypt: II. Quantitative parasitological findings at necropsy. *American Journal of Tropical Medicine and Hygiene*, **26,** 702–16.

Cheever, A. W. and Weller, T. H. (1958). Observations on the growth and nutritional requirements of *Schistosoma mansoni in vitro*. *American Journal of Hygiene*, **68**, 322–39.

Chernin, E. (1968). Interference with the capacity of *Schistosoma mansoni* miracidia to infect the molluscan host. *Journal of Parasitology*, **54**, 509–16.

Chernin, E. (1974). Some host-finding attributes of *Schistosoma mansoni* miracidia. *American Journal of Tropical Medicine and Hygiene*, **23**, 320–7.

Chernin, E. (1975). A worm's-eye view of biomedical journals. *Federation Proceedings*, **34**, 124–30.

Chernin, E., Michelson, E. H. and Augustine, D. L. (1956). Studies on the biological control of schistosome-bearing snails. I. The control of *Australorbis glabratus* populations by the snail, *Marisa cornuarietis*, under laboratory conditions. *American Journal of Tropical Medicine and Hygiene*, **5**, 297–309.

Christie, J. D. and Upatham, E. S. (1977). Control of *Schistosoma mansoni* transmission by chemotherapy in St. Lucia. II. Biological results. *American Journal of Tropical Medicine and Hygiene*, **26**, 894–8.

Chu, K. Y. (1976). The validity of baseline data for measuring incidence rates of *Schistosoma haematobium* infection in the molluscicided area, UAR–0049 project. *Annals of Tropical Medicine and Parasitology*, **70**, 365–7.

Clarke, V. de V. (1966a). Evidence of the development in man of acquired resistance to infection of *Schistosoma* spp. *Central African Journal of Medicine*, **12**, 1–3.

Clarke, V. de V. (1966b). The influence of acquired resistance in the epidemiology of bilharziasis. *Central African Journal of Medicine*, 12 (6, Suppl.), 1–30.

Cline, B. L., Rymzo, W. T., Hiatt, R. A., Knight, W. B. and Berrios-Duran, L. A. (1977). Morbidity from *Schistosoma mansoni* in a Puerto Rican community: a population-based study. *American Journal of Tropical Medicine and Hygiene*, **26**, 109–17.

Cohen, J. E. (1973). Selective host mortality in a catalytic model applied to schistosomiasis. *American Naturalist*, **107**, 199–212.

Cook, J. A., Baker, S. T., Warren, K. S. and Jordan, P. (1977a). A controlled study of morbidity of schistosomiasis mansoni in St Lucian children, based on quantitative egg excretion. *American Journal of Tropical Medicine and Hygiene*, **23**, 625–33.

Cook, J. A., Jordan, P. and Bartholomew, R. K. (1977b). Control of *Schistosoma mansoni* transmission by chemotherapy in St Lucia. I. Results in man. *American Journal of Tropical and Medicine and Hygiene*, **26**, 887–93.

Cummins, J. G. (1972). Economic implications of schistosomiasis. In "Proceedings of a Symposium on the Future of Schistosomiasis Control", (Ed. M. J. Miller), pp. 24–9. Tulane University, Tulane.

Dalton, P. R. (1976). A socio-ecological approach to the control of *Schistosoma mansoni* in St Lucia. *Bulletin of the World Health Organization*, **54**, 587–95.

Deom, J. (1975). The role of the World Health Organization. In "Man-Made Lakes and Human Health" (Eds. N. F. Stanley and M. R. Alpers), pp. 387–400. Academic Press, London and New York.

Edington, B. M., von Lichtenberg, F., Nwabuebo, I., Taylor, J. R. and Smith, J. H. (1970). Pathologic effects of schistosomiasis in Ibadan, Western State of Nigeria. I. Incidence and intensity of infection; distribution and severity of lesions. *American Journal of Tropical Medicine and Hygiene*, **19**, 982–5.

Farid, M. A. (1975). The Aswan high dam development project. In "Man-Made Lakes and Human Health", (Eds. N. F. Stanley and M. P. Alpers), pp. 89–102. Academic Press, London and New York.

Farid, Z., Miner, W. F., Higashi, G. I. and Hassan, A. (1976). Reversibility of lesions in schistosomiasis: a brief review. *Journal of Tropical Medicine and Hygiene*, **79**, 164–5.

Farooq, M. (1963a). Importance of determining transmission sites in planning bilharzia control. Field observations from the Egypt-49 project area. *American Journal of Epidemiology*, **83,** 603–12.

Farooq, M. (1963b). A possible approach to the evaluation of the economic burden imposed on a community by schistosomiasis. *Annals of Tropical Medicine and Parasitology*, **57,** 323–31.

Farooq, M. (1964). Medical and economic importance of schistosomiasis. *Journal of Journal of Tropical Medicine and Hygiene*, **67,** 105–12.

Farooq, M. and Mallah, M. G. (1966). The behavioral pattern of social and religious water contact activities in the Egypt-49 Bilharziasis project area. *Bulletin of the World Health Organization*, **35,** 377–87.

Farooq, M., Hairston, N. G. and Samaan, S. A. (1966a). The effect of area-wide control on the endemicity of bilharziasis in Egypt. *Bulletin of the World Health Organization*, **35,** 369–75.

Farooq, M., Neilson, J., Samaan, S. A., Mallah, M. B. and Allam, A. A. (1966b). Prevalence of bilharziasis in relation to personal attributes and habits. *Bulletin of the World Health Organization*, **35,** 293–318.

Fenwick, A. (1972). The costs and a cost-benefit analysis of an *S.mansoni* control programme on an irrigated sugar estate in northern Tanzania. *Bulletin of the World Health Organization*, **47,** 573–8.

Fenwick, A. and Figenschou, B. H. (1972). The effect of *Schistosoma mansoni* infection on the productivity of cane cutters on a sugar estate in Tanzania. *Bulletin of the World Health Organization*, **47,** 567–72.

Ferguson, F. F. (1977). "The Role of Biological Agents in the Control of Schistosome-Bearing Snails". US Department of Health, Education and Welfare, Public Health Service, Communicable Diseases Center, Atlanta, Georgia.

Fine, P. E. M. and Lehman, J. S. jr. (1977). Mathematical models of schistosomiasis: report of a workshop. *American Journal of Tropical Medicine and Hygiene*, **26,** 500–4.

Forsyth, D. M. (1969). A longitudinal study of endemic urinary schistosomiasis in a small East African community. *Bulletin of the World Health Organization*, **40,** 771–83.

Forsyth, D. M. and Bradley, D. J. (1966). The consequences of bilharziasis. Medical and public health importance in North-west Tanzania. *Bulletin of the World Health Organization*, **34,** 715–35.

Gazaverli, M., Khalil, H. A. and Gazayerli, I. M. (1971). Pathology of schistosomiasis haematobium (urogenic bilharziasis). *In* "Pathology of Protozoal and Helminthic Diseases", (Ed. Marcial-Rojas), Ch. 18, pp. 439–49. Williams and Wilkins, Baltimore.

Gilles, H. M., Zaki, A. A-Z., Soussa, M. H., Samaan, S. A., Soliman, S. S., Hassan, A. and Barbosa, F. (1973). Results of a seven-year snail control project on the endemicity of *Schistosoma haematobium* infection in Egypt. *Annals of Tropical Medicine and Parasitology*, **67,** 45–65.

Gönnert, R. and Andrews, P. (1977). Praziquantel, a new broad-spectrum anti schistosomal agent. *Zeitschrift für Parasitenkunde*, **52,** 129–50.

Gordon Smith, C. E. (1976). Medicine in a developing tropical environment. *Transactions of the Royal Society of Tropical Medicine and Hygiene*, **70,** 1–9.

Gratz, N. G. (1974). Urbanization and filariasis. World Health Organization unpublished working document, WHO/Fil/74.119.

Hansen, E. L. (1976). Application of tissue culture of a pulmonate snail to culture larval *Schistosoma mansoni*. *In* "Invertebrate Tissue Culture" (Eds. E. Kurstak and K. Maramorosch), pp. 87–97. Academic Press, London and New York.

Holmes, R. (1977). [Quotation cited from review of novel by Grameci]. *Harper's Magazine*, October 1977, p. 88.

Hussein, M. F. (1973). Animal schistosomiasis in Africa: a review of *Schistosoma bovis* and *Schistosoma mattheei*. *Veterinary Bulletin*, **43**, 341–7.

Husting, E. L. (1970). Sociological patterns and their influence on the transmission of bilharziasis. *Central African Journal of Medicine*, **16** (Suppl.), 5–10.

International Bank for Reconstruction and Development (1975). "Health Sector Policy Paper". IBRD, Washington.

Islam, K. S. (1975). Schistosomiasis in domestic ruminants in Bangladesh. *Tropical Animal Health Proceedings*, **7**, 244.

James, C., Webbe, G. and Nelson, G. S. (1977). The susceptibility to praziquantel of *Schistosoma haematobium* in the baboon (*Papio anubis*) and of *S. japonicum* in the vervet monkey (*Cercopithecus aethiops*). *Zeitschrift für Parasitenkunde*, **52**, 179–94.

Jobin, W. R., Brown, R. A., Velez, S. P. and Ferguson, F. F. (1977). Biological control of *Biomphalaria glabrata* in major reservoirs in Puerto Rico. *American Journal of Tropical Medicine and Hygiene*, **26**, 1018–24.

Jordan, P. (1972a). Epidemiology and control of schistosomiasis. *British Medical Bulletin*, **28**, 55–9.

Jordan, P. (1972b). Schistosomiasis and disease. *In* "Proceedings of a Symposium on the Future of Schistosomiasis Control" (Ed. J. Miller), pp. 17–22. Tulane University, New Orleans, La.

Jordan, P. (1974). Incidence rates of *Schistosoma haematobium* infection, UAR-0049 project. *Annals of Tropical Medicine and Parasitology*, **68**, 243–4.

Jordan, P. (1975). Schistosomiasis—epidemiology, clinical manifestations and control. *In* "Man-Made Lakes and Human Health", (Ed. N. F. Stanley and M. P. Alpers), pp. 35–50. Academic Press, London and New York.

Jordan, P. (1977). Schistosomiasis—research to control. *American Journal of Tropical Medicine and Hygiene*, **26**, 877–86.

Jordan, P., Woodstock, L., Unrau, G. O. and Cook, J. A. (1975). Control of *Schistosoma mansoni* transmission by provision of domestic water supplies. *Bulletin of the World Health Organization*, **52**, 9–20.

Jordan, P., Woodstock, L. and Cook, J. A. (1976). Preliminary parasitological results of a pilot mollusciciding campaign to control transmission of *Schistosoma mansoni* in St Lucia. *Bulletin of the World Health Organization*, **54**, 295–302.

Kloetzel, K. (1962). Splenomegaly in schistosomiasis mansoni. *American Journal of Tropical Medicine and Hygiene*, **11**, 472–6.

Lawrence, J. A. and Condy, J. B. (1970). The developing problem of schistosomiasis in domestic stock in Rhodesia. *Central African Journal of Medicine*, **16** (Suppl.), 19–22.

Lehman, J. S., jr., Mott, K. E., Morrow, R. H. jr., Muniz, T. M. and Boyer, M. H. (1976). The intensity and effects of infection with *Schistosoma mansoni* in a rural community in northeast Brazil. *American Journal of Tropical Medicine and Hygiene*, **25**, 285–95.

Lepes, T. (1976). Present major activities in tropical medicine on a global scale. *Tropenmedizin und Parasitologie*, (Suppl.), 1–10.

Lipes, J. K. and Hiatt, R. A. (1977). Determinants of human water-contact patterns in urban Puerto Rico with special reference to schistosomiasis. *Boletin de la Asociacion medica de Puerto Rico*, **69**, 35–44.

Lucas, A. O., Adeniyi-Jones, C. C., Cockshott, W. B. and Gilles, H. M. (1966). Radiological changes after medical treatment of vesical schistosomiasis. *Lancet*, **1**, 631–3.

Lum, H. K. and Heyneman, D. (1972). Intramolluscan inter-trematode antagonism and its possible role in biological control. *In* Advances in Parasitology (Ed. B. Dawes), Vol. 10, pp. 191–268. Academic Press, London and New York.

Macdonald, G. and Farooq, M. (1973). The public health and economic importance of schistosomiasis. *In* "Epidemiology and Control of Schistosomiasis", (Ed. N. Ansari), Ch. 5, pp. 337–53, Karger, Basel.

McMullen, D. B. (1973). Biological and environmental control of snails, *In* "Epidemiology and Control of Schistosomiasis" (Ed. N. Ansari), Ch. 11, pp. 533–91, Karger, Basel.

Marcial-Rojas R. A. (1971). Pathology of schistosomaisis mansoni *In* "Pathology of Protozoal and Helminthic Diseases" (Ed. Marcial-Rojas), Ch. 16, pp. 373–413. Williams and Wilkins, Baltimore.

Meleney, H. E. (1954). Problems in the control of schistosomiasis. *American Journal of Tropical Medicine and Hygiene*, **3,** 209–18.

Miller, M. J. (ed.) (1972). "Proceedings of a Symposium on the Future of Schistosomiasis Control" Statement of Final Plenary Session, p. 3, Tulane University, New Orleans La.

Minners, H. A. (1977). Editorial. Tropical Medicine—new vigor. *Science*, **196,** 1275.

Miyake, M. (1971). Pathology of schistosomiasis japonicum. *In* "Pathology of Protozoal and Helminthic Diseases" (Ed. Marcial-Rojas), Ch. 17, pp. 414–433. Williams and Wilkins, Baltimore.

Myrdal, G. K. (1972). Discussion comments. *In* "The Careless Technology", (Eds. M. T. Farvar and J. P. Milton), pp. 146–7. Natural History Press, Garden City, New York.

Narin, F. and Shapiro, R. T. (1977). The extramural role of the NIH as a research support agency. *Federation Proceedings*, **36,** 2470–6.

Obeng, L. E. (1975). Health problems of the Volta Lake system. *In* "Man-Made Lakes and Human Health" (Eds. N. F. Stanley and M. P. Alpers), pp. 221–30. Academic Press, New York.

Olivier, L. J. (1974). The economics of human parasitic infections. *Zeitschrift für Parasitenkunde*, **45,** 197–210.

Ongom, V. L. and Bradley, D. J. (1972). The epidemiology and consequences of *Schistosoma mansoni* infection in West Nile, Uganda. I. Field Studies of a community at Panyagoro. *Transactions of the Royal Society of Tropical Medicine and Hygiene*, **66,** 835–51.

Paperna, I. (1969). Studies on the transmission of schistosomiasis in Ghana. IV. Transmission of *Schistosoma haematobium* in the forest and savannah zones of south east Ghana. *Ghana Medical Journal*, **8,** 35–46.

Paperna, I. (1970). Study of an outbreak of schistosomiasis in the newly formed Volta Lake in Ghana. *Zeitschrift für Tropenmedizin und Parasitologie*, **21,** 411–25.

Pellegrino, J., Lima-Costa, F. F., Carlos, M. A. and Mello, R. T. (1977). Experimental chemotherapy of schistosomiasis mansoni. XIII. Activity of praziquantel, an isoquinoline-pyrazino derivative, on mice, hamsters and Cebus monkeys. *Zeitschrift für Parasitenkunde*, **52,** 151–68.

Pesigan, T. P., Farooq, M., Hairston, N. G. *et al.* (1958a). Studies on *Schistosoma japonicum* infection in the Philippines. I. General considerations and epidemiology. *Bulletin of the World Health Organization*, **18,** 345–55.

Pesigan, T. P., Hairston, N. G., Jauregui, J. J., *et al.* (1958b). Studies on *Schistosoma japonicum* infection in the Philippines. II. The molluscan host. *Bulletin of the World Health Organization*, **18,** 481–578.

Pesigan, T. P., Farooq, M., Hairston, N. G., *et al.* (1958c). Studies on *Schistosoma japonicum* infection in the Philippines. III. Preliminary control experiments. *Bulletin of the World Health Organization*, **19,** 223–61.

Reinecke, R. K. (1970). The epizootiology of an outbreak of bilharziasis (*Schistosoma mattheei*) in Zululand. *Central African Journal of Medicine*, **16,** (Suppl.), 10–12.

Richards, C. S. (1970). Genetics of a molluscan vector of schistosomiasis. *Nature, London*, **227,** 806–10.

Richards, C. S. and Merritt, J. W., jr. (1972). Genetic factors in the susceptibility of juvenile *Biomphalaria glabrata* to *Schistosoma mansoni* infection. *American Journal of Tropical Medicine and Hygiene* **21**, 425–34.

Sadun, E. H. (1972). Control by immunization: problems and prospects. *In* "Proceedings of a Symposium on the Future of Schistosomiasis Control" (Ed. M. J. Miller), pp. 49–55, Tulane University, New Orleans, La.

Salisbury, H. E. (1977). China's leaders view last 10 years as "lost". *New York Times*, 5 November 1977, p. 3.

Sasa, M. (1972). Epidemiology of filariasis and schistosomiasis in Asia and the Pacific: a review. *In* "Research in Filariasis and Schistosomiasis" (Ed. M. Yokogawa), Vol. 2, pp. 3–20. University of Tokyo and University Park Press, Baltimore.

Schultz M. G. (1977). Parasitic diseases. *New England Journal of Medicine* **297**, 1259–61.

Scott, J. A. (1938). The regularity of egg output of helminth infestations, with special reference to *Schistosoma mansoni*. *American Journal of Hygiene*, **27**, 155–75.

Senft, A. W. and Weller, T. H. (1956). Growth and regeneration of *Schistosoma mansoni in vitro*. *Proceedings of the Society for Experimental Biology and Medicine*, **93**, 16–19.

Smith, J. H., Kamel, I. A., Elwi, A. and von Lichtenberg, F. (1974). A quantitative postmortem analysis of urinary schistosomiasis in Egypt. I. Pathology and pathogenesis. *American Journal of Tropical Medicine and Hygiene*, **23**, 1054–71.

Smith, J. H., Elwi, A. and Kamel, I. A. (1975). A quantitative post-mortem analysis of urinary schistosomiasis in Egypt. II. Evolution and epidemiology. *American Journal of Tropical Medicine and Hygiene*, **24**, 806–22.

Smithers, S. R. (1976). Immunity to trematode infections with special reference to schistosomiasis and fascioliasis. *In* "Immunology of Parasitic Infections" (Eds. S. Cohen and E. H. Sadun), Ch. 20, pp. 296–332. Blackwell, Oxford.

Stibbs, H. H., Chernin, E., Ward, S. and Karnovsky, M. L. (1976). Magnesium emitted by snails alters swimming behaviour of *Schistosoma mansoni* miracidia. *Nature, London*, **260**, 702–3.

Stoll, N. R. (1947). This wormy world. *Journal of Parasitology*, **33**, 1–18.

Sturrock, R. F. and Upatham, E. S. (1973). An investigation into the interactions of some factors influencing the infectivity of *Schistosoma mansoni* miracidia to *Biomphalaria glabrata*. *International Journal of Parasitology*, **3**, 35–41.

Thomas, L. (1974). "The Lives of a Cell", p. 118. Viking Press, New York.

Thomas L. (1977a). On the science and technology of medicine. *Daedalus*, **106**, 35–46.

Thomas, L. (1977b). Biomedical science and human health: the long range prospect. *Daedalus*, **106**, 163–71.

United States Government, Schistosomiasis Delegation (1977). Report of the American schistosomiasis delegation to the People's Republic of China. *American Journal of Tropical Medicine and Hygiene*, **26**, 427–62.

United States Government, Agency for International Development (1972). "Population Program Assistance", AID, Washington.

Unrau G. O. (1975). Individual household water supplies in rural St. Lucia as a control measure against *Schistosoma mansoni*. *Bulletin of the World Health Organization*, **52**, 1–8.

von Lichtenberg, F. (1975). Schistosomiasis as a worldwide problem: pathology. *Journal of Toxicology and Environmental Health*, **1**, 175–84.

von Lichtenberg, F., Edington, G. M., Nwabuebo, I., Taylor, J. R. and Smith, J. H. (1971). Pathologic effects of schistosomiasis in Ibadan, Western State of Nigeria. II. Pathogenesis of lesions of the bladder and ureters. *American Journal of Tropical Medicine and Hygiene*, **20**, 244–54.

Waddy, B. B. (1975). Research into the health problems of man-made lakes, with special reference to Africa. *Transactions of the Royal Society of Tropical Medicine and Hygiene*, **69,** 39–50.

Warren, K. S. (1973a). The pathology of schistosome infections. *Helminthological Abstracts*, **42,** 591–633.

Warren, K. S. (1973b). Regulation of the prevalence and intensity of schistosomiasis in man: Immunology or ecology. *Journal of Infectious Diseases*, **127,** 595–609.

Warren, K. S. (1973c). "Schistosomiasis. The Evolution of a Medical Literature. Selected Abstracts and Citations, 1852–1972", Massachusetts Institute of Technology Press, Cambridge.

Warren, K. S. and Hoffman, D. B. jr. (1976). "Schistosomiasis. III. Abstracts of the complete literature 1963–1974." Hemisphere Publishing Co, Washington, D.C.

Warren, K. S. and Newall, V. A. (1967). "Schistosomiasis. A Bibliography of the World's Literature from 1852 to 1962". Vol. I—Keyword Index; Vol. II—Author Index. Western Reserve Press, Cleveland.

Webbe, G. (1972). Control of schistosomiasis in Ethiopia, Sudan, and East and West African countries. *In* "Proceedings of a Symposium on the Future of Schistosomiasis Control" (Ed. M. J. Miller), pp. 115–21. Tulane University, New Orleans, La.

Webbe, G. and James, C. (1977). A comparison of the susceptibility to praziquantel of *Schistosoma haematobium, S. japonicum, S.mansoni, S.intercalatum*, and *S.mattheei* in hamsters. *Zeitschrift fur Parasitenkunde*, **52,** 169–77.

Weisner, J. B. (1977). Quoted by Robert Cook in the *Boston Globe*, 7 June 1977.

Weller, T. H. (1975). Schistosomiasis: its significance in a changing ecology. *Journal of Toxicology and Environmental Health*, **1,** 185–90.

Weller, T. H. (1976). Manson's schistosomiasis: frontiers *in vivo, in vitro*, and in the body politic. *American Journal of Tropical Medicine and Hygiene*, **25,** 208–16.

Weller, T. H. and Wheeldon, S. K. (1970). Cell cultures from helminthic tissues. *Journal of Parasitology*, **56,** (4), 365.

Woodruff, A. W. (1969). Problems in the control of tropical diseases. *Biotechnology and Bioengineering Symposium*, **1,** 201–09.

World Health Organization (1973). Schistosomiasis control. *WHO Technical Report Series*, no. 515.

World Health Organization, Expert Committee on Bilharziasis (1953). First Report. *WHO Technical Report Series*, no. 65.

Wright, W. H. (1968). Schistosomiasis as a world problem. *Bulletin of the New York Academy of Medicine*, **44,** 301–22.

Wright, W. H. (1972). A consideration of the economic impact of schistosomiasis. *Bulletin of the World Health Organization*, **47,** 559–66.

Wright, W. H. (1973). Geographic distribution of schistosomes and their intermediate hosts. *In* "Epidemiology and Control of Schistosomiasis", (Ed. N. Ansari), Ch. 3, pp. 32–249. Karger, Basel.

Yokogawa, M. (1974). Epidemiology and control of schistosomiasis japonica. *In* "A Symposium on the Epidemiology of Parasitic Diseases" (Ed. M. Sasa), pp. 83–99. International Medical Foundation, Japan.

Yokogawa, M., Sano, M., Kojima, S., Araki, K., *et al.* (1972). Schistosoma infection among dairy cows in the Tone River basin in Chiba Prefecture. *In* "Research in Filariasis and Schistosomiasis" (Ed. M. Yokogawa), Vol. 2, pp. 87–93. University of Tokyo, and University Park Press, Baltimore.

Discussion

Dr Warren said that Professor Chernin's elegant lecture had covered the field very broadly; he asked, as time was pressing, that any questions should take a similarly broad view.

Professor Bruce-Chwatt in relation to the St Lucia programme, asked what was the general opinion regarding Weisbrod's report, which had queried the socio-economic impact of schistosomiasis on the population of St Lucia.

Professor Chernin replied that there had been much criticism of Weisbrod's book, and the principles on which it was based. There was no record of schistosomiasis on St Lucia before the late 1920s; successive data indicate that the intensity and prevalence of infection have risen steadily. In recent years some 200-odd cases of hepatosplenic schistosomiasis had been reported, and he had no doubt that without disease control, that figure would rise. Many people would doubt very seriously the premise on which the Weisbrod book was based.

Dr Warren said that he had been working on St Lucia at the time the Weisbrod team was there, and the subsequent report had been based on the wrong premises. At the time no-one had realized that there was a great deal of hepatosplenic disease but it had been recently pointed out that St Lucia had as much hepatosplenic disease in relation to prevalence and intensity of schistosomiasis as anywhere in the world.

Professor Chernin pointed out that the book still appeared in bibliographies, and unfortunately might be read by people who were unable to evaluate it.

Dr Warren introduced the next speaker, Dr S. R. Smithers, saying that Dr Smithers and his group at Mill Hill, London, were considered by many to have made the greatest contribution to knowledge of immunity in schistosomiasis of any group in the world, and he knew of no finer study on the ecology of schistosomiasis than that based on Dr Smithers' early work carried out in the Gambia.

11. Immunology and Schistosomiasis

S. R. Smithers

Introduction

The partnership between schistosomiasis and immunology can be likened to the relationship between man and woman. All of us are aware of our changing attitude to the opposite sex as we progress from childhood to maturity. In childhood, boys and girls express little interest in each other; they prefer the company of their own sex. During adolescence, however, these attitudes begin to change; each sex develops its own special features, which are clearly of great interest to their opposite number. It becomes clear that they have much to offer each other; it might even be said that they cannot do without each other. Courtship begins, and although early courtship may be uneasy and there may be several failures, there is an eventual long-lasting relationship.

Twenty years ago, in their comparative childhood, schistosome parasitologists and immunologists had little to offer each other. Apart from expressions of mild curiosity, there was little meaningful communication between the two. Since that time, both disciplines have shown some remarkable developments and, where there has been adequate contact, a tentative and then a growing awareness of each other's presence has become evident. Parasitologists were the first to appreciate the delights the immunologists had to offer; those immunologists who had been successfully wooed, realize that the reverse is also true. Now the two have formed a relationship which I trust will be long and rewarding.

The least successful partnership between schistosome parasitology and immunology is to be found in the field of immunodiagnosis, where the parasitologist has leaned heavily on the techniques of the immunologist, but contributed little to the partnership. The most satisfying relationship so far, has been in immunopathology, where both parasitologists and immunologists have each made essential and interdependent contributions to a flourishing field. The latest relationship, in the area of protective immunity, has all the signs of developing into a durable, stimulating and highly prolific partnership.

Immunodiagnosis

Fifty years have passed since Hamilton Fairly first used the intradermal test in the diagnosis of schistosomiasis and there has been an even longer period since the Japanese workers applied the complement fixation test to the diagnosis of this disease (Kagan and Pellegrino, 1961). By the end of 1960 numerous descriptions of these techniques had appeared in the literature but a clear evaluation and comparison of the results was impossible because the procedure used and the preparation of antigens was not standardized. During the 1950s, the discovery of specific reactions between serum from infected hosts and live cercariae (Vogel and Minning, 1949) or schistosome eggs (Oliver-Gonzalez, 1954) gave hopes for more sensitive and practical diagnostic procedures. About the same time, Kagan (1955) adapted the indirect haemagglutination test for the diagnosis of schistosomiasis.

It is surprising to recall that although the fluorescent antibody technique was first used to demonstrate pneumococcal antigen in tissues in 1942 (Coons *et al.*, 1942) and Ouchterlony described his technique of double diffusion in gel in 1953, neither of these new tools was developed for practical application in schistosome diagnosis until the 1960s (Sadun *et al.*, 1961; Capron *et al.*, 1966).

In recent years, as more sensitive methods for detecting antibodies were developed, several new techniques were adopted. Among these are the radioimmunoassays, using radiolabelled anti-immunoglobulin to detect antibody (Schinski *et al.*, 1976) and enzyme immunoassays (Voller *et al.*, 1976). The latter are based on the use of antigens that are linked to an insoluble carrier surface, either plastic tubes in the "ELISA" (enzyme-linked immunosorbent assay) technique (Huldt *et al.*, 1975), or Sepharose beads in the "DASS" (defined antigen substrate spheres) method (Deelder and Streefkerk, 1975). The surface is used to "capture" the relevant antibodies in the serum and the resulting complex is detected by an enzyme-labelled anti-immunoglobulin. The degradation of the enzyme substrate measured photometrically is proportional to the concentration of antibody in the sera.

It is my belief, however, that modern immunodiagnosis of schistosomiasis provides no further information about the parasitological or immune state of the host than did the early complement fixation and intradermal tests. Although the sensitivity and convenience of methods for detecting antibodies has improved, there has been a continuing use of undefined antigens. Thus a conglomeration of antigens from extracts of adult worms, cercariae, eggs and even infected snail tissue have detected a wide and indeterminate antibody response. As a result, all diagnostic assays are limited; they cannot indicate the species of schistosome involved, nor can they distinguish the presence of an active infection from one previously experienced but now cured. Although present-day serological tests may have a limited use in sophisticated laboratories and possibly in epidemiological studies, the species of the schistosome, the presence of an active infection and an estimate of worm burden, can be determined only by detecting parasite eggs in faeces or urine. Thus immunodiagnosis has little relevance to everyday practice of medicine in endemic rural areas of the Third World.

New developments are needed which will enable simple immuno-diagnostic procedures (1) to demonstrate the presence of an active infection, (2) to identify the species of schistosome involved, (3) to quantify the worm and egg load of an individual, (4) to determine the effectiveness of chemotherapeutic treatment, (5) to reveal the degree of granuloma formation around the egg, and (6) to measure the level of protective immunity.

Continuing efforts to produce more sensitive methods for detecting antibodies will not result in satisfying the criteria described above. Emphasis should now be directed to the isolation of those specific antigens which have relevance to the host/parasite relationship. Surface antigens of the young schistosomula, for example, might detect antibodies which are functional in protective immunity; antigens of the egg could reveal quantitative information on egg load or estimate the severity of granuloma formation; certain antigens may detect anti-antibodies which rapidly disappear from the circulation following loss of infection. There is an obvious need to apply the latest techniques of protein and carbohydrate immunochemistry to antigen isolation for application to immunodiagnosis of schistosomiasis.

A beginning has already been made; Senft and Maddison (1975) have used an enzyme from the intestinal tract of the adult schistosome, isolated by affinity chromatography, as an antigen for intradermal testing. The antigen appears to be species specific and to induce fewer false–positive reactions than crude adult worm extract, although its sensitivity is low. Affinity chromatography has also been used by Pelley *et al.* (1976) to purify antigens from the schistosome egg. One antigen designated MSA_1 is the principal antigen involved in granulomatous hypersensitivity; when labelled with ^{125}I and used in a radioimmuno-assay to detect antibody in 5 μl of patients' serum, it shows high sensitivity, a degree of species-specificity (Pelley *et al.*, 1977), and the serological response to this antigen suggests that it is related to the intensity of infection and chemotherapeutic cure (R. P. Pelley, personal communication).

A simple method for the detection of antigen or immune complexes in the blood or urine of patients would facilitate and accelerate the evaluation of chemotherapeutic treatment, and is probably the only approach to estimating the worm burden of an individual. Schistosome antigen was first detected in a patient's urine 20 years ago (Okabe and Tanaka, 1958) and more recently, circulating antigen in the sera of experimental animals has been partially characterized (Gold *et al.*, 1964; Nash *et al.*, 1974). The development of new and sensitive assays of detecting immune complexes (World Health Organization, 1977) has enabled workers to demonstrate unequivocally the presence of circulating immune complexes in the sera of schistosome patients (Smith *et al.*, 1977; Bout *et al.*, 1977). Investigations on circulating immune complexes are at an early stage; before their immunodiagnostic significance can be evaluated it will be necessary to relate their presence to the intensity of infection and possibly to distinguish one from another (complexes with worm antigen, for example, may correlate with infection in a different way than do complexes with egg antigen). The tools are available for investigations of this kind in both human and experimental models, and the new enzyme immunoassays combined with improved antigen isolation appear to offer one suitable approach.

Immunopathology

The 20 years of activity which has centred on the immunopathogenesis of schistosomiasis has been amply rewarded. In the 1950s there was no clear demonstration that the egg was responsible for inducing a granulomatous reaction in the portal areas of the liver. Some investigators had suggested that the presence of dead worms, worm toxins, and even malnutrition, were responsible factors (Warren, 1972). Today there is no question that the host's immunological reaction to the schistosome egg is the essential factor in the pathogenesis of hepatosplenic schistosomiasis and the prospect of regulating this reaction to the benefit of the host is now the principle aim. This satisfactory outcome of two decades of research has been due to the marriage of sound basic parasitology to the immunological tools and concepts which have become available during that period.

The stimulus for this study was initially provided by Warren and his colleagues who introduced the lightly infected mouse as an experimental model of hepatosplenic schistosomiasis. They established that hepatosplenomegaly, portal hypertension and oesophageal varices were seen only in animals with egg-producing bisexual infections. Deficient diets, parasite toxins and the presence of dead worms were unaccompanied by any gross manifestation of the disease (Warren, 1963).

The elements of the egg that are necessary to induce granuloma formation were investigated by von Lichtenberg, using an original method in which living or dead eggs, plastic spheres, miracidia, or egg-shell were injected into the microvasculature of the lungs. His findings indicated that pulmonary granuloma formation is the result of a gradual and continual release of antigen from the egg (von Lichtenberg, 1962). These two fundamental parasitological observations enabled a liaison with immunology to begin.

Andrade and his colleagues were the first to use the fluorescent antibody technique to study the granuloma and were able to demonstrate the presence of parasite antigen and antibody in the lesion (Andrade *et al.*, 1961). von Lichtenberg (1964), also using fluorescent antibody, demonstrated the sequestration of antigen in the granuloma centre and the accelerated destruction of antigen in granuloma of sensitized mice.

The concepts of immunology were now to be fully integrated into these studies. Warren, with a number of different co-workers, utilized the Lichtenberg lung model to investigate the aetiology of the granuloma. Eggs were injected into the tail veins of mice, the lungs removed at various time-intervals thereafter, and the reactions around the eggs measured. It was shown that, after sensitization to schistosome eggs given intraperitoneally, mice exhibit an accelerated and augmented granuloma formation to eggs introduced into the lungs by intravenous injections. The reaction is specific in cross-sensitization experiments with *Ascaris* eggs and with different species of schistosomes, and sensitization could be adoptively transferred between histo-compatible mice with lymph-node or spleen cells, but not passively transferred with serum. These three important criteria, sensitization, specificity and passive transfer, established that the schistosome-egg granuloma is an immunological response. Moreover, the ability to transfer the sensitization with cells but not with serum indicated that this response was of the cell-mediated type, and a series of experiments in which the granuloma were suppressed by agents which suppressed cell-mediated but not humoral response confirmed this finding (Warren, 1972).

Following the demonstration of the immunological aetiology of the granuloma, attempts were made to isolate from the eggs the antigens responsible for the host reaction. The initial study, showing that a saline extract of homogenized eggs (SEA) was capable of sensitizing mice to granuloma formation (Boros and Warren, 1970), has culminated in the application of modern immunochemical techniques, i.e. gel filtration, polyacrylamide gel electrophoresis, affinity chromatography, ion exchange chromatography and radioimmunoassay, to the isolation and characterization of the prominent antigens in SEA. Pelley and his colleagues (Pelley *et al.*, 1976; Hamburger *et al.*, 1976) have isolated a major immunopathologically active antigen designated MSA_1; it is a glycoprotein of molecular weight 137 000 and exhibits a degree of stage and species-specificity consistent with the granulomatous response to *S.mansoni*.

Although granuloma formation is responsible for the disease process in schistosomiasis, it appears that this immune response has the vital function of sequestering harmful and toxic products released from the egg (von Lichtenberg, 1964). Thus mice which are unable to form granulomas following artificial depletion of T-lymphocytes by thymectomy or after treatment with anti-lymphocyte serum (ALS), die more quickly (Buchanan *et al.*, 1973). In contrast, congenitally athymic (nude) mice which develop small granulomas show a decrease in morbidity compared with their infected heterozygous thymus-bearing litter-mates (Hsu *et al.*, 1976).

These results might have been foreseen from previous basic parasitological observations which showed that, during the course of chronic schistosomiasis, mice showed a lessening in the size of newly formed granulomas and an improvement in the clinical parameters of hepato-splenic disease (Andrade and Warren, 1964; Warren, 1966). Thus to maintain a healthy status it is necessary for the host to curb the intense anti-egg responsiveness of early infection whilst retaining the essential function of the granuloma.

The suppression of the cell-mediated response to the egg has been confirmed in human *schistosomiasis mansoni* patients, where the lymphocyte blastogenic response to SEA in the chronically infected is diminished, although the response to other schistosome antigens gains in strength as chronic infections are established (Colley *et al.*, 1977).

The realization that the immune response to the schistosome egg is regulated under natural conditions and leads to spontaneous modulation of granuloma formation has revitalized activity in this field. The mechanisms involved in immunoregulation, including the role of antibodies, suppressor cells and immune complexes are now under intense investigation (Colley, 1976). We shall need to understand more about immunoregulation in man, not only in *schistosomiasis mansoni*, but in *S.japonicum* and *S.haematobium* infections; is it favourable or unfavourable to the host? There appears to be no reason why these questions should not be resolved well within the next decade. It should then be possible to decide whether manipulation of the immunoregulatory mechanisms could play a therapeutic role in alleviating the severe pathology associated with the disease.

Protective Immunity

The glittering prize, a schistosoma vaccine, is unlikely to be won without a thorough understanding of the antigens and mechanisms involved in protective immunity. Immunization against schistosomes would have been accomplished long ago if there were rapid development of effective immunity following a natural infection. Diseases which are controlled by vaccination, such as smallpox, poliomyelitis, diphtheria, usually induce an absolute resistance in patients fortunate enough to recover. After exposure to schistosomes, however, man and most experimental animals remain infected for long periods. The chronic nature of the disease implies that the parasite has evolved mechanisms which counter the host's immune response. An understanding of host effector mechanisms and parasite escape mechanisms is therefore a necessary pre-requisite before a rational approach towards developing an effective vaccine can be made. Protective immunity is a difficult and challenging area of schistosome research; although there has been substantial progress over the past 20 years, there is no indication that vital break-throughs have yet been made.

Only in recent years has it been possible to apply immunological expertise to the study of protective immunity. Progress so far has relied largely on investigations of a parasitological nature. The situation is similar to that seen in immunopathology where sound basic investigations of parasitology were essential before one could usefully turn to the immunologists for help.

In 1953, Vogel and Minning published their classic paper on acquired resistance of *Macaca rhesus* to *Schistosoma japonicum*. After 14 years of investigation these workers have concluded that infected monkeys develop a powerful resistance to reinfection, that resistance would develop in the absence of egg deposition and that, in the immune host, the schistosomula of a challenge infection are largely destroyed in the lungs. They were unable to demonstrate a role for antibody in this immunity, either by passive transfer experiments or by correlating the resistant state with complement fixation tests, the *cercarienhüllenreaktion*, or intra-dermal tests. They also failed to immunize against infection by injecting homogenized adult worm material.

Vogel and Minning's observations indicated that monkeys took from several months to several years to develop substantial protective immunity. Subsequent investigations on *S.mansoni*-infected rhesus monkeys by Smithers and Terry (1965) showed clearly, however, that immunity developed more rapidly. A partial resistance to challenge was evident only two or four weeks after infection, and solid resistance was demonstrated at 16 weeks. These observations were important because they illustrated that adult worms of the primary infection were still present and active during and after the destruction of a challenge infection. Clearly, whatever the nature of the immune response which prevented the schistosomula from maturing, this response did not destroy established adult worms nor prevent them from laying eggs. This situation, an immunity in the presence of an active infection, was called con-comitant immunity (Smithers and Terry, 1969). The term was bor-rowed from the tumour immunologists where an analogous situation had been described in tumour-bearing animals (Gershon *et al.*, 1967).

The subsequent finding that the adult worm provides the major stimulus to immunity (Smithers and Terry, 1967) focused attention on an important and hitherto neglected concept of schistosome immunity. If the adult worms induce an immunity which destroys invading schisto-somula, how do the adults evade the immune response which they themselves have engendered?

The concept of concomitant immunity thus enabled researchers in this field to appreciate more clearly the complexity of the host/parasite relationship and helped to define two crucial questions which have pro-vided the incentive for all subsequent studies on protective immunity. These are:

(1) what is the basis of the immune mechanism which destroys new invading parasites; and
(2) how do the older worms of an established infection circumvent the host's immune response?

To deal first with question (2): there are two fundamental findings relating to the surface of the schistosome which will have significant bearing on the answers to this question. First, experiments in which worms from a donor host were transferred into a recipient of a different species immunized against red blood cells (rbc) of the donor, demon-strated an intimate association of host or host-like molecules with the plasma membrane of the schistosome (Smithers *et al.*, 1969; Cioli and Neis, 1972; Boyer *et al.*, 1977; Erickson *et al.*, 1973). In the presence of antiserum against rbc of the donor, the tegument is rapidly destroyed and the worms are killed. This observation also illustrated that the surface of the worm is not an inert structure but is susceptible to damage in the presence of the right antibody.

Further investigations have shown that host antigens are related to the blood-group substances of the host and, *in vitro* at least, they appear to be acquired as glycolipids (Goldring *et al.*, 1976; Goldring *et al.*, 1977a). A. E. Butterworth, however, discusses some very latest work (see p. 155) which shows that proteins may also be involved in the host antigen phenomenon. It is suggested that the acquisition of host anti-gens by the worm serves to mask foreign antigens at the schistosome surface and thus enables the parasite to evade the immune response (Smithers *et al.*, 1969). Although this theory is supported by circum-stantial evidence (McLaren *et al.*, 1975; Goldring *et al.*, 1977b), direct proof of the protective function of host antigens is still awaited.

Secondly, a unique character of the schistosome tegument was described by Hockley and McLaren (1973). In the definitive host, the surface of the worm consists of a double plasma membrane comprising two lipid bilayers. This new membrane is formed rapidly, within three hours of cercarial penetration. It is present in all blood flukes so far examined, including those from fish and turtles, but it is absent from other trematodes (McLaren and Hockley, 1977). This observation suggests that the double membrane is an adaptation to the sanguinous habitat and may be concerned with evasion of the immune response. Wilson and Barnes (1977) believe that the outer bilayer of the double membrane has a short half-life and suggest that increased membrane turnover may be a mechanism countering antibody attack. Freeze fracture studies on this complex membrane have demonstrated an increase in the number of intramembranous particles in the outer leaflet of the double membrane at a time when the parasite is migrating through the lungs, i.e. when the parasite is apparently not recognized by the host as foreign (McLaren *et al.*, 1978). The significance of these findings is still under investigation.

The potential for answering the first question has similarly received a boost from two rather more technical advances in parasitology. The first was the adaptation of the technique for culturing schistosomes *in vitro* to immunological studies. Clegg's culture system (Clegg, 1965) was used by Clegg and Smithers (1972) to study the effect of serum from immune monkeys on schistosomes *in vitro*. Previously, there had been no evidence of antibody damage to adult worms cultured in immune serum, but, now aware of the ability of the older worm to evade the host response, these workers studied the effect of immune serum on young schistosomula newly transformed from cercariae. They found that in the presence of antibody and complement, the schistosomula were killed; in contrast, older schistosomula recovered from the skin or lungs of mice, or cultured in normal serum for a few days, were not susceptible to the lethal effect of this antibody.

These findings have formed the basis for several other *in vitro* studies, all of which have demonstrated various antibody-dependent cellular cytotoxic mechanisms effective against the young schistosomula (see Smithers and Terry, 1976). Although it is difficult to evaluate the relevance of *in vitro* phenomena with the protective response *in vivo*, the *in vitro* approach has provided valuable indications of possible *in vivo* mechanisms and it will continue to be used and developed in the future.

The second advance was to change the experimental animal model. The rhesus monkey had provided valuable data, but for further progress it was necessary to use more convenient animals. The wealth of immunological information on mice and rats and the availability of inbred strains of these rodents, made them the obvious choice. The development of rapid assays of protective immunity by the lung-recovery technique (Perez *et al.*, 1974; Sher *et al.*, 1974), or by radio-labelling worms of the challenge infection (Phillips *et al.*, 1977), illustrated how conveniently these hosts could be used as models for schistosome immunity.

From work with the mouse and rat models, several new features of schistosome immunity have come to light. In these hosts concomitant immunity is developed as rapidly as in the rhesus monkey. The target of the host's immune response are the invading schistosomula of the challenge infection (Sher *et al.*, 1974; Phillips *et al.*, 1977). Interestingly, it may be only for a brief period during their early development that the schistosomula are susceptible to immune attack (Sher, 1977; Smithers *et al.*, 1977). Immunity is thymus-dependent (Sher, 1977) and passive transfer experiments have indicated that IgG antibodies are involved (Phillips *et al.*, 1975; Sher *et al.*, 1977). A requirement for a cellular component has also been demonstrated with possibly the eosinophil playing a major role (Mahmoud *et al.*, 1975; von Lichtenberg *et al.*, 1977). There is no space for discussion of these important findings in detail, but the contribution by A. E. Butterworth (see p. 160) covers some of the latest work in this area.

Thus in 1977 we have in use the essential *in vivo* and *in vitro* model systems and we have acquired sufficient basic information to be able to discuss protective immunity at a level necessary to arouse the interest and seek the cooperation of the immunologists—perhaps even to lure them into the field. With their help, we can expect to identify the controlling mechanisms and the cellular and humoral elements of the host's immune response to schistosomes; and with their collaboration we should succeed in identifying the mechanisms used by the worm to circumvent immunity. Within the next decade adequate information about the protective response should be at hand to allow an assessment of whether or not vaccination against this miserable and increasingly prevalent disease is an attainable goal.

References

Andrade, Z. A., Paronetto, F. and Popper, H. (1961). Immunocytochemical studies in schistosomiasis. *American Journal of Pathology*, **39**, 589–98.

Andrade, Z. A. and Warren, K. S. (1964). Mild prolonged schistosomiasis in mice: alterations in host response with time and the development of portal fibrosis. *Transactions of the Royal Society of Tropical Medicine and Hygiene*, **58**, 53–7.

Boros, D. L. and Warren, K. S. (1970). Delayed hypersensitivity-type granuloma formation and dermal reaction induced and elicited by a soluble factor isolated from *Schistosoma mansoni* eggs. *Journal of Experimental Medicine*, **132**, 488–507.

Bout, D., Santoro, F., Carlier, Y., Bina, J. C. and Capron, A. (1977). Circulating immune complexes in schistosomiasis. *Immunology*, **33**, 17–22.

Boyer, M. H., Kalfayan, L. J. and Ketchum, D. G. (1977). The host antigen pheno-menon in experimental murine schistosomiasis: III. Destruction of parasites transferred from mice to hamsters. *American Journal of Tropical Medicine and Hygiene*, **26,** 254–7.

Buchanan, R. D., Fine, D. P. and Colley, D. G. (1973). *Schistosoma mansoni* infection in mice depleted of thymus-dependent lymphocytes: II. Pathology and altered pathogenesis. *American Journal of Pathology*, **71,** 207–18.

Capron, A., Vernes, A., Biguet, J., Rose, F., Clay, A. and Adenis, L. (1966). Les précipitins sériques dans les bilharzioses humaines et experimentales à *Schistosoma mansoni, S.haematobium* et *S.japonicum*. *Annales de parasitologie humaine et comparee*, **41,** 123–87.

Cicoli, D. and Neis, R. (1972). Antigens dell'ospite in *Schistosoma mansoni*. *Parassitologia*, **14,** 73–9.

Clegg, J. A. (1965). *In vitro* cultivation of *Schistosoma mansoni*. *Experimental Parasitology*, **16,** 133–47.

Clegg, J. A. and Smithers, S. R. (1972). The effects of immune rhesus monkey serum on schistosomula of *Schistosoma mansoni* during cultivation *in vitro*. *International Journal of Parasitology*, **2,** 79–98.

Colley, D. G. (1976). Adoptive suppression of granuloma formation. *Journal of Experimental Medicine*, **143,** 696–700.

Colley, D. G., Cook, J. A., Freeman, G. L., Bartholomew, R. K. and Jordan, P. (1977). Immune responses during human schistosomiasis mansoni: I. *In vitro* lymphocyte blastogenic responses to heterogeneous antigenic preparations from schistosome eggs, worms and cercariae. *International Archives of Allergy and Applied Immunology* (in press).

Coons, A. H., Creech, H. J., Jones, R. N. and Berliner, E. (1942). The demonstration of pneumococcal antigen in tissues by the use of fluorescent antibody. *Journal of Immunology*, **45,** 159–70.

Deelder, A. M. and Streefkerk, J. G. (1975). *Schistosoma mansoni*: immunohisto-peroxidase procedure in defined antigen substrate spheres (DASS) system as serologic field test. *Experimental Parasitology*, **37,** 405–10.

Erickson, D. G., Beattie, R. J., Yamaguchi, S., Miyasaka, E. and Williams, J. E. (1973). Host-parasite relationship in schistosomiasis mansoni and japonica in rhesus monkeys: interhost worm transfers. *Japanese Journal of Parasitology*, **22,** 307–14.

Gershon, R. K., Carter, R. L. and Kondo, K. (1967). On concomitant immunity in tumour-bearing hamsters. *Nature, London*, **213,** 674–6.

Gold, R., Rosen, F. S. and Weller, T. H. (1969). A specific circulating antigen in hamsters infected with *Schistosoma mansoni*. Detection of antigen in serum and urine and correlation between antigenic concentration and worm burden. *American Journal of Tropical Medicine and Hygiene*, **18,** 545–51.

Goldring, O. L., Clegg, J. A., Smithers, S. R. and Terry, R. J. (1976). Acquisition of human blood group antigens by *Schistosoma mansoni*. *Clinical Experimental Immuno-logy*, **26,** 181–7.

Goldring, O. L., Kusel, J. R. and Smithers, S. R. (1977a). *Schistosoma mansoni*: in *vitro* studies of the origin of host-like antigens on the schistosomular surface. *Experimental Parasitology*, **43,** 82–93.

Goldring, O. L., Sher, A., Smithers, S. R. and McLaren, D. J. (1977b). Host antigens and parasite antigens of murine *Schistosoma mansoni*. *Transactions of the Royal Society of Tropical Medicine and Hygiene*, **71,** 144–8.

Hamburger, J., Pelley, R. P. and Warren, K. S. (1976). *Schistosoma mansoni* soluble egg antigens. Determination of the stage and species-specificity of their serologic reactivity by radioimmunoassay. *Journal of Immunology*, **117,** 1561–6.

Hockley, D. J. and McLaren, D. J. (1973). *Schistosoma mansoni*: changes in the outer membrane of the tegument during development from cercaria to adult worm. *International Journal of Parasitology*, **3**, 13–25.

Hsu, C. K., Hsu, S. H., Whitney, R. A. and Hansen, C. T. (1976). Immunopathology of schistosomiasis in athymic mice. *Nature, London*, **262**, 397–8.

Huldt, G., Lagerquist, B., Phillips, T., Draper, C. C. and Voller, A. (1975). Detection of antibodies in schistosomiasis by enzyme-linked immunosorbent assay (ELISA). *Annals of Tropical Medicine and Parasitology*, **69**, 483–8.

Kagan, I. G. (1955). Haemagglutination after immunization with schistosome antigens. *Science*, **122**, 376–7.

Kagan, I. G. and Pellegrino, J. (1961). A critical review of immunological methods for the diagnosis of bilharziasis. *Bulletin of the World Health Organization*, **25**, 611–74.

von Lichtenberg, F. (1962). Host response to eggs of *Schistosoma mansoni*: I. Granuloma formation in the unsensitized laboratory mouse. *American Journal of Pathology*, **41**, 711–31.

von Lichtenberg, F. (1964). Studies on granuloma formation: III. Antigen sequestration and destruction in the schistosome pseudotubercle. *American Journal of Pathology*, **45**, 75–94.

von Lichtenberg, F., Sher, A. and McIntyre, S. (1977). A lung model of schistosome immunity in mice. *American Journal of Pathology*, **87**, 105–24.

McLaren, D. J., Clegg, J. A. and Smithers, S. R. (1975). Acquisition of host antigens by young *Schistosoma mansoni* in mice: correlation with failure to bind antibody *in vitro*. *Parasitology*, **70**, 67–75.

McLaren, D. J. and Hockley, D. J. (1977). Blood flukes have a double outer membrane. *Nature, London*, **269**, 147–9.

McLaren, D. J., Hockley, D. J., Goldring, O. L. and Hammond, B. J. (1978). A freeze fracture study of the developing tegumental outer membrane of *Schistosoma mansoni*. *Parasitology*, **76**, 327–48.

Mahmoud, A. A. F., Warren, K. S. and Peters, P. A. (1975). A role for the eosinophil in acquired resistance to *Schistosoma mansoni* infection as determined by anti-eosinophil serum. *Journal of Experimental Medicine*, **142**, 805–13.

Nash, T. E., Prescott, B. and Neva, F. A. (1974). The characteristics of a circulating antigen in schistosomiasis. *Journal of Immunology*, **112**, 1500–7.

Okabe, K. and Tanaka, T. (1958). A new urine precipitation reaction for schistosomiasis japonica, a preliminary report. *Kurume Medical Journal*, **5**, 45–52.

Oliver-Gonzales, J. (1954). Anti-egg precipitins in the serum of humans infected with *Schistosoma mansoni*. *Journal of Infectious Diseases*, **95**, 86–91.

Ouchterlony, O. (1953). Antigen-antibody reactions in gels: IV. Types of reactions in co-ordinated systems of diffusion. *Acta Pathologica et Microbiologica Scandinavica*, **32**, 231–40.

Pelley, R. P., Pelley, R. J., Hamburger, J., Peters, P. A. and Warren, K. S. (1976). *Schistosoma mansoni* soluble egg antigens: I. Identification and purification of three major antigens and the employment of radioimmuno-assay for their further characterization. *Journal of Immunology*, **117**, 1553–60.

Pelley, R. P., Warren, K. S. and Jordan, P. (1977). Purified antigen radio-immunoassay in serological diagnosis of schistosomiasis mansoni. *Lancet* 8042 **ii**, 781–5.

Perez, H., Clegg, J. A. and Smithers, S. R. (1974). Acquired immunity to *Schistosoma mansoni* in the rat: measurement of immunity by the lung recovery technique. *Parasitology*, **69**, 349–59.

Phillips, S. M., Reid, W. A., Bruce, J. I., Hedlund, K., Colvin, R. C., Campbell, R., Diggs, C. L. and Sadun, E. H. (1975). The cellular and humoral response to

Schistosoma mansoni infections in inbred rats: I. Mechanisms during initial exposure. *Cellular Immunology*, **19,** 99–116.

Phillips, S. M., Reid, W. A. and Sadun, E. H. (1977). The cellular and humoral response to *Schistosoma mansoni* infection in inbred rats: II. Mechanisms during re-exposure. *Cellular Immunology*, **28,** 75–89.

Sadun, E. H., Anderson, R. I. and Williams, J. S. (1961). Fluorescent antibody test for the laboratory diagnosis of schistosomiasis in humans by using dried blood smears on filter paper. *Experimental Parasitology*, **11,** 117–20.

Schinski, V. D., Clutter, W. C. and Murrel, K. D. (1976). Enzyme and ^{125}I-labelled anti-immunoglobulin assays in the immunodiagnosis of schistosomiasis. *American Journal of Tropical Medicine and Hygiene*, **25,** 824–31.

Senft, A. W. and Maddison, S. E. (1975). Hypersensitivity to parasite proteolytic enzyme in schistosomiasis. *American Journal of Tropical Medicine and Hygiene*, **24,** 83–9.

Sher, A. (1977). Immunity against *Schistosoma mansoni* in the mouse. *American Journal of Tropical Medicine and Hygiene*, 26, (suppl.) 20–8.

Sher, F. A., Mackenzie, P. E. and Smithers, S. R. (1974). Decreased recovery of invading parasites from the lungs as a parameter of acquired immunity to schistosomiasis in the laboratory mouse. *Journal of Infectious Diseases*, **130,** 626–33.

Sher, A., Smithers, S. R., Mackenzie, P. and Broomfield, K. (1977). *Schistosoma mansoni*: immunoglobulins involved in passive immunization of laboratory mice. *Experimental Parasitology*, **41,** 160–6.

Smith, M. D., Verroust, P. J., Morel-Maroger, L., Geniteau, M. and Coulard, J. P. (1977). A study of the presence of circulating immune complexes in schistosomiasis. *Transactions of the Royal Society of Tropical Medicine and Hygiene*, **71,** 343–8.

Smithers, S. R. and Terry, R. J. (1965). Naturally acquired resistance to experimental infections of *Schistosoma mansoni* in the rhesus monkey (*Macaca mulatta*). *Parasitology*, **55,** 701–10.

Smithers, S. R. and Terry, R. J. (1967). Resistance to experimental infection with *Schistosoma mansoni* in rhesus monkeys induced by the transfer of adult worms. *Transactions of the Royal Society of Tropical Medicine and Hygiene*, **61,** 517–33.

Smithers, S. R. and Terry, R. J. (1969). Immunity in schistosomiasis. *Annals of the New York Academy of Sciences*, **160,** 826–40.

Smithers, S. R. and Terry, R. J. (1976). The immunology of schistosomiasis. *In* "Advances in Parasitology" (Ed. B. Dawes), vol. 14, pp. 399–422. Academic Press, London and New York.

Smithers, S. R., Terry, R. J. and Hockley, D. J. (1969). Host antigens in schistosomiasis. *Proceedings of the Royal Society, Ser. B.*, **171,** 483–94.

Smithers, S. R., McLaren, D. J. and Ramalho-Pinto, F. J. (1977). Immunity to schistosomes: the target. *American Journal of Tropical Medicine and Hygiene*, **26,** (suppl.) 11–19.

Vogel, H. and Minning, W. (1949). Hullenbildung bei Bilharzia-Cercarien im serum bilharzia-infizierter Tiere und Menschen. *Zentralblatt für Bakteriologie*, Abt. Orig. **153,** 91–105.

Vogel, H. and Minning, W. (1953). Uber die erworbene Resistenz von Macacus rhesus gegenüber *Schistosoma japonicum*. *Zeitschrift für Tropenmedizin und Parasitologie*, **4,** 418–505.

Voller, A., Bidwell, D. E. and Bartlett, A. (1976). Enzyme immunoassays in diagnostic medicine. Theory and practice. *Bulletin of the World Health Organization*, **53,** 55–65.

Warren, K. S. (1963). The contribution of worm burden and host response to the development of hepatosplenic schistosomiasis mansoni in mice. *American Journal of Tropical Medicine and Hygiene*, **12,** 34–9.

Warren, K. S. (1966). The pathogenesis of "clay-pipe stem cirrhosis" in mice with chronic *Schistosomiasis mansoni*, with a note on the longevity of schistosomes. *American Journal of Pathology*, **49,** 477–89.

Warren, K. S. (1972). The immunopathogenesis of schistosomiasis: a multi-disciplinary approach. *Transactions of the Royal Society of Tropical Medicine and Hygiene*, **66,** 417–34.

Wilson, R. A. and Barnes, P. E. (1977). The formation and turnover of the membranocalyx on the tegument of *Schistosoma mansoni*. *Parasitology*, **74,** 61–71.

World Health Organization (1977). The Role of Immune Complexes in Disease. *WHO Technical Report Series*, No. 606.

Discussion

Professor Cohen asked what was the current belief about the emergence of immunity in exposed populations.

Dr Smithers said that there was little information about immunity in man. Work being carried out in the Gambia was showing, contrary to previous belief, that a concomitant immunity developed in *S.haematobium* infections after about four or five years; there appears to be rapid turnover of worm population and in the young if transmission was interrupted, then children rapidly lost most of their adult worm population. It seemed that in the early years of infection, immunity did not play a great part.

Dr Warren recalled that it had once been generally assumed that immunity was a controlling factor, but from more recent knowledge it seemed that exposure was not constant. Examination of available information on immunity and schistosomiasis in man, showed no definitive evidence that man developed immunity to any of the three species. In passive transfer studies in man involving both antibody and transfer factor, it had not been possible to demonstrate any immunity.

Regarding the longevity of *S.haematobium*, it was known from single case reports that worms of all three species could live as long as 20 or 30 years and it had been generally assumed that this was the average life-span. However, studies in California had suggested that the average life-span of *S. mansoni* was about seven years, and unpublished information from the US Naval Medical Research Unit in Cairo had reported a significant decline in egg-output over a six-month period, from patients hospitalized for long periods of time with *S.haematobium* infection. So it was possible that the life-span of *S.haematobium* might be less than one year.

Dr Smithers said that the study of immunity as a significant factor in the control of schistosomiasis was difficult to perform, because immunity found in man was not simple. Concomitant immunity would mean that an infected individual would also be resisting cercarial challenge. There was a great need for more studies on human immunity in the field.

Dr M. Taylor (*Winches Farm Field Station, St Albans*) was interested in Dr Smithers' views on effective acquired resistance in man, and felt that some observations on bovine schistosomiasis might have a bearing on the question.

A field study in endemic, enzootic area of *S.bovis* infection in the Sudan was being carried out. Plotting the relationship between the age of the animal and intensity of infection, as measured by faecal egg counts, had shown similar results to human investigations, although the age at which the decline in intensity began was much lower in domestic animals. In cattle, 100% of animals were infected by the time they were 18 months old, then both prevalence and intensity declined markedly. This pattern was found in human schistosomiasis, but the situation differed in that it was unlikely that the decline found in cattle was due to a decline in water contact. The hypothesis that older animals were acquiring a protective resistance was tested experimentally, by removing older, almost uninfected (as judged by faecal egg output) animals from the endemic area (Kosti), to the laboratory in Khartoum. They were challenged with 70 000 *S.bovis* cercariae, which was sufficient to kill similar animals of the same zebu breed from a non-endemic area, Kuku. The Kuku animals, following challenge, developed enormous egg counts, whereas Kosti-challenged animals had a very slight increase in egg output, of perhaps a hundredth of the challenged controls. Kosti controls— animals with light infections that were not challenged—showed virtually no increase in egg output. Haemoglobin concentrations in the Kuku animals declined to fatal levels in 14 weeks post challenge, while Kosti animals that were challenged behaved similarly to Kosti controls. These results were reflected in other clinical and pathophysiological measurements. Briefly, this gave a clear indication that animals with low egg outputs, chronically exposed in a natural situation, developed an extremely strong resistance to an artificial challenge situation. Dr Taylor suspected that this also happened in man, but it could not be shown experimentally.

Dr Warren said that although experiments in cattle were interesting, it was difficult to extrapolate the data to man. In regard to water contact, for instance, Jordan had shown on St Lucia that decline in egg output parallelled decline in water contact in man, whereas cattle maintained close water contact throughout their lives. Each animal species has a different reaction in terms of immunity to schistosomiasis and it was very difficult to extrapolate from one animal species to another.

Dr Smithers commented on the inability to demonstrate passive transfer in man. He pointed out that it was not possible to demonstrate passive transfer with serum of immunity in a rhesus monkey, but that the rhesus monkey developed a tremendous immunity to schistosoma infection.

Dr Christina James (*Winches Farm Field Station, St Albans*) said that Dr Taylor's observations could be supported by a report on canal cleaners in Egypt. People without previous exposure to schistosomiasis who came into the area and were employed as canal cleaners became ill, whereas those who had carried on such work for many years did not.

Dr Warren said he understood there were certain flaws in the reasoning in this report, in that canal cleaners who had been working for many years were the survivors. The report raised many questions and it would be interesting to read precise details; unfortunately it had as yet only appeared in abstract form.

Dr M. H. Boyer (*Harvard School of Public Health*) echoed Dr Warren's caution about species differences in schistosomiasis. He said that Dr Smithers' experiments on concomitant immunity in rhesus monkeys had been repeated in a mouse model, which had shown nowhere near the level of concomitant immunity as had been found in the rhesus monkey.

Dr Smithers said that he understood there was variation even between mouse strains.

Dr Warren said another study regarding canal cleaners in Leyte in the Philippines demonstrated that canal cleaners who were exposed to infection did not show raised antibodies; however, if rabbits infected with *S. japonicum* were exposed to further infection there was an increase in antibody levels. What this meant, Dr Warren did not know.

Dr C. A. Wright (*British Museum, London*) pointed to a possible parallel between the Kosti cattle and the canal cleaners. Original work on the pathology of *S. bovis* had used the Kosti strain because it was from an area where the disease in cattle was lethal. It was possible that the picture seen here, in the cattle which had survived, parallelled the situation with the canal cleaners.

Dr A. O. Lucas (*World Health Organization, Geneva*) felt that there was too much pessimism about inducing immunity in man. He pointed out that one of the best immunizing agents in public health was the tetanus toxid, but all available evidence showed that natural infection with tetanus did not induce immunity in man. Occasionally man could induce something artificially which Nature could not, and he hoped that schistosomiasis would be the next good example.

He asked Dr Smithers if the immunologists could produce a test which would show previous contact with schistosomiasis, even though the worms might be dead. Some available tests became negative after a time; he would like to see one test to show that worms were present and alive, and another test to show that they had been there but were not now present.

Dr Smithers thought that a skin test would do this; he agreed with Dr Lucas that when enough was known about the mechanism and evasion of the immune response of the worms, it would become possible to induce immunity artificially.

Dr Warren said that one of the reasons why immunity was not developing might be related to the ecology. The exposure of most people and the worm burdens of most people were so low that the amount of antigen present might not be enough to induce immunity. Once the relevant antigens were available, sufficient antigen plus the newer adjuvants could be successful in inducing immunity. He added that most workers in the field felt that they were learning a tremendous amount about immunity in experimental animals that was relevant to man, despite the apparent pessimism of earlier comments, and that this session on immunity should end on a highly optimistic note.

Moving on to the next presentations, Dr Warren said that Dr Smithers exemplified the generation of specialists called immunological parasitologists, but that the next two contributions were from the new generation of parasitological immunologists—that is, immunologists who had been attracted to the field as a challenge for immunology, and who had been applying to it their quite formidable techniques and talents. The first speaker, Dr Anthony Butterworth, had trained at Cambridge University under Professor R. R. A. Coombs, had worked in Nairobi for many years, and was now working with Professor John David's group at Harvard on the immunology of schistosomiasis.

12. Cell Biology and Schistosomiasis

A. E. Butterworth

The title of this article is perhaps a little misleading, as the discussion is restricted solely to one problem which may be expressed in terms of cell biology: it is that the migrating schistosome is foreign to the host and should, like any other antigenic material, be eliminated. S. R. Smithers has shown that this is sometimes, but not always, the case. The adult worms of a primary infection can survive even in hosts which are immune to superinfection; and, furthermore, in many hosts immunity to re-infection is incomplete. We can therefore view this topic from two opposing aspects. First, what are the mechanisms by which some parasites successfully evade the host's immune response; and, secondly, in those instances in which a host succeeds in destroying the parasite, what are the mechanisms by which it achieves this?

Three conditions may be required for an effective immune response against any parasite.

(1) The parasite must present an antigen to the host; the host must be capable of responding to this antigen; and the antigen must be expressed on the parasite not only during the induction of the response but also during its expression.

(2) The effector mechanism elicited in response to the parasite must be capable of inducing sufficient damage to prevent further maturation or replication of that parasite.

(3) Additional responses may also be required to allow early access of the effector mechanism to the site of the invading parasite. Equally, the effector mechanism must not be blocked, or otherwise rendered ineffective, either by simultaneous events occurring within the host or by changes induced by the parasite.

In other words, one may expect to have a delicate balance established between a changing parasite on the one hand and an interacting multiplicity of host responses on the other hand, which may or may not lead to the destruction of the parasite. Each of these points is considered in turn, the second in greatest detail.

Presentation of Parasite Antigen to the Host

The basic point about antigen presentation is that, although the adult worm of a primary infection is a good inducer of an effective immune response, it is itself protected from that response. This protection is acquired soon after skin penetration, and appears to depend, at least in part, on the passive uptake by the migrating schistosomulum of a coating of host material.

In the experiments of Smithers and his colleagues (Clegg *et al.*, 1971; Goldring *et al.*, 1976; Goldring *et al.*, 1977), it was shown that young schistosomula cultured *in vitro* would acquire erythrocyte alloantigens (see Table 1). When human red cells were used, it was found that

Table 1

Selective acquisition of "host antigens" by schistosomula

Acquired	Not acquired
ABH	MNS
Lewis	Rhesus
	Duffy
ABH from non-secretor serum	ABH from secretor saliva
Forssman	
H-2K products	Ly 1
H-2I products	Thy 1
Mouse alloantigens unrelated to H-2	H-Y
	C3
	Ig
	Albumin

References: Clegg *et al.*, 1971; Goldring, *et al.*, 1976, 1977; A. Sher, B. F. Hall and M. A. Vadas, personal communication; Dean and Sell, 1972.

antigens of the ABO and Lewis systems, which can exist as glycolipids, were taken up; whereas other antigens, such as those of the MNS, rhesus and Duffy systems, were not. Furthermore, ABH antigens were taken up from the serum of non-secretor individuals, in which they exist as glycolipids, but not from the saliva of secretor individuals, in which they exist as glycoproteins. Finally, it was shown that megalolipid extracts of erythrocytes, with blood-group antigen determinants, would serve as a source of host antigen.

These findings led to the tentative conclusion that only glycolipids would serve as a source of host antigen. Very recently, however, A. Sher, B. F. Hall and M. A. Vadas (1977, personal communication) have found that antigens known only to exist as glycoproteins are also taken up. The system they have used involves the recovery of schistosomula from the lungs of inbred mice, between five and six days after intravenous injection of schistosomula prepared *in vitro*. This is followed by indirect immunofluorescence to detect uptake of host antigens on the surface of the schistosomula, using highly specific antisera raised in congenic animals. A considerable degree of selectivity is demonstrable in this system, as revealed by the lack of uptake of many common constituents both of serum and of cells. However, products of both the K and the I regions of the mouse major histocompatibility complex (MHC) *are* acquired by the worm. Although it has been argued by one group that the antigenic determinant of the I-coded product is oligosaccharide in nature (Parish *et al.*, 1976), it is generally agreed that the whole molecule is a glycoprotein (Cullen *et al.*, 1974); while for the K- and D- coded products, the antigen determinants are associated with the protein part of the molecule (Schwartz *et al.*, 1973). Thus, it is now apparent that glycoproteins, as well as glycolipids, can be taken up by the worm. Furthermore, as discussed later, one possible explanation for the absence of demonstrable cytotoxic T-cell activity against schistosomula was that these organisms had no host MHC products in association with their own antigens, an association which in other systems is necessary for the expression of T-cell cytotoxicity (Zinkernagel and Doherty, 1974; Doherty *et al.*, 1976). This argument is now invalid, at least in its simplest form, and alternative explanations must be sought.

Acquisition of host antigen, as Smithers mentions, has been shown to be associated with a decreased ability of antischistosomular antibodies to bind to the organism (McLaren *et al.*, 1975), while Sher (1977) has found that schistosomula cultured *in vitro* in the presence of a source of host antigen are protected from attack after intravenous injection into immune mice. In other words, the coat of host material is probably sufficient to mask the worm's own antigenic determinants. However, acquisition of host antigens may not be the only mechanism by which the worm evades attack. For example, Dean (1977) has recently postulated, from metabolic inhibition studies on schistosomula cultured *in vitro* in defined media, that a change occurs in the membrane soon after skin penetration which is unrelated either to the acquisition of host antigen or to subsequent membrane turnover, and which is sufficient to protect the worm. Along different lines, we have recently begun to investigate the differential susceptibility of individual schistosomula to attack in an *in vitro* system mediated by antibody and nonspecific effector cells. Fresh schistosomula cultured in the presence of antibody and of a large excess of effector cells frequently show an "all-or-none" effect. Either they are completely ensheathed with effector cells and are dead, or they are free of more than one or two attached cells and are alive. This phenomenon has previously been recorded by Dean *et al.* (1974) in a complement-dependent cell-mediated cytotoxic system in the rat. One obvious possible explanation is that some individual parasites are failing to express on their surface antigens recognizable by the particular antiserum used, as a result either of genetic heterogenetity within the parasite population or of phenotypic heterogeneity with respect to membrane structure after skin penetration. Alternatively, it might be postulated that the organism is in some way either actively preventing adherence, or allowing adherence but subsequently repairing itself and sloughing off the effector cell. With the *in vitro* techniques now available, this whole field is open to more detailed study.

Effector Mechanisms Capable of Damaging the Susceptible Parasite

Let us turn now to the second condition for immunity listed: namely that, given that there is a phase when at least some of the challenge organisms are susceptible to attack, the host response must be capable of damaging those organisms. Smithers has already described the results from experiments *in vivo*, which so far indicate that antibody-dependent cell-mediated effector mechanisms are active in protection. This article concentrates instead on studies *in vitro*, considering in particular the nature of the cells which are capable of mediating damage, and the mechanism by which they do so.

One general point should be made about these experiments from the start. This is that they tell one nothing directly about the mechanism of immunity *in vivo*. The simple demonstration that a particular response is mounted by a host and can damage a parasite *in vitro* does not necessarily imply that this response is effective *in vivo*. A good example of this is the first effector mechanism that was studied *in vitro*, involving damage to schistosomula by a "lethal" IgG antibody together with large amounts of complement. This activity was originally demonstrated (Clegg and Smithers, 1972) in immune rhesus monkeys and later (Smith and Webbe, 1974; Perez *et al.*, 1974) in rats, baboons and man. The time-course of appearance of lethal antibody in infected rhesus monkeys coincided approximately with the development of immunity, suggesting on a correlative basis that the two might be associated. However, later work (Sher *et al.*, 1974) showed that although rats could be immunized with partially purified adult-worm antigens to produce high titres of lethal antibody, these rats were not immune to challenge. In other words, lethal antibody—at any rate on its own—is insufficient to account for protection.

This type of experiment emphasizes the importance of testing directly any mechanism demonstrated *in vitro* for its relevance to immunity *in vivo*. Within this clearly-defined limitation, however, experiments *in vitro* allow a much more detailed analysis of effector mechanisms, especially cellular, than would be possible *in vivo*. In addition, of course, they offer the only way of studying potentially relevant responses in man.

The stage of the parasite chosen for studies *in vitro* has usually been the young schistosomulum obtained just after skin penetration. The reason for this is clear from what has already been said; namely, that this is the stage that appears to be susceptible to immune attack. Such schistosomula can be prepared by allowing infective cercariae to penetrate an isolated preparation of mouse or rat skin; during this penetration the cercariae shed their tails, lose their water-resistant glycocalyx, and develop the double-bilayer membrane characteristic of the schistosomulum. They can then be cultured *in vitro*, and damage can be studied either by microscopical analysis at various levels, or by measuring release of a previously incorporated radioisotopic label such as ^{51}chromium. Both approaches have advantages and disadvantages. The advantages of the ^{51}Cr assay are that it is objective, and allows the handling of very large numbers of samples. A potential disadvantage is that it is recording a permeability change in the parasite which is not necessarily related to damage, although we have found that ^{51}Cr release correlates well with microscopically-detectable eosinophil-mediated damage (Glauert and Butterworth, 1977). A more serious theoretical drawback is that it is an averaging technique, indicating nothing about damage to individual schistosomula. It is therefore not suitable for use in the sort of experiment described earlier, where one is trying to analyse why some organisms within a preparation are susceptible to damage, while others are not. For this, a microscopical assay such as the methylene blue or trypan blue uptake tests are needed.

It is worth bearing in mind that the schistosomulum is a huge organism compared with targets used in more conventional systems. This has two implications. First, one would not expect intracellular killing mechanisms to be effective, of the type that play an important role in immunity against bacterial, and perhaps some protozoal, parasites. Secondly, one would expect a requirement for a much higher multiplicity of effector cells to target cells than is usual with single target cell systems—and this is indeed the case.

It may now be asked: which cellular effector mechanisms might one expect to demonstrate *in vitro*, and which have in fact been described? The first group in Table 2 are those characteristic of a classical cell-mediated response, in which the T-lymphocyte is involved in the effector arm of the response as well as in its induction. Such T-cells may be involved directly, as cytotoxic T-lymphocytes (CTL) capable of inducing direct specific damage to the parasite, or indirectly, by releasing a mediator which activates a macrophage to exert a nonspecific cytotoxic effect.

In all situations involving CTL studied so far, there has been a genetic restriction on the effector cell to target cell interaction, in that the effector cell has to recognize either allogeneic MHC products, or

Table 2

Cellular effector mechanisms active against schistosomula *in vitro*

	T-cell related
Cytotoxic T-lymphocytes	Not found
Activated macrophages	Not found
	Antibody- and complement-dependent
IgG + complement + neutrophils	Rat, guinea-pig
	Antibody-dependent complement-independent
Lymphocytic K-cells	Not found
IgG (cytophilic) + macrophages	Rat
IgE/antigen complexes + macrophages	Rat, baboon, man
IgG + eosinophils or neutrophils	Man, baboon, rat

References: Butterworth *et al.*, 1974, 1975, 1977a, 1977b; Capron *et al.*, 1975, 1977; Clegg *et al.*, 1971; David *et al.*, 1977; Dean *et al.*, 1974, 1975; A. M. Glauert, A. E. Butterworth and R. F. Sturrock, in preparation; Mackenzie *et al.*, 1977; Perez and Smithers, 1977; Perez *et al.*, 1974; Sher *et al.*, 1974; Smith and Webbe, 1974.

antigen associated with syngeneic MHC products. In the case of virus-infected target cells, for example, CTL from immune animals kill only syngeneic virus-infected targets; they fail to kill uninfected targets, nor do they kill allogeneic infected targets (Zinkernagel and Doherty, 1974). Two possible explanations have been put forward for this: (1) that the CTL recognizes an antigen composed partly of virus antigen and partly of self MHC products (the "altered self" hypothesis), or (2) that the CTL bears two independent receptors, one for the viral antigen and one for the self MHC product, both of which must interact with the target. These two possibilities have not yet been resolved; for both of them, however, the requirement for an MHC product on the target is important. In the case of schistosomula, in contrast to virus-infected host cells, there is no intrinsic reason to suspect that MHC products should be present on the surface. Hence, it was not surprising that no workers have yet succeeded in demonstrating CTL activity against schistosomula. However, the observation mentioned earlier, namely that both K and I-region products are acquired by the schistosomulum as host-antigen, invalidates this simple view. It is still possible, of course, that the MHC product is not present on the schistosomulum in the right way for recognition by a CTL or that the CTL, even though it can recognize a schistosomulum, is intrinsically unable to kill it. On the other hand, it is also possible that CTL could be formed and could be perfectly effective, but that their induction is suppressed in naturally-infected animals. This would be much more interesting from the point of view of attempting to induce an effective CTL response *in vivo*, and we have started a series of experiments to resolve the various possibilities.

A second T-cell-related system, in which macrophages are activated by a T-cell mediator, or lymphokine, to exert a non-specific cytotoxic effect, has been extensively studied as a mechanism for killing tumour cells *in vitro*. It has not yet been described as a mechanism effective against schistosomula—mainly because, as far as I know, nobody has yet looked for it.

Turning now to the antibody-dependent cell-mediated systems, these are more likely to be relevant *in vivo* from the observations mentioned earlier, namely, that immunity can be transferred with serum but depends on the presence in the recipient of a radiosensitive cell. These reactions can be divided into two categories: those which depend on the presence of complement, and those which are able to work in the absence of complement. One reaction has been described which is entirely dependent on complement. This involves damage mediated by rat neutrophils, but not eosinophils or macrophages, in the presence of an IgG antibody from immune animals (Dean *et al.*, 1974; Dean *et al.*, 1975). In this system, the neutrophils cause an enhanced and accelerated destruction of schistosomula by comparison with schistosomula incubated with antibody and complement alone. There is no clear evidence, however, that the antibody differs from the complement-dependent lethal antibody mentioned earlier.

Several other systems exist in which the presence of complement is not an absolute prerequisite for the demonstration of damage, although there is the possibility that complement may enhance the effect in some cases. The classical antibody-dependent, complement-independent system, involving damage mediated by an Fc receptor-bearing lymphocyte (K-cell), appears to be ineffective, as discussed later. Macrophages, however, have been shown to mediate damage in two reactions. The first involves an IgG antibody from immune rats, which is cytophilic for normal rat macrophages, and which enables these macrophages to adhere to and kill schistosomula (Perez and Smithers, 1977). This antibody can be separated from lethal antibody on QAE Sephadex, and there is a good correlation between the rise and decline of activity and the rise and decline of immunity.

A second macrophage-mediated reaction (Capron *et al.*, 1975; Capron *et al.*, 1977) is extremely unusual, in that it implicates IgE in macrophage responses. In this reaction, two stages are involved. The first is an alteration in macrophage function, resembling activation, induced by pre-incubation with IgE-containing immune complexes from rat serum. The second stage is an IgE-dependent interaction of these altered macrophages with the schistosomulum, associated with adherence and damage. There appears to be an IgE requirement in both stages; and the time-course of the development of the ability to induce this effect in the serum of infected rats parallels the time-course of development of immunity.

Finally, damage detectable by the ^{51}Cr-release assay can be induced by an IgG antibody from infected humans or baboons, together with either neutrophils or eosinophils from normal individuals (Butterworth *et al.*, 1974; M. A. Vadas, T. R. David and A. E. Butterworth, unpublished data). Recently, a similar effect has been demonstrated in rats (Mackenzie *et al.*, 1977). The involvement of eosinophils in this reaction is particularly interesting in view of the long-known association of eosinophilia with helminth infection, and of several observations which implicate the eosinophil in immunity *in vivo*. These are that ablation of eosinophils in mice abolishes both actively acquired and passive immunity (Mahmoud *et al.*, 1975); and that cellular infiltrate around dying schistosomula in the skin and lungs of immune mice is predominantly eosinophilic in composition, in contrast to normal animals in whom a neutrophil response predominates (von Lichtenberg *et al.*, 1976). Two main points are now considered concerning this reaction: first, the nature of the effector cell, and, secondly, the mechanism whereby it damages the schistosomulum.

Our initial observation was that heat-inactivated sera from infected humans or baboons, in the presence of mixed peripheral blood leukocytes from normal individuals, would induce a release of chromium from labelled schistosomula which was markedly greater than the background level of release observed in the presence of serum alone, effector cells alone, or medium alone (Butterworth *et al.*, 1974). When we set out to fractionate the effector cell by density gradient centrifugation, we found to our surprise that a granulocyte-rich fraction was far more active than a mononuclear-rich fraction containing lymphocytes and monocytes. The more the lymphocytes are purified, the less the activity, even though these cells can still be demonstrated to be cytotoxic for chicken red blood cells. This finding, which has been consistent between all workers in the field, implies that the mechanisms whereby the lymphocytic K-cell damages mammalian or avian target cells are not active against schistosomula, and raises the question of whether lymphocytes under any circumstances can be induced to exert a cytotoxic effect on these organisms.

We then attempted to identify the particular granulocyte responsible for mediating damage in this system. First, we found that pretreatment of unpurified peripheral blood leukocytes with anti-eosinophil serum and complement reduced subsequent cytotoxicity to a greater extent than did pretreatment with an anti-neutrophil serum, suggesting that eosinophils were a major component of the reaction (Butterworth *et al.*, 1975). Next, the effect of eosinophil-enriched cell preparations, obtained by density centrifugation from the blood of *eosinophilic* patients, was tested either fresh or after overnight culture (Butterworth *et al.*, 1977a). These cells were shown to be active, and in some cases they were considerably more active than unpurified cells from normal individuals. In the experiment shown in Table 3, for example, eosinophils of 96 % purity were obtained from a patient with marked eosinophilia of unknown origin. These cells when tested immediately after preparation were as active as unpurified cells from a normal individual; and after culture for one day, there was enhancement of

Table 3
Cytotoxic activity of purified eosinophils from an eosinophilic patient

	Percentage ^{51}Chromium release from labelled schistosomula				
	+Ab				−Ab
	2500:1	500:1	100:1	20:1	2500:1
Normal buffy coat					
(3% eosinophils)	42	38	26	22	22
96% fresh eosinophils	47	35	27	23	23
98% cultured					
eosinophils	40	37	37	32	22
	Antibody: 21			Medium: 15	

Ab antischistosomular antibody.
Cells from a patient with 75% eosinophilia of unknown origin were prepared from dextran-sedimented peripheral blood by centrifugation over Hypaque. These cells were tested either fresh or after overnight culture for their ability to induce release of ^{51}chromium from labelled schistosomula, in the presence or absence of antischistosomular antibody, at various effector-to-target ratios. Dextran-sedimented peripheral blood leukocytes from a normal individual were included for comparison.
Reference: A. E. Butterworth, unpublished data.

activity in comparison with fresh normal cells. In other words, some eosinophils can be demonstrated to have a very marked cytotoxic potential.

In our early experiments, we failed to detect an effect of mixed neutrophil and mononuclear cells which had been depleted of eosinophils. In these experiments, however, the recovery of neutrophils was very poor, and it was possible that we were selecting out a small subpopulation of less dense neutrophils by the rather primitive separation techniques used. More recently, however, M. A. Vadas has developed a better technique for separating both neutrophils and eosinophils from normal peripheral blood, and has found that some neutrophils are more active than are eosinophils. Table 4 shows the results of one such experiment. Peripheral blood leukocytes from a normal individual were separated into several fractions of increasing density by centrifugation on a discontinuous metrizamide gradient. Fractions were then tested for their ability to mediate antibody-dependent damage to schistosomula. The fractions of intermediate density, highly enriched in neutrophils, were more active than the high-density eosinophil-rich fractions, even though these still showed some effect. It may be noted that the dose response curves for eosinophils were flatter than those for

Table 4
Cytotoxic activity of normal peripheral blood leukocytes fractionated by density
centrifugation

Cell fraction	Eo	Neutro	Mono	*Percentage* [51]*chromium release from labelled schistosomula*			
				+*Ab*			−*Ab*
				3200:1	*1000:1*	*320:1*	*3200:1*
Unpurified	9	76	15	48	40	32	25
21% metrizamide	0	89	11	37	40	26	18
22% metrizamide	3·5	95	1·5	39	42	29	19
23% metrizamide	89	11	0	38	25	23	18
24% + 25% metrizamide	97·5	2·5	0	35	23	22	16
				Antibody: 18		Medium: 16	

Ab antischistosomular antibody.
Cells from normal human peripheral blood were fractionated by dextran sedimentation,
followed by centrifugation at 1200 g for 45 minutes on discontinuous metrizamide gradients.
These fractions, after washing, were tested for their ability to induce release of [51]chromium
from labelled schistosomula, in the presence or absence of antischistosomular antibody, at
various effector-to-target ratios.
Reference: M. Vadas, A. E. Butterworth and J. R. David, unpublished data.

neutrophils, but that in both cases a slight effect was noted at a ratio of
320:1.

In summary, although eosinophils under some circumstances can be
demonstrated to be highly active, it can no longer be argued that they
are the only cell responsible for initiating damage, nor, indeed, that in
normal peripheral blood they are the most important component. What
this implies is that if eosinophils eventually prove to have any particular association with immunity in schistosomiasis, then it may be either
because they selectively accumulate at the site of parasite destruction or
because their functional properties are enhanced when they arrive
there. Another implication is that we might not now expect the mechanism of damage to be attributable to any functionally specific component of the eosinophil, but rather to a component which is common to
both types of granulocyte. In this context, the state of present knowledge about the mechanisms of damage may be briefly summarized
(David *et al.*, 1977a; Butterworth *et al.*, 1977b; A. M. Glauert, A. E.
Butterworth and R. F. Sturrock, in preparation) (see Table 5). In
these experiments, the effect of both purified eosinophils and unpurified
granulocyte-rich preparations has been investigated by electron
microscopy and by the use of metabolic inhibitors. Three stages appear
to be involved.

(1) An intimate contact between the effector cell and the surface of
the antibody-coated schistosomulum, not seen in control preparations

Table 5

Mechanism of granulocyte-mediated damage to schistosomula

Light and electron microscopy
(1) Adherence:
      Antibody-dependent
      Eosinophils more than neutrophils
      Progressive accumulation of cells around target
      Intimate contact established between cell and target
(2) Degranulation:
      Granule contents, containing peroxidase, appear between effector
      cell and target

Metabolic inhibitors	*Putative action on:*
(1) Inhibition of ^{51}chromium release with:	
Cytochalasins A and B: early effect, reversible by washing	Microfilaments (contact/ degranulation)
2-deoxyglucose: partially reversible by excess glucose	Glycolysis
Iodoacetate, sodium fluoride	Glycolysis
Chelating agents	Divalent cations
Aminophylline + isoproterenol	cAMP levels
Tosyl-lysyl-chloromethyl ketone	Esterases
(2) No inhibition of ^{51}chromium release with:	
Potassium cyanide, antimycin	Oxidative phosphorylation
Mitomycin C	mRNA synthesis
Cycloheximide, puromycin	Protein synthesis
Colchicine	Microtubule function
Ethanolamine hydrochloride, choline	Phospholipases
Superoxide dismutase, catalase	Superoxide, H_2O_2

References: Butterworth *et al.*, 1977b; David *et al.*, 1977; A. M. Glauert, A. E. Butterworth and R. F. Sturrock, in preparation; McLaren *et al.*, 1977; M. Robbins, J. R. David and A. E. Butterworth, in preparation; M. A. Vadas, personal communication.

without antibody. Eosinophils adhere much better than neutrophils (M. A. Vadas, personal communication), a rather unexpected finding in view of their relative paucity of Fc receptors in human blood.

(2) Degranulation of the effector cell (of which eosinophils have been studied in the greatest detail) with release of lysosomal enzymes onto the surface of the parasite (Glauert *et al.*, in preparation; McLaren *et al.*, 1977). In this context, although not necessarily causally related, it has been found that chromium release induced either by purified eosinophils or by mixed granulocytes can be inhibited by the cytochalasins A and B, by inhibitors of glycolysis, by chelating agents, and by agents which raise intracellular cyclic AMP levels. In contrast, chromium release is not inhibited by inhibitors of oxidative phosphorylation, of protein synthesis, or of mRNA synthesis. These findings suggest in-

directly that damage depends on the glycolysis-dependent release of a preformed granule molecule—a finding which is suppotred by the fine structural observations.

(3) Presentation of the preformed lysosomal effector molecule or molecules to the cell surface. The nature of these molecules, or of the factors which govern their activity at the schistosomular surface, is entirely unknown, except insofar as nonspecific esterase inhibitors such as tosyl-lysyl-chloromethylketone can inhibit damage. These may, however, have nonspecific actions on the effector cell. The formation of hydrogen peroxide or of superoxide radicals does not appear to have the importance that it does in the antibacterial action of neutrophils, since superoxide dismutase and catalase fail to inhibit chromium release (Robbins *et al.*, in preparation). Equally, inhibitors of phospholipase have no effect.

It seems probable that damage will eventually be attributable to a rather complex action of a multitude of enzymes or other factors present within the release lysosomal contents, and it is unlikely that metabolic inhibitor studies will be of much further assistance. The approaches required now are probably to study the effects of isolated granule components on the surface of the worm, and to develop new assays for detecting early changes in the parasite, and their nature. Already, however, the mechanism of damage can be seen to differ from that induced by lymphocytic K-cells, in which no degranulation occurs and which probably exert damage by a phospholipase action (Frye and Friou, 1975). It is still possible that damage is attributable to some rather specific property of the eosinophil/neutrophil series, and the importance of determining this property lies in the possibility of eventually manipulating it, both *in vitro* and conceivably *in vivo*, by the use of cell-stimulating agents of an adjuvant type.

Role of Other Responses in Allowing Access of Effector Mechanisms to the Susceptible Parasite

Most of this presentation has been concerned with two main points: first, the evasion by the maturing schistosomulum of established immune responses, with the corollary that only young schistosomula are susceptible; and secondly, a description of those mechanisms which may be active against young schistosomula. For the sake of completion, a third point may be briefly mentioned: namely, that for a mechanism to be effective *in vivo*, it must be able to reach the parasite before the parasite protects itself. In other words, what processes are available which may enhance the access of a mechanism to the parasite? And do these processes also enhance the ability of that mechanism to damage the parasite? Most cellular effector mechanisms have been studied using peripheral blood, or sometimes peritoneal, effector cells; but what we need to know now is how these cells reach the extravascular spaces in the skin, and how they behave when they arrive there.

Virtually nothing is known about this important aspect of the host response; there are various theoretical possibilities. First, a host may require a *systemic* enhancement of effector cells to express complete immunity; an example here might be the systemic eosinophilia associated with schostosomiasis. In this context, it has recently been observed that immunity in baboons shows some correlation not only with cell-dependent cytotoxic antibody levels, but also with the relative cytotoxic activity of unpurified peripheral blood leukocytes (Sturrock *et al.*, 1977). Secondly, a *local* reaction may be required at the site of the invading parasite to attract the relevant effector cell. Examples might be delayed hypersensitivity reactions with release of lymphocyte mediators, or immediate hypersensitivity reactions with release of mast cell chemotactic factors such as ECF-A (eosinophil chemotactic factor of anaphylaxis) or other vasoactive amines. In this context, depletion of vasoactive amines in mice with reserpine is associated with loss of tissue reactions against schistosomula, both after cercarial challenge and after intravenous injection of schistosomula prepared *in vitro* (A. Sher, P. W. Askenase, S. McIntyre and F. von Lichtenberg, personal communication). Finally, mediators of immediate and delayed hypersensitivity reactions, as well as enhancing effector cell access, may also increase effector cell function. The sort of observation that may be relevant here is the finding that eosinophil C3 receptors increase after incubation with ECF-A (Anwar and Kay, 1977), and that eosinophils incubated with ESP (eosinophil stimulation promoter) show an enhanced capacity to destroy schistosome eggs (S. L. James and D. G. Colley, personal communication). These possibilities are clearly speculative, but represent an avenue that might be worth following up.

Conclusions

To conclude, it is apparent that our understanding of cellular immune mechanisms in schistosomiasis has grown in recent years, partly through analysis of the mechanism of immune invasion, and partly through emphasis on the action of cells in the expression of the immune response. On the other hand, the situation is now in some ways more confused than it was before; we have too many potential effector mechanisms, each of which might be induced, enhanced or suppressed under different conditions in different host species. Given this situation, three areas now appear both important and within our competence to study:

(1) Relevance testing *in vivo* of the various effector mechanisms described *in vitro*; in experimental animals by somewhat difficult modifications of classical techniques in cellular immunology, and in man by adequately designed correlative studies.

(2) Determination of the mechanism of damage in the various *in vitro* systems; is there any common denominator, and, if so, can this be artificially enhanced by the use of adjuvant-like materials?

(3) Analysis of the mechanisms influencing entry of the effector reaction into the skin, and its efficacy therein. Is this a limiting factor in immunity and, if so, can it be artificially modified?

These questions, of course, presuppose from a practical point of view that a logical approach to the control of schistosomiasis by immunological means is a reasonable proposition. This is a postulate that cannot rationally either be asserted or denied until more fundamental information has been acquired. This circular argument renders any discussion about the relevance of any particular line of research somewhat unhelpful; we are caught in the paradox of not knowing the value of our work until we have done more of it.

References

Anwar, A. R. E. and Kay, A. B. (1977). The ECF-A tetrapeptides and histamine selectively enhance human eosinophil complement receptors. *Nature (London)*, **269**, 522–4.

Butterworth, A. E., Sturrock, R. F., Houba, V. and Rees, P. H. (1974). Antibody-dependent cell-mediated damage to schistosomula *in vitro*. *Nature, (London)*, **252**, 503–5.

Butterworth, A. E., Sturrock, R. F., Houba, V., Mahmoud, A. A. F., Sher, A. and Rees, P. H. (1975). Eosinophils as mediators of antibody-dependent damage to schistosomula. *Nature (London)*, **256**, 727–9.

Butterworth, A. E., David, J. R., Franks, D., Mahmoud, A. A. F., David, P. H., Sturrock, R. F. and Houba, V. (1977a). Antibody-dependent eosinophil-mediated damage to ^{51}Cr-labelled schistosomula of *Schistosoma mansoni*: damage by purified eosinophils. *Journal of Experimental Medicine*, **145**, 136–50.

Butterworth, A. E., Remold, H. G., Houba, V., David, J. R., Franks, D., David, P. H. and Sturrock, R. F. (1977b). Antibody-dependent eosinophil-mediated damage to ^{51}Cr-labelled schistosomula of *Schistosoma mansoni*: mediation by IgG, and inhibition by antigen-antibody complexes. *Journal of Immunology*, **118**, 2230–6.

Capron, A., Bazin, H., Dessaint, J. P. and Capron, M. (1975). Specific IgE antibodies in immune adherence of normal macrophages to *Schistosoma mansoni* schistosomules. *Nature (London)*, **253**, 474–6.

Capron, A., Dessaint, J. P., Joseph, M., Rousseaux, R., Capron, M. and Bazin, H. (1977). Interaction between IgE complexes and macrophages in the rat: a new mechanism of macrophage activation. *European Journal of Immunology*, **7**, 315–22.

Clegg, J. A. and Smithers, S. R. (1972). The effects of immune rhesus monkey serum on schistosomula of *Schistosoma mansoni* during cultivation *in vitro*. *International Journal of Parasitology*, **2**, 79–98.

Clegg, J. A., Smithers, S. R. and Terry, R. J. (1971). Acquisition of human antigens by *Schistosoma mansoni* during cultivation *in vitro*. *Nature (London)* **232**, 653–4.

Cullen, S. E., David, C. S., Shreffler, D. C. and Nathenson, S. G. (1974). Membrane molecules determined by the H-2 associated immune response region: isolation and some properties. *Proceedings of the National Academy of Sciences of the USA*, **71**, 648–52.

David, J. R., Butterworth, A. E., Remold, H G., David, P. H , Houba, V. and Sturrock, R. F. (1977). Antibody-dependent eosinophil-mediated damage to ^{51}-Cr-labelled schistosomula of *Schistosoma mansoni*: effect of metabolic inhibitors, and other agents which alter cell function. *Journal of Immunology*, **118**, 2221–9.

Dean, D. A. (1977). Decreased binding of cytotoxic antibody by developing *Schistosoma mansoni*. Evidence for a surface change independent of host antigen adsorption and membrane turnover. *Journal of Parasitology*, **63**, 418–26.

Dean, D. A. and Sell, K. W. (1972). Surface antigens on *Schistosoma mansoni*: II. Adsorption of a Forssman-like host antigen by schistosomula. *Clinical and Experimental Immunology*, **12**, 325–32.

Dean, D. A., Wistar, R. and Murrell, K. D. (1974). Combined *in vitro* effects of rat antibody and neutrophilic leukocytes on schistosomula of *Schistosoma mansoni*. *American Journal of Tropical Medicine and Hygiene*. **23**, 420–8.

Dean, D. A., Wistar, R. and Chen, P. (1975). Immune response of guinea-pigs to *Schistosoma mansoni*: I. *In vitro* effects of antibody and neutrophils eosinophils and macrophages on schistosomula. *American Journal of Tropical Medicine and Hygiene*, **24**, 74–82.

Doherty, P. C., Blanden, R. V. and Zinkernagel, R. M. (1976). Specificity of virus-immune effector T cells for H-2K or H-2D compatible interactions: implications for H-antigen diversity. *Transplantation Review*, **29**, 89–124.

Frye, L. D. and Friou, G. J. (1975). Inhibition of mammalian cytotoxic cells by phosphatidylcholine and its analogue. *Nature (London)*, **258**, 333–5.

Glauert, A. M. and Butterworth, A. E. (1977). Morphological evidence for the ability of eosinophils to damage antibody-coated schistosomula. *Transactions of the Royal Society of Tropical Medicine and Hygiene*, **1**, 291–2.

Goldring, O. L., Clegg, J. A., Smithers, S. R. and Terry, R. J. (1976). Acquisition of human blood group antigens by *Schistosoma mansoni*. *Clinical and Experimental Immunology*, **26**, 181–7.

Goldring, O. L., Kusel, J. R. and Smithers, S. R. (1977). *Schistosoma mansoni*: origin *in vitro* of host-like surface antigens. *Experimental Parasitology*, **43**, 82–93.

Mackenzie, C. D., Ramalho-Pinto, F. J., McLaren, D. J. and Smithers, S. R. (1977). Antibody-mediated adherence of rat eosinophils to schistosomula of *Schistosoma mansoni in vitro*. *Clinical and Experimental Immunology*, (in press).

McLaren, D. J., Clegg, J. A. and Smithers, S. R. (1975). Acquisition of host antigens by young *Schistosoma mansoni* in mice: correlation with failure to bind antibody *in vitro*. *Parasitology*, **70**, 67–75.

McLaren D. J. Mackenzie C. D. and Ramalho-Pinto F. J. (1977). Ultrastructural observations on the *in vitro* interaction between rat eosinophils and some parasitic helminths (*Schistosoma mansoni, Trichinella spiralis* and *Nippostrongylus braziliensis*). *Clinical and Experimental Immunology* (in press).

Mahmoud, A. A. F., Warren, K. S. and Peters, P. A. (1975). A role for the eosinophil in acquired resistance to *Schistosoma mansoni* infection as determined by anti-eosinophil serum. *Journal of Experimental Medicine*, **142**, 805–13.

Parish, C. R., Jackson, D. C. and McKenzie, I. F. C. (1976). Low-molecular-weight Ia antigens in normal mouse serum: III. Isolation and partial chemical characterization. *Immunogenetics*, **3**, 455–63.

Perez, H., Clegg, J. A. and Smithers, S. R. (1974). Acquired immunity to *Schistosoma mansoni* in the rat: measurement of immunity by the lung recovery technique. *Parasitology*, **69,** 349–59.

Perez, H. A. and Smithers, S. R. (1977). *Schistosoma mansoni* in the rat: the adherence of macrophages to schistosomula in vitro after sensitization with immune serum. *International Journal of Parasitology*, **7,** 315–20.

Schwartz, B. D., Kato, K., Cullen, S. E. and Nathenson, S. G. (1973). H-2 histocompatibility alloantigens. Some biochemical properties of the molecules solubilized by NP-40 detergent. *Biochemistry*, **12,** 2157–64.

Sher, A. (1977). Immunity against *Schistosoma mansoni* in the mouse. *American Journal of Tropical Medicine and Hygiene*, **26,** (Suppl.) 20–28.

Sher, A., Kusel, J. R., Perez, H. and Clegg, J. A. (1974). Partial isolation of a membrane antigen which induces the formation of antibodies lethal to schistosomes cultured *in vitro*. *Clinical and Experimental Immunology*, **18,** 357–69.

Smith, M. A. and Webbe, G. (1974). Damage to schistosomula of *Schistosoma haematobium in vitro* by immune baboon and human sera and absence of cross-reaction with *Schistosoma mansoni*. *Transactions of the Royal Society of Tropical Medicine and Hygiene*, **68,** 70–1.

Sturrock, R. F., Butterworth, A. E., Houba, V., Karamsadkar, S. D. and Kimani, R. (1977). *Schistosoma mansoni* in the Kenyan baboon (*Papio anubis*): the development and predictability of resistance to homologous challenge (in press).

von Lichtenberg, F., Sher, A., Gibbons, N. and Doughty, B. L. (1976). Eosinophil-enriched inflammatory response to schistosomula in the skin of mice immune to *Schistosoma mansoni*. *American Journal of Pathology*, **84,** 479–500.

Zinkernagel, R. M. and Doherty, P. C. (1974). Restriction of *in vitro* T cell-mediated cytotoxicity in lymphocytic choriomeningitis within a syngeneic or semi-allogeneic system. *Nature (London)*, **248,** 701–3.

Discussion

Dr R. M. Krause (*National Institutes of Health, Bethesda*) asked Dr Butterworth whether, in the early experiments where he had shown chromium release with cells from the schistosomula with antiserum present, he had any antigen preparations that could absorb out that antibody.

Dr Butterworth replied that whole fresh schistosomula on their own could absorb out the antibody activity. Such absorbed sera had lost the ability to react with the membranes of adult worms in frozen section, while they retained activity against the gut components of adult worms. Isolated preparations of antigens had not yet proved successful since preparations of egg antigens, as well as adult worm antigens, depleted the cell-dependent activity after simple addition to the antisera. It seemed they had prepared immune complexes which subsequently blocked effector cell activity. Clearly, isolated antigens must be put on to immunoabsorbents to absorb out the activity from the sera. So far this had proved difficult, since the antigens eluted very readily from the immunoabsorbent columns.

Dr Adel A. F. Mahmoud (*Case Western Reserve University, Cleveland*) said that it seemed there were at least three stages in the *in vitro* system; the cell attachment, the chromium release and the final damage of the schistosomula, which occurred at different time periods. Using a cell with an Fc receptor, chromium release might occur at eight hours, and whether it was a neutrophil or an eosinophil was irrelevant because the crucial question was "What happens at 24 hours? Will the antibody-coated schistosomula be destroyed by neutrophils or not?" He said there was a paper which showed that if heart muscle is cultured with an antibody against the heart muscle and an Fc receptor-bearing cell was added, whether it was a neutrophil or an eosinophil, chromium release occurred; that did not mean that either cell was destroying the heart muscle. New data, particularly on the neutrophil, might show that chromium release was dependent on Fc receptor on the cell, but that final destruction needed a specific cell.

Dr Butterworth said, firstly, that in work with purified eosinophils they had correlated chromium release with damage as detectable by phase-contrast microscopy. Correlation was good and the damage was marked; the organisms were shattered and spilt their contents.

Secondly, he did not think it was ture that any Fc receptor-bearing cell could induce chromium release, because lymphocytic K-cells failed to induce chromium release.

Thirdly, he agreed that it was difficult to distinguish between a damaged and a dead schistosomulum. The chromium release assay provided an objective measurement of damage to the parasite. Microscopical assays of destruction, although more definitive, were very subjective.

He said that any *in vitro* mechanism studied in this way was artificial, because one could not reproduce the situation where the effector cell had to arrive at the schistosomula. This was where he thought the difference between the eosinophil and neutrophil might eventually become clear. As well as being able to act, the effector cell had to be able to reach the site of action.

Dr C. E. Gordon Smith (*London School of Hygiene and Tropical Medicine*) asked if it was possible to say how many reactions were needed to kill the schistosomula, and whether they could repair themselves. He wondered whether there were any critical points where damage would cause total disruption, or if it was sufficient to make a hole in them.

Dr Butterworth did not know. He thought it possible that damage resulted from a number of effector cells spilling their contents along the surface of the schistosomula. He said that using a mixed preparation, there seemed to be an accumulation of cells at the site of the reaction. One could postulate an initial hole, insufficient in itself to cause enough damage to prevent the organism maturing, but subsequently enhanced by many other cells acting and accelerating the reaction in a non-specific way. In other words, the schistosomulum was now a classical phagocytosable particle.

Professor Cohen asked whether survivors could be selected, and if they were then uniformly survivors in a given strain of mouse or whether they might behave differently in a different strain.

Dr Butterworth said that this was an experiment which was technically just possible, but he had not yet done it. The approach so far used had been to look by direct immunofluorescence at whether the schistosomula which were not being attacked had antigen on their surface. One might predict that they did not, but results so far were insufficient to make a positive statement.

Returning to Dr Smithers' point about the question of immunity in man, he thought it was unduly pessimistic to say categorically that immunity did not exist. The problem was really to design the correct experiment to test whether or not immunity occurred in man.

He described a study which had recently been set up in Nairobi to investigate immunity, in a school of 500 children, of whom 300 were infected. Of these 300, about half came from an area far away from the infecting waterbody, which is a river, and half came from an area close to it. From evidence with experimental animals, if immunity was going to occur, it would be under conditions of high-intensity rather than low-intensity infections. After treatment, in the absence of immunity, one would predict that those with the original high prevalence and intensity of infection would become re-infected more quickly than those with the original low prevalence and intensity of infection. If immunity existed it would occur in the high-intensity group; after treatment the original low-intensity group would become infected and the original high-intensity group would not. The study had the intrinsic control of the original low-infected group. One would be controlling for transmission in the particular years studied because the low-infected group would become re-infected. Dr Butterworth thought that this was a possible approach to the question of immunity in man.

Dr Warren said that one problem with the design was that the study was in an area where there was a low exposure rate. One group, returning to this area after treatment, would have much greater water contact and, therefore, would be exposed to far more cercariae than the other group. He asked how Dr Butterworth was correcting for those factors.

Dr Butterworth said that this was the whole point of the study. In the absence of immunity one would predict that, after treatment, reinfection rates in the original high-intensity would be higher than in the other group, whereas, in the presence of immunity, reinfection rates in the original low-intensity group would be low, but detectable, and reinfection rates in the high-intensity group would be lower still.

Dr Warren asked what would be seen with partial immunity.

Dr Butterworth said that Dr Sturrock planned to carry out a catalytic curve analysis, in which he could predict re-infection rates in each of the two groups. He was predicting a rate of approximately 18 in the high-infection group and 8 in the low-infection group. It was only necessary to show a reduction of re-infection rate in the high-infection group, from the predicted re-infection rate.

Dr Mahmoud thought that at least five years was needed for observation of the children after treatment, because the rate of acquisition of infection in an endemic area was very slow. It would not be possible to perceive a change in the rate of re-infection in the two sub-populations in a shorter time.

Dr Butterworth said that the figures of 18 and 8 were calculated on the basis of two years, although five years would obviously be better. He thought the difficulty lay in the fact that immunity to re-infection might not persist for five years after treatment.

Dr Warren introduced the next speaker, Dr Mahmoud, who was currently working on immunology and haematology with respect to his interest in white blood cells and their function in parasitic infections. He had performed field work in Kenya and Egypt on the relationship between intensity of infection and disease in schistosomiasis, on more rapid means of diagnosis in the field, and on better, less toxic and more rapid means of chemotherapy for the mass treatment of schistosomiasis.

13. The Use of Chemotherapy in Schistosomiasis Control

Adel A. F. Mahmoud

Introduction

Man's attempts to treat schistosomal infection and its sequelae have not ceased since the ancient Egyptians described the endemic "aaa" syndrome or haematuria. They knew that the infection came from contact with water, and one of the prescribed methods for treatment was a shield on the external genitalia. Later the Kahun papyrus gave a detailed method for treating haematuria (Ebbell, 1927) which falls within the jurisdiction of malpractice laws as we know them now!

The era of scientific chemotherapy against schistosomiasis was unduly delayed after the discovery of the worms in 1852 (Bilharz). The first specific chemotherapeutic agent was introduced 66 years later by Christopherson (1918). One is tempted to speculate that the scientific fights launched around the turn of the century regarding the life-cycle and the species of the worm may have diverted attention from describing the clinical and pathological features of the disease and may have delayed the discovery of specific therapy. Furthermore, two other aspects of schistosomiasis lagged behind. First, the dimensions and significance of the infection as a public health problem in endemic areas is not fully appreciated. We are influenced during our training by the medical view that centres all the attention on the individual patient: our understanding of the dynamics, transmission, and management of the infection on a community level has been less than satisfactory. Second, tartar emetic—which was introduced in 1918—remained for most of the half-century that followed as a major antischistosomal therapeutic agent. Tartar emetic is an efficient drug but has to be administered under strict medical supervision and for a protracted course. It is practically of no use in the management of schistosomiasis as a public health problem in an endemic area.

This review is largely devoted to three areas which reflect major advances as far as chemotherapy of schistosomiasis is concerned.

(1) Schistosomiasis as a community problem: whom do we treat?
    (a) dynamics of the schistosome infection
    (b) the relationship of infection to disease
    (c) new quantitative field-diagnostic techniques
(2) Newer chemotherapeutic agents:
    (a) hycanthone
    (b) oxamniquine
    (c) metrifonate
    (d) praziquantel
(3) Application of chemotherapeutic agents in control schemes:
    (a) selective chemotherapy
    (b) targeted mass treatment
    (c) St Lucia experience

Finally, in considering the future of schistosomiasis control we should face the question "What is the goal of a community-oriented control programme for schistosomiasis?".

Schistosomiasis as a Community Problem

Dynamics of the Schistosome Infection
The individual patient is the basic concern of clinical medicine; however, evaluating the public health impact and the epidemiological patterns of disease in a community necessitates the utilization of additional tools. Likewise, sitting in the outpatient department of a major teaching hospital in a schistosomiasis-endemic area exposes the individual physician to a myriad of patients with hepatosplenomegaly, ascites, etc., but contributes little to the understanding of the relationship of infection to disease or the multiplicity of factors leading to the persistence of infection in the community. Only recently has a general framework of thinking about the epidemiology, pathogenesis, and morbidity of schistosomiasis in a particular community emerged. The salient features of the general framework are of prime importance in setting our goals in schistosomiasis control via chemotherapy.

Macdonald (1965) and Hairston (1965) were the first to construct models describing the epidemiology of schistosomiasis and the dynamics of its transmission. Macdonald's work established the importance of considering various probabilistic aspects of the parasite life-cycle such as probability of worm-pairing. Quantitative description of the pairing process has led to the recognition of a critical density of helminths required in some infected individuals for maintaining the parasite life-cycle. Prevalence and intensity curves in many recently studied endemic areas (Lehman, *et al.*, 1976; Ongom and Bradley, 1972; Siongok *et al.*, 1976; Warren et al., 1974) show an aggregation of worm burdens which fits a negative binomial distribution. This can simply mean that in endemic areas, most infected individuals harbour low-to-moderate worm burdens and only a small percentage of individuals have heavy worm infestation. The aggregation of worm burdens in a few members of the human species has both epidemiological and clinical implications. Epidemiologically, as the concentration of worms within a few hosts increases, their opportunity to find mates increases and consequently decreases the "breakpoint" density required for helminth maintenance. Thus, Macdonald's model can be used to identify the subpopulation of heavily infected individuals which is largely responsible for maintenance of infection in a community.

The Relationship of Infection to Disease in Schistosomiasis

The schistosomes have a complicated life-cycle with an intermediate snail host in which asexual multiplication occurs and a definitive human host in which there is sexual reproduction. It is essential to realize that each infective cercaria has less than a 50% chance to develop into only one worm, and that male and female worms in the blood vessels of man do not multiply. Along with the rate of acquisition of new infections (which has been shown to be slow) and the limited life-span of the worms, the distribution of schistosomiasis in endemic communities results in a majority with light infection and no or minimal disease. A. W. Cheever's post-mortem studies have shown a close association between worm burdens, egg counts in stools and tissues, and the extent of pathology. We, as well as other groups (Cline *et al.*, 1977; Hiatt, 1976; Lehman *et al.*, 1976; Mahmoud *et al.*, 1975; Ongom and Bradley, 1972; Siongok *et al.*, 1976; Warren *et al.*, 1974), have conducted a series of cross-sectional community-based studies in schistosomiasis-endemic areas in St Lucia, Brazil, Kenya, Puerto-Rico, Ethiopia and Egypt. All these studies confirm the negative binomial distribution of the infection and point to the close association of morbidity with the intensity of infection. Two issues are usually raised at these studies: their cross-sectional nature and the possibility of other factors involved in disease in schistosomiasis. We must realize that we are looking at the epidemiology of an infection and the resulting disease at a community level. Our data may not apply to an individual patient; in the same way the data generated from individual observations have very little epidemiological significance.

The negative binomial distribution of schistosomiasis and the close association between intensity of infection and disease allows us to identify not only the subpopulation of infected individuals responsible for maintenance of the infection in the community, but, in addition, those who are at maximal risk of developing disease.

New Quantitative Field Diagnostic Techniques

The development of the two epidemiological concepts that individuals with heavy worm burdens may be responsible for the maintenance of infection in the community and are at risk of disease resulted in a central position for the quantification of schistosome infections. A number of egg-counting techniques have been described (Bell, 1963; Bradley, 1964; Ritchie, 1948; Scott, 1957), but they are usually performed in the laboratory and are time-consuming. We have adapted a nuclepore filtration technique for field quantification of *Schistosoma haematobium* eggs in urine samples (Peters *et al.*, 1976). Table 1 summarizes some of the results.

Table 1
Field quantification of *S.haematobium* eggs in urine samples

No. of samples	10 ml aliquots interval	10 ml aliquots mean ± s.e.	1 ml aliquots interval	1 ml aliquots mean ± s.e.
63	0	0	0	0
11	1–9	3·2 ± 0·74	0	0
31	10–99	39·4 ± 5·48	1–14	4·2 ± ·57
15	100–400	166·7 ± 21·08	9–35	15·3 ± 1·74

This method proved most adaptable to field conditions; using a relatively untrained team, preparation and reading of duplicate samples were performed in less than two minutes per subject.

For stool examination in the field we have adapted the Kato technique (P. A. Peters, M. A. El Alamy, K. S. Warren and A. A. F. Mahmoud, in preparation) which allows counting of total number of eggs in smears 50 mg thick. Several improvements including reduction of the sample size to 20 mg (Table 2) led to the development of an

Table 2
Quick Kato technique: rate of clearing and proportionality of counts

Time of reading	Weight of faecal sample 10 mg	Weight of faecal sample 20 mg Mean egg count ± s.e.	Weight of faecal sample 50 mg
15 min	2·7 ± 0·8	9·8 ± 2·4	1·6 ± 0·6
1 h	2·9 ± 1·1	9·5 ± 2·4	6·3 ± 3·9
3 h	3·1 ± 1·0	9·9 ± 2·4	11·3 ± 5·4
6 h	2·1 ± 0·6	9·8 ± 2·3	19·2 ± 5·4
24 h	3·2 ± 1·0	9·7 ± 2·4	23·3 ± 5·7
48 h	2·8 ± 1·0	9·9 ± 2·3	23·9 ± 5·7

accurate, quick, and reproducible method for quantification of eggs in the stools.

Newer Chemotherapeutic Agents

The search for newer schistosomicidal drugs has progressed slowly since the introduction of antimonials in 1918. Within the last two decades, however, several major discoveries have led to a revolution in the field of chemotherapy: from multiple protracted courses of intravenous heavy metal injection we are now seeking single-dose oral or intra-muscular therapeutic agents. The importance of this progress is that chemotherapy can and does now play a central role in the control of schistosomiasis.

Niridazole, a nitrothiazole derivative, was the first oral antischisto-somal drug introduced for human use in the early 1960s (Abdalla and Saif, 1969). It was a step forward because of its oral mode of administra-tion. Niridazole, however, had the major drawback of the prolonged duration of therapy (5–10 days) which limits its usefulness in mass chemotherapeutic campaigns. Research on niridazole has recently acquired a tremendous momentum because of its potent long-acting immunosuppressive effect which may prove to be of clinical significance (Jones *et al.*, 1977; Lucas *et al.*, 1969; Mahmoud *et al.*, 1975; Webster *et al.*, 1975).

There are four antischistosomal agents that can be administered in single doses and which represent a true turning-point in the chemo-therapy of this infection.

Hycanthone
Hycanthone is a hydroxymethyl analogue of Miracil D which was the first metal-free compound used as an antischistosomal agent (Rosi *et al.*, 1965). Numerous clinical trials have been carried out in the major

Hycanthone

endemic areas for schistosomiasis and indicate the high efficacy of a single intramuscular injection of hycanthone against both *S.mansoni* and *S.haematobium*. The usual recommended dose of hycanthone is 3 mg per kg body-weight, but Cunha *et al.*, (1971) reported that 1·5 mg per kg body-weight is an effective dose and that using higher doses is of no advantage. A few studies which have involved lower doses of hycanthone have shown a pronounced reduction of worm burdens with virtual elimination of side-effects (Cook *et al.*, 1976; Rees *et al.*, 1976). Recently, Warren *et al.*, (1978) have established a dose-response to hycanthone in man using three different doses, the highest being 1·5 mg per kg (Fig. 1). This dose resulted in a 96% decrease of egg output and

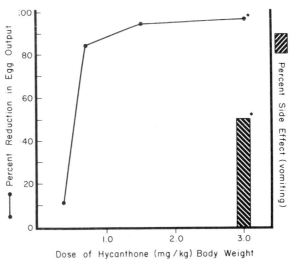

Fig. 1 Response to varying doses of hycanthone (mg per kg body-weight, abscissa), in terms of decreased Schistosoma mansoni *egg outputs in the faeces (percentage, ordinate) one month after treatment. Data were obtained from the studies of Warren* et al. *(in press).* *Results of treatment (percentage vomiting) with 3 mg per kg are from the studies of Cook* et al. *(1976).*

0·75 mg per kg in an 85% decrease. In contrast to the frequent vomiting associated with the 3 mg per kg dose (Cook *et al.*, 1976) no side-effects were observed with any of the lower doses (Warren *et al.*, 1978).

Severe adverse reactions to hycanthone are very rare. Hepatic necrosis followed by death has been reported in 20 cases, which in some instances was associated with other diseases (Katz, 1977). The controversy about hycanthone stemmed from the reports about its possible mutagenicity and carcinogenicity. Without going into the details of these arguments, it may be said that WHO and the USA-Japan panel recently convened meetings which reached the conclusion that on the basis of available data on hycanthone, no genetic effect of the drug in man could be reliably estimated, and that there was no reason for precluding its use in the clinical therapy of schistosomiasis.

Oxamniquine
Oxamniquine is a 2-aminomethyltetrahydroquinoline derivative displaying strong antischistosomal activity against *S.mansoni* only. Oxamniquine is now used orally in South America as a single dose of 15–20

$$CH_2OH, O_2N, CH_2NHCH(CH_3)_2$$

Oxamniquine

mg per kg body weight. Although extensive clinical data are not yet available, early reports of the cure rates following orally-administered oxamniquine range between 70% and 100% (Coura et al., 1973; Katz et al., 1976; Katz et al., 1977). In St Lucia J. Cook et al. (personal communication) found that oxamniquine induced a drop of between 95% and 97% in egg counts in three months. Higher doses of oxamniquine are reported to be required for treatment of *S.mansoni* in Egypt but this needs further confirmation (Z. Farid, personal communication). Side-effects of oral oxamniquine therapy are slight, manifesting mainly as dizziness and drowsiness in about 30–40% of treated individuals but disappearing within six hours. Thus, oxamniquine seems to be a very useful addition to man's arsenal against *S.mansoni* that can be used for mass chemotherapy.

Metrifonate

This organophosphorous anticholinesterase compound has recently been introduced as an effective oral schistosomicidal drug. It is only effective against *S.haematobium* infection and has been used in a dose of 7·5 mg per kg body-weight given at intervals of 14–28 days to a maxi-

$$H_3C—O, O, P, H_3C—O, CHOH—CCl_3$$

Metrifonate

Table 3

Mean *S.haematobium* urine egg-counts before and 3 months after treatment with a single oral dose of metrifonate (10 mg per kg)

No. of subjects	Initial egg count[a]		Post-treatment egg count[b]		P[c]	Percentage reduction
	Range	Mean ± s.d.	Range	Mean ± s.d.		
14	1–49	24·1 ± 14·5	0–19	4·9 ± 7·0	< ·001	80
20	50–149	101·0 ± 27·6	0–28	4·0 ± 6·8	< ·001	96
17	150–399	271·7 ± 75·3	0–89	15·5 ± 21·7	< ·001	94
21	400–2334	986·2 ± 549·8	0–108	27·0 ± 33·0	< ·001	97
72		384·5 ± 494·8		13·6 ± 23·4		96·5

[a] mean of 9 daily urines.

[b] mean of 3 daily urines in 70 subjects; 2 subjects had 2 urines.

[c] t value from paired-sample t test.

mum of three doses. Cure rates have been in the range of 60–95% in various treated populations with more than 90% drop of egg counts (Davis and Bailey, 1969; Forsyth and Rashid, 1967; Reddy *et al.*, 1975). Recently T. K. A. Siongok, K. A. Warren, J. H. Ouma and D. Smith (in preparation) experimented with single-dose metrifonate regimens. The data are summarized in Table 3.

These results show that single-dose metrifonate therapy is a potentially useful approach in mass treatment campaigns for *S.haematobium* endemic areas. The side-effects of metrifonate therapy are usually minimal. Depression of plasma and erythrocyte cholinesterase was noticed but both levels returned to normal values within a short period.

Praziquantel

Praziquantel is a newcomer, a member of the heterocyclic pyrazino-isoquinoline system. Work in progress with this drug indicates that it is effective in experimental animals when given in a single oral dose, reducing the worm burden by 95%. These experiments were conducted

Praziquantel

on several experimental animals infected with *S.mansoni*, *S.haematobium*, or *S.japonicum* (Davis and Bailey, 1969; Z. Farid, personal communication; Forsyth and Rashid, 1967; Gönnert and Andrews, 1977; James *et al.*, 1977; Reddy *et al.*, 1975; Siongok *et al.*, in preparation; Webbe and James, 1977). In primates, praziquantel in a single dose of 100 mg per kg completely cured *S.haematobium* infection, whereas a dose of 50 mg per kg given on five consecutive days cured the vervet monkey from *S.japonicum* infections. *S.mansoni* infection in the cebus monkey was cured by single oral doses of 100 mg per kg. These preliminary results from animal experiments are very promising. In fact, praziquantel is now in the stage of clinical trials in endemic areas, and the indications are very favourable that we might have a single-dose oral chemotherapeutic agent against the three species of human schistosomes.

Chemotherapy in Schistosomiasis Control

In the early and mid-1960s snail control by molluscicides was generally considered to offer the most effective and rapid means of reducing schistosomiasis transmission. Molluscicides, however, have several drawbacks and their long-term usefulness is limited. This led some endemic countries to add mass chemotherapy as an adjunct to their control programmes. The most widely used drug during the early days was tartar emetic given over a long protracted course and associated with a long list of side and toxic effects. With the introduction in 1964 of niridazole, an oral drug that is given over a relatively short period, chemotherapy on a community basis became a feasible alternative for the control of schistosomiasis.

The information on the role of chemotherapy in the control of schistosomiasis is fragmentary: here three approaches which represent important landmarks are indicated.

Selective Chemotherapy

In 1974, based on his experience in the field of schistosomiasis, Kloetzel formulated a hypothesis which he called "selective chemotherapy". The basic arguments for this hypothesis were as follows.

(a) Schistosomiasis as a disease develops in only a minority of infected individuals. This minority can be identified as those with more than 500 eggs per g faeces in the age-group 10–15 years.
(b) If chemotherapy is introduced before the age of 10 years it will effect a drastic reduction of egg-counts, and even if the patient remains in the endemic area, post-treatment levels of egg-counts will not increase to any marked extent.
(c) Field trials of this selective or preventive chemotherapy show that egg output remained low and development of splenomegaly was prevented.

Kloetzel proposed that in endemic areas treatment should be administered to those individuals with more than 500 eggs per g, in the age group 10–19 years. A combination of both criteria involves treating approximately 10% of the population with 39% reduction of egg output in the environment.

Targeted Mass Treatment

We have developed Kloetzel's concepts in several directions in our field-work in Kenya. The criteria of selecting individuals for therapy were set to parallel the results of our morbidity studies. Morbidity (hepatomegaly) in Lower Nduu, Kenya, was mainly found in those with >400 eggs per g, representing approximately one-third of the population. We have used half the recommended dose of hycanthone to treat this heavily infected population (Warren and Mahmoud, 1976). Our results are summarized in Table 4.

Table 4
Targeted mass treatment of the population of the village of Lower Nduu, Kenya

Subjects (egg output > 400 per g)	122 (mean age 14 years)	
Therapy:	Hycanthone—single intramuscular injection 1·50 mg per kg (half dose)	
Side-effects:	None	
Results	Before	4 months
Mean eggs per g faeces	1250	36
Reduction in egg output	97%	

Mainly young persons were treated, inducing 97% reduction in their egg counts; furthermore, although only 30% of the entire study population was treated, egg output into the environment was reduced by approximately 80%. Three years of follow-up examinations of the study population showed that there was no marked difference between year 1 and year 2 where the only intervention was to treat those with hepato-splenomegaly (A. A. F. Mahmoud, P. A. Peters, A. M. El Kholy, M. A. El Alamy, M. H. Wahdan, H. B. Houser, in preparation). However, by the end of the second-year survey, chemotherapy was given to 95% of those with more than 400 eggs per g. The distribution of the infection and the age-specific intensity curves were drastically changed by year 3. The change was reflected as a reduction of prevalence of the infection in the whole community and in the incidence of new infections in the younger age-group. Follow-up studies are planned over the next several years to assess the impact of our "targeted mass treatment" approach.

The St Lucia Project
In 1965 a joint programme on schistosomiasis control was initiated on the island of St Lucia to evaluate the available control methods for schistosomiasis. The chemotherapeutic agents were hycanthone (2·5 mg per kg body-weight) initially; oxamniquine was later introduced.

The results of this model project are summarized in Table 5.

Table 5

Year	Number treated	Change in incidence (%)
1973	677	18·8 → 5·4
1974	159	→ 4·1
1975	96	—

It is important to note that the impact of chemotherapy was manifested both in the incidence of new infections and the overall prevalence rates among all age-groups. Cost-effective analysis indicates that chemotherapy was the cheapest, most rapid, and most efficient method of controlling schistosomiasis on the island of St Lucia. The additional obvious advantage of chemotherapy is that it is the only available means of controlling human disease.

Summary and Conclusions

The appreciation of the following basic information on schistosomiasis in endemic areas should help in formulating a policy for its control.

(1) The dynamics of the infection in a community results in a negative binomial distribution with a small proportion of infected individuals harbouring heavy worm burdens. This subpopulation, according to the mathematical models available, is largely responsible for maintenance of the infection in a community.

(2) Morbidity studies have shown that epidemiologically disease is related to intensity of infection—again facilitating identification of a subpopulation with heavy infection which is at risk of disease.

(3) Recent developments in parasitological and serological techniques may render the identification of individuals with heavy infections as rapid as examination of a direct stool-smear.

(4) Single-dose therapeutic agents are now available.

(5) Finally, the build-up of intensity of infection in communities where mass chemotherapy has been used indicates that its rate is very slow and that these individuals may or may not need further chemotherapeutic intervention in 3–5 years.

It seems that the time is ripe for us to face the question "What is the goal of a community-oriented control programme for schistosomiasis?". The indications are that targeted chemotherapeutic programmes—based on our current knowledge of schistosomiasis as an infection and a disease and with the available schistosomicidal agents—should be the most effective parasitologically, clinically, and economically.

References

Abdalla, A. and Saif, N. (1969). *Annals of the New York Academy of Sciences*, **169,** 686.

Bell, D. R. (1963). *Bulletin of the World Health Organization*, **29,** 525.

Bilharz, T. (1852). *Zeitschrift für Wissenschaft liche Zoologie*, **4,** 53.

Bradley, D. J. (1964). *Transactions of the Royal Society of Tropical Medicine and Hygiene*, **58,** 291.

Cheever, A. W. (1968). *American Journal of Tropical Medicine and Hygiene*, **17,** 38–64.

Christopherson, J. B. (1918). *Lancet*, **ii,** 325.

Cline, B. L., Rymzo, W. T., Hiatt, R. A., Knight, W. B. and Berrios-Duzan, L. A. (1977). *American Journal of Tropical Medicine and Hygiene*, **26,** 109.

Cook, J. A. Jordan, P. and Bartholomew, R. K. (1977). *American Journal of Tropical Medicine and Hygiene*, **26,** 887.

Cook, J. A., Jordan, P. and Armitage, P. (1976). *American Journal of Tropical Medicine and Hygiene*, **25**, 602.

Coura, J. R., Argento, C. A., Figueiredo, N. de, Wanke, B. and Queiroz, G. C. de (1973). *Revista del Institute de medicina tropical de Sao Paulo*, **15** (Suppl. 1), 41.

Cunha, A. S., Carvalho, D. G. and Cambraia, J. N. S. (1971). *Revista del Instituto de medicina tropical de Sao Paulo*, **13**, 131.

Davis, A. and Bailey, D. R. (1969). *Bulletin of the World Health Organization*, **41**, 209.

Ebbell, B. (1927). *Zeitschrifte für Aegypterisch Sprache*, **62**, 16.

Forsyth, D. M. and Rashid, C. (1967). *Lancet*, **i**, 130.

Gönnert, R. and Andrews, P. (1977). *Zeitschrift für Parasitenkunde*, **52**, 129.

Hairston, N. G. (1965). *Bulletin of the World Health Organization*, **33**, 45, 163.

Hiatt, R. A. (1976). *American Journal of Tropical Medicine and Hygiene*, **25**, 808.

James, C., Webbe, G. and Nelson, G. S. (1977). *Zeitschrift fur Parasitenkunde*, **52**, 179.

Jones, B. M., Bird, M., Massey, P., Miller, D., Miller, J. J., Reeves, S. and Soloman, J. R. (1977). *British Medical Journal*, **2**, 792.

Jordan, P. (1977). *American Journal of Tropical Medicine and Hygiene*, **26**, 887.

Katz, N. (1977). *Advances in Pharmacology and Chemotherapy*, **14**, 1.

Katz, N., Grinbaum, E., Chaves, A., Zicker, F. and Pellegrino, J. (1976). *Revista del Instituto de medicina tropical de Sao Paulo*, **18**, 371.

Katz, N., Zicker, F. and Pereira, J. P. (1977). *American Journal of Tropical Medicine and Hygiene*, **26**, 234.

Kloetzel, K. (1974). *Transactions of the Royal Society of Tropical Medicine and Hygiene*, **68**, 344.

Lehman, J. S., Jr., Mott, K. E., Morrow, R. H., Jr., Muniz, T. M. and Boyer, M. H. (1976). *American Journal of Tropical Medicine and Hygiene*, **25**, 285.

Lucas, A. O., Akpom, C. A., Cockshott, W. P. and Bohrer, S. P. (1969). *Annals of the New York Academy of Sciences*, **169**, 629.

Macdonald, G. (1965). *Transactions of the Royal Society of Tropical Medicine and Hygiene*, **59**, 489.

Mahmoud, A. A. F., Mandel, M. A., Warren, K. S. and Webster, L. T. jr. (1975). *Journal of Immunology*, **114**, 279.

Ongom, V. L. and Bradley, D. J. (1972). *Transactions of the Royal Society of Tropical Medicine and Hygiene*, **66**, 835.

Peters, P. A., Mahmoud, A. A. F., Warren, K. S., Ouma, J. H. and Siongok, T. K. A. (1976). *Bulletin of the World Health Organization*, **54**, 159.

Reddy, S., Oomen, J. M. V. and Bell, D. R. (1975). *Annals of Tropical Medicine and Parasitology*, **69**, 73.

Rees, P. H., Bowry, H. N., Roberts, J. M. D. and Thuku, J. J. (1976). *American Journal of Tropical Medicine and Hygiene*, **25**, 602.

Ritchie, L. S. (1948). *Bulletin of the United States Army Medical Department*, **8**, 326.

Rosi, D., Peruzzotti, G., Dennis, E. W., Berberian, D. A., Freele, H. and Archer, S. (1965). *Nature (London)*, **208**, 1005.

Scott, J. A. (1957). *Texas Reports on Biology and Medicine*, **15**, 425.

Siongok, T. K. A., Mahmoud, A. A. F., Ouma, J. H., Warren, K. S., Muller, A. S., Handa, A. K. and Houser, H. B. (1976). *American Journal of Tropical Medicine and Hygiene*, **25**, 273.

Warren, K. S. and Mahmoud, A. A. F. (1976). *Transactions of the Association of American Physicians*, **89**, 195.

Warren, K. S., Mahmoud, A. A. F., Cummings, P., Murphy, D. J. and Houser, H. B. (1974). *American Journal of Tropical Medicine and Hygiene*, **23**, 902.

Warren, K. S., Siongok, T. K. A., Ouma, J. H. and Houser, H. B. (1978). *Lancet*, **i**, 352.

Webbe, G. and James, C. (1977). *Zeitschrift für Parasitenkunde*, **52**, 169.

Webster, L. T. jr, Butterworth, A. E., Mahmoud, A. A. F., Mngola, E. N. and Warren, K. S. (1975). *New England Journal of Medicine*, **292**, 1144.

Discussion

Dr Warren said it was exciting to realize that this information had not been available even five years ago, and that more was being constantly gathered. A key problem now was to keep the Ministries of Health in developing countries where schistosomiasis occurred, informed of the rapid developments which impinged directly on the development of more cost-effective and efficient methods of control of the disease.

Professor C. F. A. Briujning (*Institute of Tropical Medicine, Leiden*) asked Dr Mahmoud if he knew when praziquantel would become commercially available, and what the price might be.

Dr Mahmoud said that it was presently in second-stage clinical trials. Field trials would be necessary before the drug became available commercially. The price as yet was not known.

Professor L. Eyckmans (*Institute of Tropical Medicine, Antwerp*) referred to the idea held some years previously, that oxamniquine should be given by repeated intramuscular injections, in order to sterilize the female worms while keeping them alive in the circulation in order to maintain a certain level of concomitant immunity. He asked why this idea had been abandoned.

Dr Mahmoud said that oxamniquine given intramuscularly had proved so painful that it could not be used in the field as a chemotherapeutic agent. He added that the use of chemotherapy as a control method necessitated a single-dose agent. The infected population in Egypt was in the order of 30 million people; to mount a campaign involving a two-dose drug would be extremely difficult.

Regarding loss of immunity after treatment, if mice with chronic *S.mansoni* infection were challenged eight, ten or 12 weeks after successful cure of their primary infection, they were still immune. The situation in man was not yet known.

Dr Christina James expressed surprise that Dr Mahmoud had given St Lucia as an example of an area where chemotherapy alone had done a great deal of good. She had understood that St Lucia was a prime example of integrated control.

Dr Mahmoud explained that the St Lucia experiment had been carried out in separate valleys: one valley was given chemotherapy, another clean water supplies and a third molluscicides. This allowed comparison of the three methods of control, each one being considered separately. It could then be asked what would happen if all three were combined. All the approaches were successful, but he had been talking about the approach which was cheap, would effect a quicker result and which, above all, would treat sick humans. Putting a molluscicide in the water would not treat someone who had a hepatosplenomegaly.

Dr Lucas agreed with Dr Mahmoud on the value of chemotherapy in schistosomiasis. He felt it was necessary to extend some of the observations; first, to confirm the safety of the lower dose of hycanthone: second, to show the effectiveness of targeted mass treatments in other situations. *S.mansoni* was relatively easy to consider since much epidemiological work had been done to correlate the load of infection, as shown by egg output, with disease, but the decisions were not easy to make with *S.haematobium*. The demonstration that treatment altered or prevented the ultimate course of infection had not been so clearly made.

Reflecting the optimism that was felt about compounds presently being tested, Dr Lucas said that when the WHO Special Programme reviewed its plans for schistosomiasis, it was decided to accelerate the testing of existing compounds in order better to define their use, rather than concentrate on trying to find new ones.

Dr Mahmoud said that Dr Lucas' final point was really the crux of the matter. Whatever the future might bring, it was important to help the people in the endemic areas now, with present-day tools.

Referring to the problems with *S.haematobium*, he said that the quantitative estimation of *S.haematobium* eggs in the urine was not a satisfactory technique because there were many variables. In addition, they were discussing the relationship of disease to intensity of infection in a community, not a single individual, and no community studies had been carried out on *S.haematobium*. In assessing the disease an intravenous pyelogram (IVP) had to be used to study the pathology. Various studies, including work in post-mortem material, had shown a close correlation between disease and intensity of infection. If a decision had to be made, on a limited budget, as to which group to treat first, these epidemiological studies had shown that treatment should start with the heavy infections.

Dr Warren said that he and Dr Mahmoud, together with other investigators, had been working on these very questions. Using the nucleopore filtration technique, and measuring daily egg outputs in schoolchildren, they had shown that a single determination would give about 80% accuracy in deciding the intensity of infection. He said that a study recently carried out in the Mombasa area demonstrated a relationship between intensity and disease. And finally, the classical study of the effect of treatment on disease had been done by Dr A. O. Lucas, who showed that following treatment with niridazole there was a remarkable disappearance of the severe changes in the IVP, in people who had previously exhibited such changes.

Dr Christina James had been studying *S.haematobium* in the baboon, and the pathology of the urinary tract. They had treated heavily infected baboons, who had hydronephrosis and heavy granulomas of the bladder, with various compounds. In all instances, a vast regression of the pathology in all the organs was observed.

Dr Butterworth, referring to immunity after treatment, asked Dr Mahmoud about the studies carried out in Lower Nduu, in particular the cost per head of population treated, and the cost in relation to how often the treatment would have to be repeated. In the absence of knowledge about the length of time treated patients remained immune, he did not think it was yet possible to predict how often the treatments would be required. The presence or absence of immunity in the treated population would affect subsequent transmission.

Dr Mahmoud said that there were only the reports, Kloetzel's experience in Brazil and Cook's in St Lucia which tackled the problem of how quickly people would develop the same intensity of infection after chemotherapy. The reports related to people who were treated and left in the endemic area without the introduction of any other measures for the control of transmission. Over the three year follow-up period there was no appreciable build-up of infection. The level was about 10% of the original level of infection.

From a study of age-specific intensity curves, it appeared that maximum infection developed around the age of 10–15 years. From those data, together with data from Kloetzel and Cook, it seemed that the build-up of infection would be slow. No-one knew what would happen beyond three years, but extrapolation from the three-year figure gave a time of about seven or eight years.

Regarding the cost-effectiveness in the Lower Nduu studies, the drug, which would have been the most expensive part of the campaign, was a gift. He said that it depended on planning, who made the decisions and how it was handled. In Brazil, for example, oral oxamniquine could be bought from drug stores for about $8; because the Government is undertaking a mass treatment campaign, the drug obtained from the drug company cost less than $1 per individual.

Dr Warren raised the question of work on the half-dose of hycanthone. He said that the half-dose had been used by Rees in Kenya, by Cook in St Lucia, by his group in the Mombasa area and the Machakos area of Kenya. All workers had obtained the same results, that is, between 95% and 97% reduction in egg output. Cook had found 6% vomiting, but no-one else had observed this.

Dr P. O. Williams said that if he had a large estate in the Delta in Egypt, and asked Dr Mahmoud what he could do to free the people on his estate from schistosomiasis, what would Dr Mahmoud advise.

Dr Mahmoud said that the Delta had both *S.haematobium* and *S.mansoni*, which meant that Dr Williams could use hycanthone; if it became available and a single drug was wanted, then praziquantel would be effective. It would only complicate the situation if metrifonate and oxamniquine were introduced. He felt that hycanthone would be good enough, and it was available in the Delta. From available data, it would not need to be given again for at least five years. Dr Williams could treat only those people with heavy infections, and these could be identified using the Kato technique, which cost only a few cents. On the question of identification, he said the Bell technique had been used on St Lucia; it was a more elaborate stool examination technique, and the cost had been $1+ per head of protected population, which amounted to $3 or $4 per individual actually treated. In Egypt, three or four health units in rural areas now used the Kato technique.

Dr Lucas said that in his earlier comments he did not mention the cost of water in St. Lucia. It was not fair to compare the costs of water there with the cost of chemotherapy, because by providing the villagers with potable water it was hoped that more than just schistosomiasis would be controlled.

Returning to the question of hycanthone, he said that despite earlier comments, he would still like more patients to be carefully studied and followed up using hycanthone, before he could recommend its use unreservedly. In a town such as Ibadan, 10 000–15 000 schoolchildren were infected; it was not reassuring to be told that 120 rural schoolchildren showed no ill effects. The unpredictable toxicity of the parent compound should be remembered; some communities tolerated Miracil D well, and others did not. More people should be encouraged to try the drug in their own areas, to be sure that hycanthone is suitable for their own population. Dr Mahmoud agreed with these remarks.

Dr Warren said that hycanthone, in the high recommended dose of 3 mg per kg or 3·5 mg per kg had been used in millions of people. The major toxicity apart from vomiting, had been about 20 cases of liver necrosis. He understood from Andrade, in Brazil, that in doses of less than 3 mg per kg, no liver necrosis developed.

Dr H. A. Minners (*World Health Organization, Geneva*) asked if there was a known relationship between the intensity of infection and subsequent development of cancer of the bladder with *S.haematobium*, and if so, would it influence treatment?

Dr Mahmoud said that this was not known. He thought it would be easy to carry out a study in Egypt on the relationship; a longitudinal study would show who would develop cancer, when, and what sort of infection would lead to it.

Dr Gordon Smith thought that Dr Mahmoud's answers to Dr Williams were reasonable only if Dr Williams also went to the expense of erecting a very high fence around his plantation. He said it was unrealistic in the present state of knowledge to say that following any treatment regime, nothing need be done for five years, or for any other period of time. What evidence was there, he asked, that this would be sufficient to control the problem in a community for one year, or any other number of years. Where there is a great deal of population movement, unless the campaigns were on a gigantic scale, the five-year rule was somewhat misleading.

Dr Mahmoud referred to the history of smallpox in Egypt. Smallpox had been eradicated by means of vaccinating one-quarter of the population every four years for 25 years. By contrast, between 1918 and the 1960s large amounts of tartar emetic and intravenous heavy-metal injections had been used in Egypt to control schistosomiasis, without any criticism of rash treatment, although there were probably more deaths in Egypt from tartar emetic than from schistosomiasis. Dr Mahmoud did not think he was suggesting a rash approach. There were safe drugs available but, as with any drug, there was a certain degree of risk which should be minimized if possible. However, a decision to start should be taken: they could not wait for the vaccine.

He said that the data available on chemotherapy as a therapeutic measure were obtained from communities without fences. Kloetzel in Brazil had treated the children and sent them back to their community; he prevented splenomegaly, and the build-up of infection after three years was minimal. The same pattern was seen in St Lucia. If one-third of the population was treated, say, in Lower Nduu, that proportion was passing out into the environment 80% of the egg-load which was polluting the environment. Thus, the transmission in that population was being effectively reduced. If Macdonald's model was accepted, there would be a break-point below which transmission would be stopped. The break-point did not necessarily equal eradication of every single egg coming out of the infected population. His advice therefore to Dr Williams would be to treat his people and let them loose—nothing would happen.

Dr Warren then introduced Dr Christopher Wright, a world expert on the subject of flukes and snails.

14. Possibilities of Intermediate Host-Parasite Relationship Studies

C. A. Wright

My original brief was to discuss the possibilities of molluscan studies in the context of schistosomiasis research. Responsibility for the more cumbersome title is mine and reflects my views on the limited value of research on snails which is not closely associated with their role as hosts for schistosomes. Without snails there would be no schistosomiasis but, if schistosomiasis was not a major health problem there would be little interest in the few rather obscure groups of molluscs which serve as hosts for the parasites.

Without snails there would be no schistosomiasis! In this idea lay the hopes of many of those originally concerned with elimination of the disease. Programmes aimed at snail eradication (usually based upon chemical control) were planned and brought into operation. Development of these activities coincided with the euphoria of preliminary apparent successes in the insecticide control of mosquitoes. Disappointing early results in the snail field did not alter the basic approach. It was concluded, quite rightly, that the chemicals originally employed were not suited to the purpose and it was assumed that the development of new molluscicides would produce the desired results. None of the original compounds was designed for killing snails, all were simply existing toxic substances which, in laboratory tests, were found to be effective in some degree. Perseverance in screening further compounds (according to Ritchie (1973) about 7000 were tested between 1946 and 1955) eventually yielded several which, in various formulations, emerged as molluscicides of choice for general use. By this time the first signs of caution were becoming apparent. The goal of snail eradication was generally replaced by the idea of snail control and increasing emphasis was being placed upon the need for detailed taxonomic and ecological studies of snails in order to make the best use of the compounds available.

We are now able to look back on several years of experience and consider what has been achieved. Warren and Mahmoud (1976) have recently commented that although molluscicides have been the primary means of schistosomiasis control for the past thirty years they have not been strikingly successful. In the artificial environments of irrigation systems there have been reports of dramatic reductions in snail populations by planned, regular applications of molluscicides. However, in an assessment of a seven-year control project using molluscicides alone in Egypt, Gilles *et al.*, (1973) concluded that, despite evidence of consistent reduction in snail densities throughout the years, transmission of the disease was not materially influenced. They also commented on the need for more prolonged assessment periods for control schemes, suggesting four years as a minimum before legitimate conclusions could be drawn. Evaluation after shorter periods may well give premature results which are unjustifiably optimistic. There are, unfortunately, few reports available in which such rigorous follow-up has been carried out. A five-year combined molluscicide and chemotherapy scheme on two isolated crater-lake foci of *Schistosoma haematobium* in Cameroun has been subjected to detailed scrutiny by Duke and Moore (1976). The results do not provide much encouragement for the success of this approach in natural transmission sites. Not only was the cost extremely high but the conclusion was reached that Macdonald's (1965) "breakpoint" in transmission probably lies so close to total eradication as to be practically synonymous with it.

With the paucity of detailed information available on the results of mollusciciding schemes it is premature to say that this approach has failed. Nevertheless, the evidence so far is not promising and it is not unreasonable to ask yet again whether the concentration of so large a part of the resources available for schistosomiasis control on direct attacks on the snail hosts was justified. The conceptual parallels with insect-borne diseases are obvious, but little attention was given to the fundamental biological differences between these diseases and schistosomiasis (Wright, 1960b). The three most significant differences are the reversed vector roles of the hosts, the existence of free-living stages in the schistosome cycle and the hermaphrodite nature of the snails.

Failure to accept that man in the schistosomiasis cycle is the biological counterpart of the mosquito in malaria transmission led to undue emphasis on snail control and insufficient recognition of the need for attention to human behaviour and the parasite in the human host. Recent trends towards integrated control have begun to redress this imbalance but, if the biological background had been considered more fully, this approach could have been anticipated much earlier. The free-living phases of the parasites and their behaviour patterns were generally thought to be irrelevant to the matter of control. This oversight was responsible for a basic misconception concerning the benefits to be derived from reducing the density of snail populations. While contacts between infective miracidia and potentially susceptible snails were thought to be simply by chance encounter, it was reasonable to assume that there would be a straight linear relationship between snail population density and infection rate, therefore fewer snails would mean fewer infected snails. In fact, miracidia exhibit complex behaviour patterns and responses to environmental stimuli which assist in the location of their hosts. The efficiency of these mechanisms will vary in different environments and it is not possible to predict the threshold population level below which interference with transmission is achieved. Finally, the facultatively self-fertilizing hermaphrodite nature of the snail hosts for African schistosomiasis means that a single survivor from any treatment programme is a potential founder for a new population. Herein lies one of the most fundamental objections to control by molluscicides. The prospects of total eradication of snails, even in relatively small water-bodies, are remote and there is therefore a continuing long-term commitment to repetitive and expensive treatment.

To obviate this problem and to avoid the possible undesirable side-effects of the use of chemicals, various approaches to biological control have been investigated. The subject has recently been extensively reviewed by Ferguson (1976). Some of the limitations of biological control were discussed by Wright (1968) and not the least of these is again the problem of establishing what the "safe" limit of snail populations may be. Many of the agents which have been suggested for controlling snails are those which are normally malacophagous or which, in aquaria, have been found to be successfully competitive. The trouble with exclusively mollusc-eating predators is that, when they have reduced the population density of their prey, they in turn decline through lack of food and the snail population once again increases giving the well-known predator-prey cycle. Most of the successful competitors of snails which have been found in the abnormal and restricted environments of aquaria are normal elements of the freshwater fauna in natural habitats where they co-exist with the snails. While few, if any, of these animals will be really effective as control agents they undoubtedly exert some influence on the snail populations in nature. Omer-Cooper (1949) described the great abundance of snails in freshwater habitats near Mkuzi and Hluhlue in Zululand where the aquatic insect fauna had been eradicated as a side-effect of aerial spraying with DDT. He contrasted these sprayed habitats with others outside the control area where water-beetles and dragonfly nymphs were still numerous and snails far less common. The object of this spraying campaign was to eliminate insect vectors of malaria and trypanosomiasis in order to develop the area for cattle farming. It may be only coincidence that in 1964 there was an epizootic of bovine schistosomiasis around Mkuzi which resulted in the deaths of large numbers of sheep and cattle (Reinecke, 1970). This outbreak followed a year during which the rain season had been exceptional, resulting in prolongation of the snail breeding-periods and extension of transmission sites. Would the outbreak have been so severe if the aquatic insect fauna had also been able to benefit by the favourable breeding conditions? This case may provide a timely warning of the need for vigilance on the snail situation in areas where large-scale insecticide control of aquatic insect vectors is being carried out.

Particular approaches to biological control which have been considered promising include the introduction of competitive molluscan species, selection and introduction of genetically resistant stocks of host species and the use of other parasites or pathogens of both snails and larval schistosomes. All of these have their advocates and some may even prove useful in limited situations. The large ampulariid prosobranch snail *Marisa cornuarietis* appears to have had some effect in eliminating *Biomphalaria glabrata*, the host of *Schistosoma mansoni*, in parts of Puerto Rico. *Marisa* acts both as a competitor to and a predator upon the host snails (Ferguson, 1976) but there is doubt as to the precise reasons for its success. Its voracious appetite for aquatic vegetation makes it a potential hazard as an agricultural pest of flood-irrigated crops such as rice. Species of the North American planorbid genus *Helisoma* have been found to act as efficient competitors to African *Biomphalaria* in aquaria but the results of limited trials in Africa have not yet supported these findings in the field. An interesting side-effect of this competition has recently been reported by Frandsen (1976). Not only does the presence of *Helisoma* depress the growth of *Biomphalaria* but it also has a strong suppressive effect on the production of cercariae from infected *Biomphalaria*.

The use of non-susceptible strains of snails as biological control agents has been suggested on a number of occasions. Richards' (1970) account of the genetics of *Biomphalaria glabrata* stressed particularly the inheritance of susceptibility to infection with *S.mansoni* and discussed the possibility of introducing selected insusceptible stocks of the species into transmission sites. This approach to control assumes that, because parasitic infection has an adverse effect on the reproductive potential of snails, there will be a selective advantage in favour of the insusceptible individuals and that these will eventually outbreed and replace the susceptible forms. There are, however, some discouraging aspects to this otherwise ideal solution to the problem. The results of snail infection experiments leave little doubt that most natural host populations include a proportion of non-susceptible individuals. It is therefore reasonable to ask why this replacement of susceptible by non-susceptible forms has not occurred naturally. One important factor is that at any time only a very small proportion of the potentially susceptible snails will actually be infected and the remainder will be able to breed without restriction. A more obvious flaw is that schistosomes alone are unlikely to be the only parasites exerting pressure on a natural population of snails. Some of the other parasites may be equally infective to those which are susceptible to schistosomes and to those which are not. It is even conceivable that the characteristics which render a snail unsuitable as a host for schistosomes might enhance its host-potential for other trematodes. A further possible restriction in nature is that the factors which make a snail insusceptible may also affect its biological fitness so that its reproductive potential is less than that of the susceptible forms. Richards suggested that nonsusceptibility might be related to a deficiency on the part of the host to provide some essential requirement needed for parasite development. If this hypothesis is correct then such a physiological deficiency might well have an adverse effect on the snail's performance in other respects. Finally, in the long term, any tendency for a host population to evolve a high level of resistance to infection is likely to be countered by the parasite population evolving a greater efficiency in infectivity. Attention must be drawn here to the use of the term "resistance" in place of "insusceptibility" for the two are not synonymous. Insusceptibility is a passive characteristic of the snail and simply infers that it is not a suitable host with respect to a particular parasitic organism, while resistance implies an active response on the part of the host animal to an invading parasite (Wright, 1971a). Until recently the success of a trematode infection in a snail was seen solely in terms of the susceptibility of the host. Experiments using hybrid parasites whose parental stocks have mutually incompatible snail hosts have now shown that the ability of the invading parasite to evade the innate response of the host is of prime importance (Wright, 1974). Further work along these lines has shown that the innate responses of snails to invading organisms are not equally developed in related forms and this can explain why some species (or populations of species) are better able to serve as hosts for schistosomes than others (Wright, 1977). It can also be deduced from this evidence that any selection for increased resistance in the snails must have been countered by improvements in the invasive and evasive mechanisms of the parasites. If such evolution had not occurred the parasites would have died out.

The possibility of control by other parasites or pathogens of both the snail hosts and the schistosomes has also been suggested more than once. Renewed interest in the subject was stimulated by the work of Lie *et al.* (1965) and Lie *et al.* (1968) on the intra-molluscan predation of schistosome sporocysts by rediae of echinostome trematodes. In the laboratory a most elegant series of experiments showed not only that echinostome rediae can seek out and destroy the larval stages of other trematodes but also that there is a hierarchy among echinostome species in which the dominant forms are predatory upon those lower down in the "pecking order". These and subsequent experiments have contributed a great deal to our further understanding of the relationships between snail hosts and their parasites but there must be strong reservations about the utility of this approach to field control of schistosomiasis. The species of echinostome which is most effective against *S.mansoni* suffers from the extreme disadvantage of being closely restricted in its adult host requirements and the logistic problems of obtaining adequate supplies of eggs for field use would be very great. In Africa it is by no means uncommon to find heavy infestations of echinostome parasites in snail populations which are actively supporting schistosome transmission. It may be that in such situations the echinostomes are exercising a limited control on the schistosomes without which schistosome transmission would be more intense. It is also possible that other parasites with redial stages may be capable of offering some kind of competition and there are many areas where the amphistome flukes of cattle could be effecting a limitation on schistosome transmission.

A group of organisms which may offer slightly better prospects as agents for biological control of trematodes are the microsporidian protozoa. Canning (1975) has recently reviewed the species which have been reported as parasitic in platyhelminths. In heavy infestations they cause extensive damage to the intra-molluscan stages of trematodes and thus prevent the production of cercariae. Dr E. U. Canning (personal communication) has pointed out that so far the effects of only two species of microsporidia on economically important flukes have been studied. Of these, *Nosema eurytremae* has been tested against *S.mansoni* and *Fasciola hepatica* but very large doses of spores (up to 1×10^7 per snail) are needed to cause depression of cercarial output. Another species, *Unikaryon pyriformis*, has proved to be more pathogenic to *F.hepatica* but, unlike *N.eurytremae* which can be cultivated in tissue culture and in large invertebrates such as locusts, *U.pyriformis* has not so far been grown in artificial systems. Other species of microsporidia parasitize molluscs and although they appear to have acceptable levels of host restriction most have been found to be relatively non-pathogenic. The search for species with greater pathogenicity to either larval parasites or their snail hosts continues, together with more fundamental research on the mode of transmission. If these investigations meet with success then there is reason to hope that agents with acceptable levels of specificity, restricted to the target organisms, may eventually become available for use in areas where other means of control cannot be applied.

If direct attacks on the snail hosts are unlikely to succeed or to be economically realistic on a large scale, where do the best prospects for schistosomiasis control lie? In the long term the answer must undoubtedly be in environmental control coupled with effective and safe chemotherapy. Jackson (1965) made the point that first principles of public health served well to control many disease agents before the advent of modern chemicals which, in many cases, merely supplied the *coup de grâce* for diseases which were already contained. The apparent success of these chemicals then led to a reversal of the approach to control of other diseases by concentrating effort on the search for new synthetics at the expense of attention to basic environmental situations. Sandbach (1976) through tracing the historical development of schistosomiasis research and control policy, has reached very similar conclusions. Although environmental methods of control have received general approval in principle, there has been some resistance to their implementation. This resistance is probably based, at least in part, on the slowness with which such schemes are likely to take effect, also on the lack of success which has been achieved with some of the attempts already made. Some failures have been due to the provision of alternative water sources and facilities unsuited to rural situations and unacceptable to the people for whose benefit they have been provided (Wright, 1970). Other schemes have given poor results because of their limited scope which has resulted in the elimination of only some of the potential transmission sites. The Crocodile Valley scheme in the Eastern Transvaal (Pitchford, 1966, 1970) appears to have suffered less than most from these problems: it was started in 1959, most of the environmental works were completed by 1964 at a cost of about £4000 (or £1 per head of the protected population), and subsequent maintenance costs have been negligible. The most recent figures for prevalence of schistosomiasis in the area cannot be compared with the original data because the methods of examination have changed. However, direct comparison can be made with figures from adjacent unprotected irrigation systems which have been surveyed using the new techniques (R. J. Pitchford, personal communication). These results show that in the unprotected areas the prevalence rates in schoolchildren for *S. haematobium* and *S.mansoni* are 100% and 97% respectively while in the protected area they are 30% and 62%. The figures for the protected area are probably unrealistically high because they do not take into account either the arrival of newcomers or the possible acquisition by residents of infection in other places. Of greater importance than the prevalence figures are those for mean egg output in the *S.mansoni* cases as indicators of intensity of infection. In the protected area this is 270 while in the unprotected area it is more than five times as high at 1460. In terms of cost-effectiveness this must surely be the most economical control scheme ever implemented. Extension of the scheme to adjoining irrigation areas would undoubtedly reduce the prevalence and intensity even further and the situation would then be ripe for Jackson's *coup de grâce* when suitable chemotherapy is available.

In the light of the lack of success of direct snail control measures and the obvious advantages of the environmental approach it might well be asked if there is any point in further research on snails. The answer is emphatically "yes", provided that such work is concentrated upon their role as hosts for trematodes. There are still large areas of Africa where virtually nothing is known about schistosomiasis transmission and these areas will need to be surveyed. Until it is possible to implement environmental control schemes, palliative measures such as "hot-spot" control of intensive transmission sites by molluscicides will have to be used. For both of these purposes adequately trained personnel, capable of identifying probable host snails, will be required and these people will need to be backed up by specialists in centres with long experience of the problems involved. There is also ample evidence of differences between strains of schistosomes. These differences may manifest themselves in variations in their pathological effects or, possibly, in their responses to chemotherapy. Because strains of the parasites have evolved in parallel with their snail hosts (Wright, 1960a, 1962) further studies on these problems must be carried out with adequate background knowledge of the snails concerned. Some examples of the work already done in these fields and an indication of some of the problems which are known to exist will illustrate the need for further work.

In North Africa and the Middle East *S.haematobium* is transmitted by snails of the *Bulinus truncatus* complex while in Africa south of the Sahara the parasite uses members of the *B.africanus* group. The parasites from North Africa cannot normally develop in *B.africanus* group snails and those from south of the Sahara cannot as a rule use *B.truncatus*. There are, therefore, two kinds of *S.haematobium* with largely separate geographical distributions. However, snails of the *B.truncatus* complex are known from areas where the North African strain of parasite does not yet occur. They have been found in Angola (Wright, 1963), Ethiopia (Brown and Wright, 1972) and Kenya (Brown and Wright, 1974), and in laboratory experiments snails from all these areas have been shown to be capable of acting as hosts for the north African strain of *S.haematobium*. If this strain should be introduced into these areas (or others where such potential hosts have not yet been found) it could easily become established and complicate this existing situation. In West Africa the snail hosts for both forms of *S.haematobium* occur and the two parasite strains are also found. In Ghana there is some evidence to suggest that hybridization has taken place. The barrier to cross-infection between the *B.truncatus* and *B.africanus* group snails has to some extent broken down (Paperna, 1968) and, in experimental infections in hamsters,

S.haematobium of Ghanaian origin is more infective, grows and matures more rapidly and reaches larger maximum size than other strains of the parasite (Wright and Knowles, 1972). All of these characteristics are suggestive of hybridization (Wright and Southgate, 1976). Both McCullough (1962) working in Ghana and Cowper (1963) in Nigeria suggested that the more serious cases of *S.haematobium* infection which they encountered might be attributable to the strain of parasite carried by the *B.truncatus* group host (*B.rohlfsi*). This in itself is an important suggestion worthy of further investigation but, with recent information about the characteristics of hybrid schistosomes in experimental animals, the possibility of greater pathogenicity of hybrids in human hosts should not be overlooked.

Other malacological contributions have helped to explain apparent anomalies in the distribution and epidemiology of schistosomiasis. At the same time that *B.truncatus* snails capable of transmitting North African *S.haematobium* were demonstrated in Ethiopia it was also shown that the majority of *Bulinus* populations in the highland areas are not suitable hosts. All these snails were at one time thought to belong to a single somewhat polymorphic species but they are now known to be members of a polyploid complex with different chromosome numbers (Brown and Wright, 1972). Only the tetraploid forms are readily susceptible to infection by *S.haematobium* while the diploids, hexaploids and octoploids are not. The possibility that *B.forskali* may be a potential host for *S.haematobium* has frequently been suggested in many areas. It has now been shown that there is a complex of apparently relic related species (*B.bavayi*, *B.beccarii*, *B.cernicus* and *B.senegalensis*), whose distribution is peripheral to that of *B.forskali*, and all of these species are proven hosts for *S.haematobium* (Wright, 1971b). The situation is also complicated by the role of *B.forskali* as intermediate host for *S.intercalatum* in the Lower Guinea forest area (Wright *et al.*, 1972) and for *S.bovis* in Kenya (Southgate and Knowles, 1975). The demonstration by Brygoo and Moreau (1966) that the principle intermediate host for *S.haematobium* on Madagascar is *Bulinus obtusispira* led to some apprehension in parts of the African Continent. This species was thought to belong to the *B.tropicus* group which is widely distributed in southern and eastern Africa but no member of which had been implicated in transmission of human schistosomiasis. Despite its lack of distinctive morphological features *B.obtusispira* was subsequently shown by immunological methods to be an aberrant member of the *B.africanus* group (Wright, 1971b). A recent addition to the aberrant members of the *B.africanus* group is a new species found in temporary rain-pools in the Lower Tana River area of Kenya (Brown and Wright, 1978). The systematic position of this species was not clear from its morphological characters but biochemical and immunological data leave no doubt as to its affinities. In laboratory experiments it has been shown to be susceptible to infection by a number of schistosome species and it is probable that it is responsible for transmission of schistosomiasis to the nomadic people of the area and their cattle. This discovery of a new species of potential snail host in an area already under development for irrigation purposes serves to emphasize the continuing need for detailed taxonomic studies employing modern techniques.

Several such studies are currently in hand. They include investigations into the affinities of those southern African diploid members of the *B.tropicus* complex which have morphological features similar to the tetraploid *B.truncatus* (Schutte, 1966). There have been isolated reports of successful laboratory infections of some populations oι these snails with *S.haematobium* and it is therefore important to establish their potential as possible hosts, particularly if they are likely to be involved in new irrigation developments. Another area of interest concerns the West African tetraploid *B.rohlfsi* which has successfully colonized Lake Volta but which does not appear to have become established in Lake Kainji. It has been known for some time that Ghanaian populations of this species have a distinctive electrophoretic pattern of their egg-proteins (Wright, unpublished data) and recent results also show that there are some unusual enzyme genotypes present in samples from the Volta Lake. Other studies are being carried out on the distribution of some enzyme genotypes in the *B.africanus* group (Wright and Rollinson, in press) and in the *B.forskali* group where accumulated data on the egg-proteins suggest that the nominate species may consist of a complex of forms.

These general investigations serve as an essential background to the kind of monitoring work which will become increasingly important in the future. So far no attempts have been made to follow up snail control schemes to determine what changes in the genetic constitution of the populations occur under the selection pressure of molluscicides. Modern electrophoretic methods of enzyme analysis should make this feasible and similar monitoring of schistosome populations should be undertaken where intensive chemotherapy is being carried out. Studies of this kind are also desirable where major development works are being undertaken, for environmental modifications may result in the creation of habitats suitable for snails not previously present in the area and they may also attract people from other places carrying different strains of schistosomes. Two situations in which changes have been brought about in schistosome populations either by chemical intervention or agricultural development have recently been described from Cameroun and both merit brief summary here.

The control project at the Barombi lakes foci of *S.haematobium* involved the use of a molluscicide (N-tritylmorpholine) and the drug niridazole (Duke and Moore, 1976). In one of the two lakes there were two species of *Bulinus* present, *B.rohlfsi*, the principal host for the parasite, and *B.camerunensis* which was only rarely found to be infected. *B.rohlfsi* was reasonably sensitive to the molluscicide and its population density was drastically reduced. *B.camerunensis* proved to be much more difficult to control, even by increased dosage of the chemical at more frequent intervals of application. During the one-year follow-up after three years of control measures had ended it was found that the infection rate in *B.camerunensis* was three times as great as it had been in the pre-control period. At least two factors were probably operating to influence this result. The primary pressure would have been removal of the principal intermediate host, thus giving a selective advantage to those parasites capable of developing in *B.camerunensis*. The second factor relates to the first in that chemotherapy in the human population would have been exerting a direct pressure upon the parasite population. There is evidence that the strain of *S.haematobium* in this focus has at some time undergone a certain amount of hybridization with *S.intercalatum*. Earlier work on the effects of niridazole on various schistosome species has shown that *S.intercalatum* is less susceptible to the drug than is *S.haematobium*. This treatment, therefore, would be likely to favour those parasites carrying *S.intercalatum* genes. *B.camerunensis*, although only slightly susceptible to the Cameroon strain of *S.haematobium* is, under experimental conditions, an excellent host for *S.intercalatum*. Thus the dual selection pressures of mollusciciding and chemotherapy appear, in this situation, to have resulted in a marked change in the local strain of parasite.

In 1968 a survey of 500 schoolchildren in the town of Loum in Cameroon revealed an overall infection rate of 54·2% with *S.intercalatum* and this was the only species of schistosome found. In 1972 a number of children in the town were found to be passing schistosome eggs in their urine and these eggs ranged in size and shape from those of *S.intercalatum* to those of *S.haematobium*. Laboratory breeding experiments proved that hybridization between the two parasite species was taking place. Field surveys showed that the snail hosts for both parasites (*B.forskali* for *S.intercalatum* and *B.rohlfsi* for *S.haematobium*) were present in the water-courses in the town and their distribution corresponded closely to that of the two parasite species and their hybrid. *S.haematobium* has been known from foci within 20 kilometres of Loum for some years but, despite continual movement of people, did not become established in the town until 1972. Unfortunately there are no records of the snail fauna before this time but the pattern of distribution of *B.rohlfsi* in 1973 suggested that it was actively colonizing the lower reaches of the streams and spreading upward. *B.forskali* is more tolerant of shaded conditions than is *B.rohlfsi* and the invasion of this second species into the area has almost certainly been facilitated by forest clearance for agricultural development. Once *B.rohlfsi* became established it was possible for *S.haematobium* transmission to occur and for the process of hybridization with the endemic *S.intercalatum* to begin. Observations made in 1973 and subsequent laboratory studies suggest that the hybrid parasite has certain biological advantages over both of the parental species and that it will probably replace *S.intercalatum* in due course. Because *S.haematobium* is dominant to *S.intercalatum* the hybrid resembles *S.haematobium* in general characteristics but retains those features of *S.intercalatum* which are advantageous to it (Southgate *et al.*, 1976; Wright and Southgate, 1976).

These two examples of changes in schistosome populations brought about by human intervention were relatively easily identified. In both cases two species of parasite and two species of snail host were involved and the changes were recognizable by direct observation. The recent report by Jelnes (1977) of the apparent development of molluscicide resistance in Iranian *Bulinus truncatus* was also discovered by straightforward comparative experiment. However, more subtle changes resulting from hybrid introgression between strains of parasites or genetic shifts in snail populations are almost certainly happening in many areas all the time. Detection of changes of this kind requires detailed laboratory experimentation backed up by the refinements of modern biochemical techniques. If the interim methods for schistosomiasis control are to be effective, they will depend to a great extent upon precise knowledge of the parasites and their hosts and of any induced changes which may occur in either.

References

Brown, D. S. and Wright, C. A. (1972). On a polyploid complex of freshwater snails (Planorbidae: *Bulinus*) in Ethiopia. *Journal of Zoology, London*, **167**, 97–132.

Brown, D. S. and Wright, C. A. (1974). *Bulinus truncatus* as a potential intermediate host for *Schistosoma haematobium* on the Kano Plain, Kenya. *Transactions of the Royal Society of Tropical Medicine and Hygiene*, **68**, 341–2.

Brown, D. S. and Wright, C. A. (1978). A new species of *Bulinus* (Mollusca: Gastropoda) from temporary freshwater pools in Kenya. *Journal of Natural History*, **12**, 217–29.

Brygoo, E. R. and Moreau, J. P. (1966). *Bulinus obtusispira* (E. A. Smith, 1886). Hôte intermediaire de la bilharziose a *Schistosoma haematobium* dans le nord-ouest de Magadascar. *Bulletin de la Societe de pathologie exotique*, **59**, 835–9.

Canning, E. U. (1975). The microsporidian parasites of Platyhelminths; their morphology, development, transmission and pathogenicity. *Miscellaneous Publications of the Commonwealth Institute of Helminthology*, **2**, 1–32.

Cowper, S. G. (1963). Schistosomiasis in Nigeria. *Annals of Tropical Medicine and Parasitology*, **57**, 307–22.

Duke, B. O. L. and Moore, P. J. (1976). The use of a molluscicide, in conjunction with chemotherapy, to control *Schistosoma haematobium* at the Barombi Lake foci in Cameroon. *Zeitschrift für Tropenmedizin und Parasitologie*, **27**, 297–313, 489–504, 505–8.

Ferguson, F. F. (1976). "The Role of Biological Agents in the Control of Schistosome-Bearing Snails", pp. 1–107. US Department of Health, Education and Welfare, Center for Disease Control, Atlanta, Georgia.

Fransden, F. (1976). The suppression, by *Helisoma duryi*, of the cercarial production of *S.mansoni*-infected *Biomphalaria pfeifferi*. *Bulletin of the World Health Organization*, **53**, 385–90.

Gilles, H. M., Zaki, A. A-A., Soussa, M. H., Samaan, S. A., Soliman, S. S., Hassan, A. and Barbosa, F. (1973). Results of a seven-year snail control project on the endemicity of *Schistosoma haematobium* infection in Egypt. *Annals of Tropical Medicine and Parasitology*, **67**, 45–65.

Jackson, J. H. (1965). Bilharziasis: an approach to the control of an endemic disease with particular reference to Natal and Zululand. *South African Medical Journal*, **39**, 152–8.

Jelnes, J. E. (1977). Evidence of possible molluscicide resistance in *Schistosoma* intermediate hosts from Iran. *Transactions of the Royal Society of Tropical Medicine and Hygiene*, **71**, 451.

Lie, K. J., Basch, P. F. and Umathevy, T (1965). Antagonism between two species of larval trematodes in the same snail. *Nature (London)*, **206**, 422–3.

Lie, K. J., Basch, P. F., Heyneman, D., Beck, A. J. and Audy, J. R. (1968). Implications for trematode control of interspecific larval antagonism within snail hosts. *Transactions of the Royal Society of Tropical Medicine and Hygiene*, **62**, 299–319.

McCullough, F. S. (1962). Observations on *Bulinus (Bulinus) truncatus rohlfsi* (Clessin) in Ghana: I. The distribution of the snails and their role in the transmission of *Schistosoma haematobium*. *Annals of Tropical Medicine and Parasitology*, **56**, 53–62.

Macdonald, G. (1965). The dynamics of helminth infection with special reference to Schistosomes. *Transactions of the Royal Society of Tropical Medicine and Hygiene*, **59**, 489–506.

Omer-Cooper, J. (1949). Does destruction of water insects cause increase of trematode disease? *Entomologist's Monthly Magazine*, **85**, 157–8.

Paperna, I. (1968). Susceptibility of *Bulinus (Physopsis) globosus* and *Bulinus truncatus rohlfsi* from different localities in Ghana to different local strains of *Schistosoma haematobium*. *Annals of Tropical Medicine and Parasitology*, **62**, 13–26.

Pitchford, R. J. (1966). Findings in relation to schistosome transmission in the field following the introduction of various control measures. *South African Medical Journal*, suppl. (8 October 1966), 2–16.

Pitchford, R. J. (1970). Control of bilharziasis by rural management. *Central African Journal of Medicine*, **16** (suppl.), 31–3.

Reinecke, R. K. (1970). The epizootiology of an outbreak of bilharziasis in Zululand. *Central African Journal of Medicine*, **16** (suppl.), 10–12.

Richards, C. S. (1970). Genetics of a molluscan vector of schistosomiasis, *Nature (London)*, **226**, 806–10.

Ritchie, L. S. (1973). Chemical control of snails. *In* "Epidemiology and Control of Schistosomiasis (Bilharziasis)", (Ed. N. Ansari), pp. 458–532. Karger, Basle.

Sandbach, F. R. (1976). The history of schistosomiasis research and policy for its control. *Medical History*, **20**, 259–75.

Schutte, C. H. J. (1966). Observations on two South African bulinid species of the truncatus group (Gastropoda, Planorbidae). *Annals of Tropical Medicine and Parasitology*, **60**, 106–13.

Southgate, V. R. and Knowles, R. J. (1975). The intermediate hosts of *Schistosoma bovis* in Western Kenya. *Transactions of the Royal Society of Tropical Medicine and Hygiene*, **69**, 356–7.

Southgate, V. R., van Wijk, H. B. and Wright, C. A. (1976). Schistosomiasis at Loum, Cameroun; *Schistosoma haematobium*, *S.intercalatum* and their natural hybrid. *Zeitschrift für Parasitenkunde*, **49**, 145–59.

Warren, K. S. and Mahmoud, A. A. F. (1976). Targeted mass treatment: a new approach to the control of schistosomiasis. *Transactions of the Association of American Physicians*, **89**, 195–204.

Wright, C. A. (1960a). Relationships between trematodes and molluscs. *Annals of Tropical Medicine and Parasitology*, **54**, 1–7.

Wright, C. A. (1960b). Some ecological aspects of the control of trematode diseases. World Health Organization, Geneva (unpublished working document, WHO/Bilharz/29, 5 August 1960).

Wright, C. A. (1962). The significance of infraspecific taxonomy in bilharziasis. *In* "Bilharziasis", (Eds G. E. Wolstenholme and M. O'Connor), pp. 103–20. Churchill, London.

Wright, C. A. (1963). The freshwater gastropod mollusca of Angola. *Bulletin of the British Museum (Natural History)*: (zool.), **10**, 447–528.

Wright, C. A. (1968). Some views on biological control of trematode diseases. *Transactions of the Royal Society of Tropical Medicine and Hygiene*, **62**, 320–4.

Wright, C. A. (1970). The ecology of African schistosomiasis. *In* "Human Ecology in the Tropics" (Eds J. P. Garlick and R. W. J. Keay), pp. 67–80, Pergamon, Oxford.

Wright, C. A. (1971a). "Flukes and Snails", pp. 1–168. George Allen and Unwin, London.

Wright, C. A. (1971b). *Bulinus* on Aldabra and the subfamily Bulininae in the Indian Ocean area. *Philosophical Transactions of the Royal Society, London*, (Ser. B), **260**, 299–313.

Wright, C. A. (1974). Snail susceptibility of trematode infectivity? *Journal of Natural History*, **8**, 545–8.

Wright, C. A. (1977). Co-evolution of African schistosomes and bulinid snails. *In* "Medicine in a Tropical Environment", (Ed. J. H. S. Gear), pp. 291–302. Balkema, Cape Town.

Wright, C. A. and Knowles, R. J. (1972). Studies on *Schistosoma haematobium* in the laboratory: III. Strains from Iran, Mauritius and Ghana. *Transactions of the Royal Society of Tropical Medicine and Hygiene*, **66**, 108–18.

Wright, C. A. and Rollinson, D. Analysis of enzymes in the *Bulinus africanus* group (Mollusca: Planorbidae) by isoelectric focusing. *Journal of Natural History* (in press).

Wright, C. A. and Southgate, V. R. (1976). Hybridization of schistosomes and some of its implications. *In* "Genetic Aspects of Host-Parasite Relationships", (Eds A. E. R. Taylor and R. Muller), pp. 55–68. Blackwell, Oxford.

Wright, C. A., Southgate, V. R. and Knowles, R. J. (1972). What is *Schistosome intercalatum* Fisher, 1934? *Transactions of the Royal Society of Tropical Medicine and Hygiene*, **66**, 28–64.

Discussion

Dr Williams referring again to his hypothetical Delta estate, asked for advice. He said that in China the parasite *S. japonicum* had been dealt with by controlling the snail and he wondered whether his Egyptian workers could deal with snails in a similar manner.

Dr Wright said that Chinese snails were dioecious—they had separate sexes—whereas all the African and South American species which transmitted schistosomes were hermaphrodites. This made it easier to control the Oriental species; added to which, the reproductive rate was much lower than in the planorbid snails. A further point was that the Chinese snails were amphibious, and could be destroyed by being dug into the ground, while all the African species were aquatic. He felt that if Dr Williams' workers could hand-pick every snail they found in the canals there would be some effect, but the problems in trying to eradicate them were endless.

Dr F. C. Robbins (*Case Western Reserve University*) asked Dr Wright whether, if those planning a new dam or irrigation scheme were to ask him whether anything could be done to avoid an increase in the incidence of schistosomiasis, he could offer any helpful advice.

Dr Wright referred to the Crocodile Valley Scheme, which was an excellent example of the production of a layout in an irrigated estate which had made a dramatic impact on schistosomiasis. It had been done with the minimum expenditure and the application of practical knowledge. The scheme covered a large area and had been quite successful. If the owners of adjacent estates had co-operated, this measure of success would have been greatly increased.

IV. Epidemiological and Environmental Approaches

15. New Epidemiological and Environmental Approaches to Tropical Infections

David J. Bradley

The preceding papers have considered the classic ways of attacking tropical infections—by chemotherapy, by immunization, and by vector control. They are at varying stages of development and have had varied field success, but discusson of them can be handled readily by considering first the tools and then their application. This is a valid distinction because, although an immense amount of sophisticated scientific work goes into the devising and production of a new vaccine or chemo-therapeutic agent, the output is a substance in a container. The user needs to understand almost nothing of the processes which led to its production and can concentrate on a quite separate and rather simple set of guidelines for its use.

Environmental approaches, whether directed towards vector control or the improvement of water supplies and faecal disposal, cannot be considered in this tidy dichotomous manner whereby we in the West can pursue our scientific way with a fairly clear conscience, separately from operational field-work. Rather, the techniques and tools themselves are relatively simpler, but the details of their application are more complex and an attempt to handle them as two separate issues will prove disastrous. One might add parenthetically that even for the chemotherapeutic agents, vaccines and insecticides, a less sharp dichotomy is highly desirable, but others may take up that issue.

Origins of Present Environmental Approaches

Environmental methods of control antedate all others, and come before discovery of the parasites or vectors in some cases. But the present revival of interest in environmental methods may be ascribed to three main changes in our perception of the world in the last two decades and outside the field of health.

First is what has been termed the "environmental revolution" and can conveniently be dated from the publication of Carson's (1962) book "Silent Spring". Its preoccupation with pollution was originally a developed-country phenomenon but the views put forward received a warmer welcome from Third World countries than might have been expected. It has had an effect on the tropics in two additional ways. Technical consultants on many Third World problems are of western origin and therefore cannot help but reflect the prevailing ethos of their home countries. In this way consultants outside the medical field have contributed to the distrust of insecticides in particular. However, western malariologists have particularly pointed out that the relative risk of malaria greatly exceeds that of DDT in many developing countries. The other indirect effect of the environmental concerns of recent years has been through lending institutions concerned with the Third World. The pressures on them lead to environmental codes derived from industrial-country concerns being attached to their lending. This has many consequences, one of them being the very active part that the World Bank group has played in schistosomiasis control.

The second change in our view of the world is the appreciation that "small" may be "beautiful" and a concern for simpler technologies, which for western countries is linked to Schumacher's (1973) book, but gained impetus from the visits of those from other countries to mainland China and from the realization that conventional approaches to many health problems had negligible chances of reaching large populations in the Third World for generations to come.

Thirdly, the recent rise in the price of oil, by its effects on the cost of producing insecticides and the transportation costs involved in vector control operations, has made the expense of pesticidal control too great for many countries.

These non-medical issues, which have combined with the spread of resistance to chlorinated hydrocarbon insecticides by anopheline mosquitoes and to 4-aminoquinolines by maleria parasites, have led to a general disenchantment with chemical means of vector control and worries over chemotherapy. The turn to environmental approaches has therefore been more a reaction against other methods than for positive reasons or new discoveries. It is a return to the methods of the past largely, with the originality mainly in the social setting of implementation rather than in the technology. In particular, the present enthusiasm for environmental control is in the local self-help context, whereas much of its past success has been in a highly authoritarian centralized system.

Therefore we consider the operation of environmental control in the past, some technical innovations, and research bearing on their use for the future. Environmental methods are rarely used alone, and thus raise issues of control strategy which will be approached in relation to epidemiological modelling.

Success in Environmental Approaches

Four examples will illustrate the key issues in environmental methods of tropical disease control. The original work by Watson (1903) in Malaysia at the beginning of the century was crucial to progress in malaria control. Simple drainage applied with determination largely freed two areas of malaria, but this did not work elsewhere. The reason was that a different vector species that bred elsewhere was involved. Ecological studies of the vectors led to the concept of "species sanitation". Essentially the tools of control by destroying mosquito habitats are simple, but great expertise is needed for their successful application.

The control of *Aëdes* by Gorgas illustrates the same need of strong administration, backed up by appropriate legislation, and detailed ecological work. A specific advance used in the Panama work by Gorgas (1915) was to put out numerous oviposition sites and then destroy the eggs, rather than simply destroying breeding-habitats. The advance was technically simple, but to perceive its application was more difficult.

Among recent schistosome control approaches, that of Japan has a major environmental component, the use of concrete linings in irrigation canals. The capital cost is very high, maintenance low, and the measures appear to have contributed to lowered transmission, though the method was not tested in isolation from other control techniques. By contrast, the Chinese methods have a very high labour requirement but low capital cost. They have required an intense degree of community discipline and the re-dug canals will need a great deal of maintenance.

Micro-epidemiological and Behavioural Studies

Three recent studies, as yet unpublished, show the issues which arise on a smaller scale within environmental projects—two do not deal with malaria or schistosomiasis but raise issues of clear relevance to their control.

Fenwick *et al.* (1973) have been relating human behaviour to transmission of *Schistosoma mansoni* in the Gezira and are finding great seasonal variations in the points of major water-contact by villagers. Thus, if a form of focal environmental control of snails were to be attempted, the concept of a "focus" would need to be far more dynamic than has appeared in the literature so far, and effective control would be more difficult than anticipated.

The study of water supplies in Lesotho by Feachem and his colleagues (1978) has clearly shown that the limiting difficulties lie in operation and maintenance rather than in construction so far as the small community is concerned. Enthusiasm to contribute funds and labour to construction or other one-off procedures can be generated relatively readily, whereas the steady source of funds and the organization to keep it running effectively is beyond the ability of many small communities without specific enabling legislation and much assistance. (The one community that was entrusted with the maintenance of its own water supply in the United Kingdom did not succeed in doing so.) These findings were corroborated by studies of health-care services in a West African country where again the problems of maintenance proved the chief difficulty at community level.

These studies, both recent and much older, point clearly to several crucial issues for environmental control of tropical disease. When a low-capital method is used, maintenance requirements are likely to be very high. If they are to be met, either a fairly sophisticated organization is needed or else unusually strong community discipline—whether imposed from outside or by the political ethos.

Major issues in environmental control, given the detailed epidemiological basis, are thus in the behavioural and operational areas. In addition, numerous technical aspects of items such as pumps, taps and latrines provide scope for development and for adaptation to local needs and resources.

Infective Systems

The preceding sections have shown the complexity of environmental control, particularly in rural communities. Complete success is unlikely. In the case of malaria, some anopheline breeding-sites are likely to remain after small-scale environmental interventions. What effect will this partial success, or reduction of mosquito density, have on malaria? The same sort of question applies to environmental snail control or excreta management in schistosomiasis. If other methods are used to supplement environmental ones, what is the best strategy? The life-cycles of tropical vector-borne infections are too complicated for the public health worker to relate the effects of vector changes to changes in the disease in man intuitively, and epidemiological models have been devised to give a sense of proportion. Macdonald's (1957) malaria model was the first of real value in this connection and essentially provided convincing and useful explanations of the differences between larviciding and residual imagocides in their effects on malaria incidence, and of the varying ease of malaria control by attack on the vectors in different places. The concept of the basic case reproduction rate, which could be calculated from mainly entomological parameters, showed the immense excess of transmission (by a factor of up to several thousand) over that needed to maintain endemicity. The excess, under equilibrium conditions, was absorbed by host immune responses either at gametogenesis or early in infection. It followed that where the basic case reproduction rate was very high, it could be much reduced, such as by control of anopheline breeding-places, without appreciable effect on the pattern of human malaria. This has immense implications for environmental control that are dealt with below. While Macdonald's model explained these two central issues in the macro-epidemiology of malaria, it was far less useful in the detailed prediction of what would happen in specific control schemes.

The advances since Macdonald's time have partly consisted in clarifying his model, which contained one major inconsistency between the logic of its assumptions and its mathematical formulation and, of great practical relevance, developing a more detailed model incorporating human immunity: Macdonald's had ommitted imunity for practical purposes and was at its best in explaining epidemics and disappearing malaria rather than smaller perturbations from equilibrium endemicity. The model developed on the Garki, Nigeria, situation by Dietz *et al.* (1974), and partly field-tested there and in south-west Kenya, is less elegant than Macdonald's in that it is a complex computer-based one with definition of the transition probabilities rather than an analytical one. It has the advantages of realism and gives a remarkably good fit to observational data. The demonstration that the data from Garki on inter-village variation are only explicable by a greater degree of exophily on the part of *Anopheles gambiae* than had previously been postulated is an indication of the power of the model. It also has an implication for environmental control: if, as Molineaux (1978) recently showed, the analysis is best considered in terms of a proportion of the mosquitoes escaping all insecticide and effectively almost none of those exposed to insecticide transmitting, then to a first-order approximation the residual insecticide is acting as a determinant of m, the density of mosquitoes, rather than of their longevity. Under such circumstances, larviciding and residual imagociding are reducing mosquito populations in an analogous manner, and environmental measures are more "competitive" as an approach to control. In other words, with a partly exophilic mosquito population, habitat reduction is a useful method, especially if cost and lack of technical expertise excludes any form of ultra-low-volume spraying out of doors.

In malaria, epidemiological models would seem a useful guide to action. They are much more advanced than in schistosomiasis where not only are models at a much earlier stage of development but also the system is twice as complex (with four rather than two stages to the cycle). More crucial still, we do not yet have a clear picture of the degree or pattern of human immunity to the schistosomiases: there is cumulatively convincing data that it is not negligible in *S.japonicum* and *S.haematobium* but more than that is not yet known with confidence. On the other hand it is a helminthiasis, and available epidemiological patterns show that the excess of transmission over that needed for survival cannot be of the same magnitude as in holoendemic malaria. It follows that in schistosomiasis, intermediate host reduction is more likely to achieve some degree of disease control than is vector control in holoendemic malaria, provided that it is directed at those snails that are actually providing the cercariae which are coming into contact with people.

With a heavily regulated parasite population, as occurs in holo-endemic stable malaria, the degree of mosquito density reduction may be a thousandfold if appreciable control of disease in man is to be achieved, whereas in areas of unstable malaria a fivefold reduction may arrest transmission. When environmental control is being encouraged it follows that expectations must be matched to the epidemiological pattern. In particular, in sub-Saharan Africa the sort of environmental control of anopheline mosquitoes that can be achieved with reasonable determination is likely to reduce anophelines a good deal, quite possibly reduce transmission of Bancroftian filariasis almost to vanishing point, and have very little effect on human malaria.

There is therefore complementarity between epidemiological models and environmental approaches. Whereas the technology for environmental change is simple, compared with drug or vaccine development, the epidemiological basis for effective control needs to be more complete. At present we are scarcely beginning to face up to these issues in relation to programmes based in rural communities.

References

Carson, R. (1963). "Silent Spring". London, Hamish Hamilton.

Dietz, K., Molineaux, L. and Thomas, A. (1974). A malaria model tested in the African savannah. *Bulletin of the World Health Organization*, **50,** 347–57.

Feachem, R. G., Burns, E., Cairncross, S., Cronin, A., Cross, P., Curtis, D., Khan, M. K., Lamb, D. and Southall, H. (1978). "Water, Health and Development: an Interdisciplinary Evaluation". Tri-Med Books, London.

Gorgas, W. (1915). "Sanitation in Panama". New York and London.

Macdonald, G. (1957). "The Epidemiology and Control of Malaria". Oxford University Press, London.

Molineaux, L. (1978). Entomological parameters in the epidemiology and control of vector-borne diseases. *In* "Proceedings of the Medical Entomology Centenary Symposium, London". Royal Society of Tropical Medicine and Hygiene, London.

Schumacher, E. F. (1973). "Small is Beautiful". Abacus, London; Harper and Rowe, USA.

Watson, M. (1903). The effect of drainage and other measures on the malaria of Klang, Federated Malay States. *Journal of Tropical Medicine and Hygiene*, **6**, 349–53.

16. New Environmental Approaches to Schistosomiasis

J. Stauffer Lehman

What is environmental control of schistosomiasis? What is schistosomiasis? Is it important? We do not have the answers to these questions, nor are we likely to have them. We may have to bite on the bullet, in fact, accepting that schistosomiasis is one of the major scourges of mankind, but let us look at what can be done to prevent its further spread.

When the United Nations talks about spending $0·4 billion to prevent the spread of deserts, all I can think of is that for every acre of desert that is prevented, a new acre of schistosomiasis is likely to be created, for irrigation necessarily may have to be used in such schemes. In that light, the amount of money spent on schistosomiasis by the Edna McConnel Clark Foundation is, indeed, small. However, we are a results-oriented foundation and the disease lends itself to attack by somebody willing to take an interest in it and to provide results leading to its control or prevention.

New irrigation schemes may account for much of the new endemicity. Schistosomiasis can easily be prevented by lining the walls of new irrigation ditches with concrete, thereby depriving the snail vector of its ecologic niche. High water velocity is another means of prevention, but erosion factors in earthen irrigation ditches usually determine velocity, not the extension of the disease. Man-made lakes are another problems, and perhaps a relatively insoluble one. The snails and infected people thrive on the shores of man-made lakes, and the Volta Lake is only one case in point. Even if a vaccine or a magic bullet were available today, I doubt that we have the delivery mechanisms to get them to the people who need them most—the poorest people, rural people with no political leverage to speak of. This problem of delivery systems will break us as we confront many of the world's diseases, and tropical diseases come most to mind. It is ironic that in this year when smallpox may be eradicated, schistosomiasis is increasing because it is an infection so closely related to development, and we cannot obstruct the development of poor countries. Some would say that safe water and sanitation are the obvious answers, but it would be misleading to suggest them as a cure-all for all water-borne diseases. Rural people deserve safe water and sanitation and it is hoped that such advances will take place. However, who is to pay for them, who will maintain them, and when will they come about? We are caught on the horns of a dilemma: to stop development, or to stop the spread of schistosomiasis. Neither seems likely, and so we must find ways of prevention through means which are cheap, reliable and safe. In many instances this will require drugs, but we do not know how to use the new drugs, nor even how to control snails. Maybe we should think about controlling the spread of schistosomiaisis through safe design of new development projects, which will obviously need the interest of and monetary input by major development agencies. This work cannot and should not be left to the foundations and those interested in the disease itself.

To date, there has been only a modest effort to control schistosomiasis and those interested in development may have to consider ways in which its spread can be halted at politically acceptable cost. Because schistosomiasis will never have a very high priority in the eyes of health administrators or of development planners, I doubt that we as individuals can influence its continued spread. Research on the disease should, however, continue, as it may offer solutions to the problem. Biological control may prove to be of importance in reducing the prevalence of schistosomiasis.

New methods of irrigation, which were developed because of their cost-effectiveness, such as overhead irrigation and tunnel drainage, promise to affect the spread of schistosomiasis because they do not provide the ecological niches that the snails require.

Another method which may prove acceptable is to keep people away from water, but it is still not known which people go into water, nor why they do so. For some occupational groups such as fishermen, the association is evident, but it may prove impossible to keep small children out of water, especially in geographically hot regions. The St Lucia experience attributes much to the creation of the laundry-shower unit, and these in all probability have been quite important. However, provision of capital structures will require health education to teach people why they are being removed from the water and this is expensive. It may be that Governments will be unwilling or unable to provide support for this type of activity. It therefore seems that schistosomiasis will be with us for a long time to come. Current research should identify those people likely to develop disease due to this tropical infection, and should explore means for controlling it.

Another species has just been discovered, the Mekong schistosome, now identified as *Schistosoma mekongi*. This, together with *S.mansoni*, *S.haematobium* and *S.japonicum*, will continue to provide problems for both scientists and development planners alike. Each demographic and geographic area may have to be treated separately, and individual solutions may be needed. A dialogue between development planners and those interested in controlling the spread of schistosomiasis may be the most important event for the future. It is hoped that such a dialogue, which has begun already, will continue, and will be recognized as a valuable way of controlling the disease environmentally. Research will continue. Ways of preventing the spread of schistosomiasis should be tested, and acceptable methods of limitation found for each endemic area. No new words on schistosomiasis have been spoken recently, but it is receiving wide attention, which should go far towards providing the basis for control of the disease.

Discussion

Professor Woodruff said that both speakers had emphasized the difficulties that environmental approaches met at the level of politics and economics. He had had personal experience of the difficulties caused by the rising price of oil some years ago in the Sudan. Not only had the price of insecticides increased, but there were queues for oil at all petrol and other stations. This had resulted in Sudanese villagers being unable to get oil to pump water into the header tanks which, in turn, meant that they went into the canals to get domestic water supplies. This increased exposure, together with a lack of insecticides, led to a great deal of dissemination of disease.

He appreciated the point about delivery systems still needing to be developed, even if the "magic bullet" were available. This increased the importance of chemotherapy.

He asked whether further pressure could be brought to bear on the World Bank to influence politicians in the schistosomal and other areas, to give loans for development, and Dr Stauffer Lehman confirmed that this pressure was important.

Dr Lucas said that for some of the infections under discussion, manageable environmental intervention could bring about reasonable results. An excellent example was the way in which safe water contact could eliminate a high proportion of the non-obligatory exposure to schistosomiasis. Also, in certain situations, modest types of intervention could produce good results with malaria. He felt that available tools were not being utilized, and many people were being unnecessarily exposed to unsafe water. Regardless of the expense of installation and maintenance, the long-term goal of providing safe water contact for all peoples of the world should not be forgotten. He did not know whether it was possible to get anywhere near the goal of "health for all by the year 2000", but the "three Hs"—"health, habitat and habit"—should be borne in mind; it was not possible to separate them.

Professor Janssens (*Institute of Tropical Medicine, Antwerp*) said that for decades there had been tools available for control, and there was no doubt that the risks from their use were much less for the environment than from the use of new and better tools which were available today. He thought the key word was given by Professor Bradley—"maintenance". Without maintenance there was no control. It was said that for maintenance, behaviour must be changed, but he did not believe that this could be achieved by sociologists, economists and health educators. He thought the problem was simply one of under-development. If the people of any area were not in a position where their social situation enabled them to understand what was meant by behaviour, then no matter how good the tools, there was no hope for improvement.

Dr C. Pant (*World Health Organization*) referred to the complexities of environmental manipulation for the control of malaria, in contrast to which the control strategy for eradication was simple, and yet the eradication programme failed. The shortage of malariologists and entomologists had been pointed out; malaria was rife in Turkey and in India. In view of these difficulties, he wondered how Professor Bradley saw the approaches to control in the immediate future.

Professor Bradley said that first of all, although there were difficulties and complexities in environmental approaches to control, he was not totally pessimistic. The approaches might be complex, but nevertheless they provided opportunities.

Regarding malaria in India, he said that in the past, very high degrees of environmental control had been reached; for instance he knew of one estate where malaria was eliminated almost completely. Since that had been accomplished before DDT was discovered, and before chloroquine was available, he saw no reason why it should not be done again. Essentially it depended on the people concerned. If sufficient organization was put into a step-by-step, gradual build-up of a control programme, it was possible, even without modern tools, to achieve a substantial degree of malaria control in a country like India where, in many places, the basic case-reproduction rate was not large. It was not the same problem as in sub-Saharan Africa. If the anopheline population was reduced to 10%, this would have a considerable effect on malaria in many of these places. He felt that since this could be achieved without the use of agents such as chloroquine and DDT, then the additional, judicious use of modern agents in current situations, meant that the prospect was not hopeless. It did, however, require considerable organization, which could not be provided by people in lavoratories.

Dr Thomas asked Professor Bradley what kind of information was required in order to make schistosomiasis models into useful guides to action.

Professor Bradley replied that a model was an hypothesis about a complex situation. In the case of malaria there had been generations of models, which had been taken into the field to see whether they could provide explanations. In the case of schistosomiasis, no major model had ever been tested in the field. The fact that a model looked mathematically satisfactory, did not involve algebraic errors, and followed logically from the assumptions, merely showed that it was mathematically consistent, not that it was a useful guide to action, because important variables might have been omitted. Therefore, until the schistosomiasis models had been tested in the field, it was not known whether they would work and it would be foolish to treat them as guides to action. What was needed essentially was detailed field verification of a mathematical model and preferably one more sophisticated than those currently available.

Another problem was that with models which were comprehensible and usable—Macdonald's being the best example—some of the assumptions made were extremely unstable. One example was the assumption that worms were spread randomly, which applied to most of the schistosome models. If the assumption was varied by saying that the worms were clumped (and it was known from autopsy data of Cheever, and from field observations that this was so), several of the fundamental conclusions of Macdonald's model broke down. In particular the concept of the break-point became extremely tenuous if it was assumed that schistosomes were clumped.

The more sophisticated mathematical models were so complex that he doubted whether they could be operated in the field. A model of intermediate complexity was needed, with its verification in the field. Without such field work, models ceased to produce useful conclusions.

Dr W. Ormerod said he had been considering similarities and differences between malaria and schistosomiasis. The differences were obvious, but one important similarity came to mind. Both malaria and schistosomiasis were found in two distinct situations. First, where the organisms and host, vectors and parasites, and the disease were ecologically balanced in stable populations. In those circumstances, he felt that care should be taken in trying to eradicate the organism; interference in such situations could make the lot of man worse than it had been previously.

The second situation was where there were new outbreaks of the disease, and that in this situation all possible tools should be used in trying to eradicate it.

Professor Bradley agreed with Dr Ormerod's words of caution about considering the implications of actions, but did not accept his dichotomy. He thought that in ecological balances, Nature was careless of how she achieved an equilibrium: the price of an ecological balance in the case of holoendemic malaria might be an extremely high infant death-rate. The situation of a high death-rate equilibrium did not seem to contribute significantly to human happiness.

V. Strategies for the Future

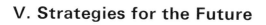

17. The View from the Third World

G. Lobe Monekosso

It is obvious that no-one can speak on behalf of more than two-thirds of the world's population or of their expectations in the area of knowledge described by experts in non-tropical countries as "tropical medicine". In this symposium we have been dealing with malaria and schistosomiasis, critically analysing the new tools provided by modern biomedical science and the prospects of alleviating or preventing disease. What I have to say is based on my personal experience; for although I have had the good fortune to visit institutions in all the major continents over the past twenty years, and have been privileged to meet some of the finest minds in tropical medicine, my experience is limited essentially to black Africa. In the Third World there are widely varying degrees of socio-economic development; my statement should therefore be considered as only "one" view of that enormous world.

Let me start by saying that the major health problems of tropical communities (infections and malnutrition) are related to and inseparable from socio-economic underdevelopment; long-term solutions must be sought in the amelioration, by the governments of tropical countries, of the quality of human life, in health education and the control of the habitat. In fact the discipline "tropical health" should be concerned as much with the participation of health workers in development as in immunology, vaccines, chemoprophylaxis, protein substitutes, etc., putting at the disposal of the world's millions the fruits of modern health technology. Here I will deal successively with the needs of the Third World (especially black Africa) in the areas of training, service and research in tropical medicine.

Amelioration of Health Services

In what manner and to what extent would appropriate attitudes, skills and knowledge in the domain of tropical medicine (tropical pathobiology, epidemiology and therapeutics) contribute to the amelioration of health services? In most areas of the world, viral, bacterial, protozoal and helminth infections dominate the scene. As many as 75% of ambulatory patients and over 30% of hospitalized patients may be suffering from infective disease. It is obvious that "tropical medicine" should not be a monopoly of a few specialists, but an integral part of all medical and health practice. Training of health personnel in this discipline will contribute significantly to the amelioration of health services in tropical countries.

In addition, the health infrastructure inherited from the colonial era should be reorganized with a view to creating a health service that would respond to the needs and aspirations of the new society. How this should be done is often disputed. Should we build huge 1000-bed hospitals in the capital cities or construct numerous tiny dispensaries in rural areas? Responsible health officials in the Third World are quite clear in their views. It is a "simple matter" of ensuring primary, secondary and tertiary care for all, using a comprehensive network of health institutions, with a broad base of primary health centres going up to the well-equipped apex of the pyramid—the specialized medical centre. Tropical medicine would find its place at all these levels, but especially at the village health centre and small district hospitals.

Implementation of this simple concept, accepted by the majority of African countries, requires detailed painstaking continuing health-services research; analysis of the tasks of health workers, including definition of new roles and categories; the siting of static health units in relation to geography, population size, communications, socio-cultural factors, and the utilization of traditional health institutions, and so on.

Training of Health Personnel

It is generally admitted that the shortage of qualified health personnel, qualitative and quantitative, is one of the principal obstacles to the organization of effective community health services in many third world countries. In view of the importance of the subject certain guidelines are reiterated here.

(1) All categories of health personnel (professional, intermediate and auxiliary) should receive their basic training in their own country or within the region (geographic/socio-economic) to which their country belongs.

(2) Health sciences establishments which train one or more of the three principal levels of health personnel (mentioned above) should co-ordinate their activities so as to constitute multidisciplinary student

health teams for practical field assignments. This would facilitate their integration into health teams at the end of their studies. Integrated multiprofessional health sciences centres are ideal for this purpose.

(3) In order to promote rapid socio-economic development, health sciences institutions should ensure that their graduates are adapted for devoted service in their countries. Health team leaders should be capable of integrating themselves into broader community development teams (including agriculturists, engineers, teachers, etc.) especially within the context of primary health care in rural communities.

(4) Academic buildings should be designed and equipped in such a manner as to facilitate the attainment of the educational objectives stated above. They should not be designed in isolation (ivory towers) but should be functional and should complement existing hospitals.

(5) Adequate technical facilities should be provided for the *practical* teaching of biomedical, clinical and socio-medical disciplines, which represent the three principal groups of attitudes, skills and knowledge indispensable for the training of all health workers.

(6) Student selection should be organized in such a manner that both newcomers and existing health staff could be recruited to all teaching programmes. Students must attain highest possible academic entry qualifications consistent with the tasks they will be called upon to perform after graduation. The competence of health workers and their upward mobility should be ensured not by facilitating their entry into new programmes but by organizing refresher courses (continuing education).

(7) The participation of practising professional and intermediate health personnel in teaching (especially practical demonstrations) should be vigorously encouraged. They will help the full-time academic staff in ensuring relevance of teaching programmes.

(8) There should be continuous co-operation and dialogue between the educators and the users of health manpower. No system of education and training of physicians, nurses, and other health personnel will have an impact on the community if it is completely divorced from health services organization.

(9) International co-operation is an imperative necessity of our times. Action programmes at the national level should be strengthened by carefully designed exchanges between Third World countries themselves, and between them and the developed countries. The final objective of such co-operation should be mutual respect and mutual understanding.

(10) In the specific area of tropical health it is obvious that this discipline or group of disciplines should be integrated in all training programmes at the appropriate intellectual and technical level, for physicians, nurses and auxiliaries. It is, by its nature, one of the most fruitful areas of international co-operation.

Medical Research Programmes

Now that health sciences education and strengthening of health services are accepted by Third World countries as major priorities, it is appropriate that interest in medical research be further stimulated. Research is at present undertaken in universities and medical faculties, as well as in established research institutes. Research workers are relatively few in number, they are often isolated, and function independently and generally in an unco-ordinated manner.

Tropical medical research falls into three broad interrelated categories: biomedical laboratory-based research, clinical hospital-based research, and medico-social, community-based research.

The majority of competent research workers are foreign to the country or to the region; so that the principal problem of medical research (including research in tropical medicine) is the strengthening of the research capability of Third World countries. This takes us back to the question of training: who is to be trained?; what types of medical research workers are needed and in what numbers?; what types of training programmes are required and how can they be evaluated?; what are the existing potential opportunities for training?

Medical research workers will include:

(1) research physicians, doctors of medicine, and other high-level professionals, with additional training in research methodology and carefully selected laboratory, clinical and epidemiological skills;

(2) research officers with a basic university education in one of the physical, biological or the social sciences, with additional training in carefully selected aspects of human biology and medicine;

(3) research assistants; senior laboratory technicians, nurses, medico-social workers, etc., trained in or possessing certain carefully determined skills which make them indispensable members of the research team.

Training programmes will include:

(1) short intensive periods of training (one to three weeks) for senior postgraduate students or established workers, designed to achieve a specific limited objective, a new technique, a review of existing knowledge, etc.;

(2) organized courses (medium duration) (one to three trimesters). Here the aim is to study the whole or part of a major discipline and obtain a postgraduate diploma or Master's degree;

(3) formal (long) research training, two to four years, designed to produce competent medical researchers, leading perhaps to a Ph.D. degree.

Opportunities for training in tropical medical research include the following:

(1) at undergraduate level, special one-year programmes for medical students leading to B.Sc. Honours degrees (in English-speaking universities); or undergraduate M.D. theses with basic research training (in French-speaking universities);

(2) junior posts as assistant lecturers or research assistants in universities or research institutes (in-service/on-the-job training);

(3) postgraduate medical research fellowships for post-doctoral students; leading to an advanced degree and/or highly specialized training, usually in a developed country.

Organization of Medical Research

As stated earlier, research is organized mainly by national universities and foreign-assisted research institutes.

Many countries now have or are in the process of establishing medical research councils, some of which are arms of a National Scientific Research Council. These have a co-ordinating role in bringing together all workers—foreign or national, university, institute or independent—to draw up priorities for medical research, agree on areas needing support and disburse limited research funds. Medical research priorities in tropical Africa include tropical infective disease (such as malaria, filariasis, schistosomiasis), malnutrition, haemoglobinopathies, the promotion of maternal and child health, operational health services research, study of medicinal plants and African traditional medical practices.

With these priorities in mind, and especially the need to strengthen the research capability of the African region, it is proposed to establish in collaboration with the World Health Organization, a network of research institutions in black Africa with a view to facilitating international co-operation in medical research especially tropical diseases and health-services research. The network will comprise three types of institutions—principal, special and peripheral centres.

Regional centres would be multinational in character, built by the host country, with or without bilateral or multilateral assistance, supported/co-ordinated by WHO, staffed and equipped to ensure teaching and research activities on a broad front. It is expected that there would be one multidisciplinary/principal centre for each of the two major language groups—English and French; and possibly a third co-ordinating bilingual centre. They will emphasize research methodology.

National centres: there would be several special centres, including most of the existing specialized centres dedicated to the study of one disease (e.g. leprosy, onchocerciasis, etc.) or one group of health problems (e.g. nutrition, cancer, genetics). These centres would be staffed and equipped either by external aid or national funds or both.

Peripheral centres would be created as appropriate within the framework of national research programmes; they would complement principal and special centres since the results of their research would be tested there. They would provide the indispensable link between fundamental biomedical and health services research.

Strategies for the Future

The Third World is deeply interested in current research on malaria, schistosomiasis and other tropical diseases; its scientists are anxious to be associated with this exciting venture. These studies are of more than academic interest or scientific curiosity. When one has vivid memories of disquieting malarial paroxysms, has seen teenagers report with terminal haematuria, a classmate excluded from school because of leprosy, or village life paralysed by a guinea-worm outbreak, not to mention epidemics of poliomyelitis, meningitis or smallpox, the matter becomes a challenge and merits a declaration of war by the international scientific community. It is unthinkable that we should enter the year 2000 without routing the enemy.

Where do we start? I believe we should start with unfinished battles. Ensure that the fruits of modern technology reach our masses; poliomyelitis, measles, tetanus and other excellent vaccines are not yet available to the children of the Third World, either because of costs, logistic difficulties or simple parental unbelief. Kwashiorkor is still prevalent in spite of our elegant biochemical knowledge. There are other unfinished battles—we have nearly abandoned research on parasitic diseases of the poor, possibly because of inadequate financial returns for expensive research. We still have very unpleasant drug regimes. Even when the knowledge, money, medicines and equipment are put graciously at our disposal we may lack trained personnel for disease control. Sometimes we do not know how to apply the remedy in the local situation. How long should a child born into a holoendemic malarial area continue with chemoprophylaxis—5, 10, 25 or 50 years?

An integrated holistic approach is vital if we are to win our unfinished battles. We need a careful review and remodelling of our health care delivery to cater for all our needs, not just a series of perfect models for leprosy, yaws, tuberculosis, etc. We need to devise affordable primary care, accessible secondary health care and selective tertiary care; with preventive, curative and promotive medicine at all levels. We need to train health personnel who will adapt themselves to, and be capable of adapting, existing health services. Their training should be integrated, preferably in a health-team setting, in order to facilitate their finding solutions to our complex health problems. Research, especially applied research, should be undertaken in the context of health-care delivery if results are to be readily applicable. Indeed training, services and research should be one continuum for reasons of economy, efficiency and realism. In this global approach there would be ample room for systematic piecemeal attack on "small" problems or fragments of major problems. In either event we should have no illusions—malaria and schistosomiasis will not yield as easily as smallpox appears to have done. Drastic changes in life-style and victory in the fight against under-development are pre-requisites to success.

And the new tools? Scientists in the Third World wish to see a dramatic increase in their numbers; they would like to see technical collaboration by which answers would be obtained more quickly— delicate, complex and expensive instruments are abundant in the de-veloped world, and there is a multitude of trained minds and hands; Third World countries still have notoriously complex, highly prevalent and disabling biomedical problems and there is a shortage of skilled manpower. Examples of fruitful collaboration are many and this should be intensified and perhaps better organized. There is no need to wait for an army of Third World scientists before continuing our fight against tropical diseases. What we must avoid is chasing technological feats of excellence—biomedical illusions. To avoid these the research priorities established by the developing countries should be respected. And it is in this context and the global approach that we welcome the new WHO initiatives in tropical diseases research.

18. What the World Health Organization Plans to Do

Adetokunbo O. Lucas

For many years the World Health Organization has given support to research on various aspects of health problems in the context of the efforts to control disease and improve health. In the area of parasitic diseases, between 1969 and 1976 some 700 research grants were awarded to scientists who were working on various aspects of these diseases. In addition, WHO's research programme includes field projects on the epidemiology and control of malaria, schistosomiasis, filariasis and trypanosomiasis. The 27th World Health Assembly passed a resolution calling for the intensification of research into tropical diseases. Following extensive consultations, a Special Programme for Research and Training in Tropical Diseases was initiated by WHO and co-sponsored by the United Nations Development Programme. The aims and mechanisms of the operation of this programme have been documented and the documentation widely circulated. This presentation includes a brief summary of the main features of the Programme with up-to-date information about its activities during this initial stage of implementation.

Objectives, Scope and Rationale of the Programme

To Develop the Improved and New Tools Needed to Control Tropical Diseases
Improved and new tools for disease control must be specifically suited to prevent, treat and control the target tropical diseases in those countries affected by them and must be applicable with minimal skills or specialized supervision, at a cost that can be borne by the affected countries, and in a manner permitting their integration into the health services of developing countries.

To Strengthen the Biomedical Research Capability of Tropical Countries
Training in the biomedical sciences and institutional support in various forms will assist the tropical developing countries to play a major role in the specification, development and testing of new tools. This involvement will ensure that the tools are effective and applicable for control of the target diseases in the affected countries and at the same time increase the biomedical research and disease-control capabilities of these countries.

Diseases Selected
The six diseases initially included in the Special Programme are: malaria, schistosomiasis, filariasis (including onchocerciasis), trypanosomiasis (including African sleeping sickness and South American Chagas' disease), leishmaniasis and leprosy. These diseases were selected on the basis of three major criteria: (a) the public health importance of the disease; (b) the inadequacy of the available tools to bring the diseases under rapid control; (c) promising leads indicating that research would be fruitful.

Research and Development

The research and development operations of the Special Programme focus upon the improvement and development of drugs (chemotherapy and chemoprophylaxis); vaccines; new approaches to the control of vectors; simple, reliable, sensitive and inexpensive diagnostic tests; and an epidemiological and operational basis for the application of improved and new tools.

The research is focused upon specific objectives and involves investigators from all relevant areas of the biomedical, physical and social sciences. Epidemiological and operational research serves to provide the basis for the specifications of the required tools and to assess their effectiveness. The research therefore ranges from the most sophisticated laboratory investigations to the use of simple diagnostic tests in the field. The research and development inter-links with related sectors such as nutrition, economics and education.

The Special Programme will bring tools to the point of proven effectiveness and then make them available to national health services for widespread application.

Scientific Working Groups (SWGs) are the *modus operandi* for research and development activities of the Special Programme. An SWG comprises all the scientists who plan and/or carry out research on a given aspect of the Programme. Members of the Group define the research objectives, devise a strategic plan to achieve them, carry out the research according to the plan, and review the plan and the research as the work progresses. Members of the Group participate in one or more of these activities according to their individual interests and expertise. The Steering Committee of an SWG manages and guides the Group's activities towards the objectives.

Individual SWGs are formed according to needs identified by the Programme's Scientific and Technical Advisory Committee (STAC) and are disbanded when they have achieved their objectives or proved to be impracticable. Figure 1 charts SWG progress.

The SWG framework for research has a definite beginning and end which are linked by a precise strategic plan. To develop such a framework and operate an SWG, the scientists must describe:

(a) the detailed objective(s) of the SWG, e.g. the specifications for a malaria vaccine applicable and effective in rural sub-Sahara Africa;

(b) the current state of the art in relation to the objective(s);

(c) the problems which remain to be solved, i.e. the gaps in knowledge;

(d) the possible research approaches and disciplines for solution of these problems, as well as the feasibility, sequence and cost of the activities, or projects, in each line of research;

(e) a clear strategic plan including each research approach and its line(s) of research, leading towards the final objectives.

The final objective(s) of an SWG rarely change, but the feasibility and priority of various lines of research may change as progress is made, new information is obtained, or new problems emerge. Changes in feasibility and priority of a line of research may result in the phasing-out of one line and/or the adoption of an entirely new approach. Such decisions are reflected in the strategic plan of research which remains the basis for the operation of the SWG.

In addition to the SWGs on the six diseases, groups have been established to deal with four inter-disciplinary areas—epidemiology, biological control of vectors, basic biomedical technology and socio-economic aspects.

Pilot activities were commenced in 1974, but the full implementation of the Programme began in 1977 following a December 1976 meeting at which various co-operating parties endorsed the scope and operation of the Programme. Substantial financial resources were also pledged and provided through voluntary donations by a number of governments, agencies and foundations.

It may be useful to review the current activities of the Programme as illustration of its mechanisms, although it is too early to attempt an evaluation of this effort after only a year of operation. The following review is compiled of excerpts from the first Annual Report of the Special Programme (document TDR/AR(1)/77.1–16).

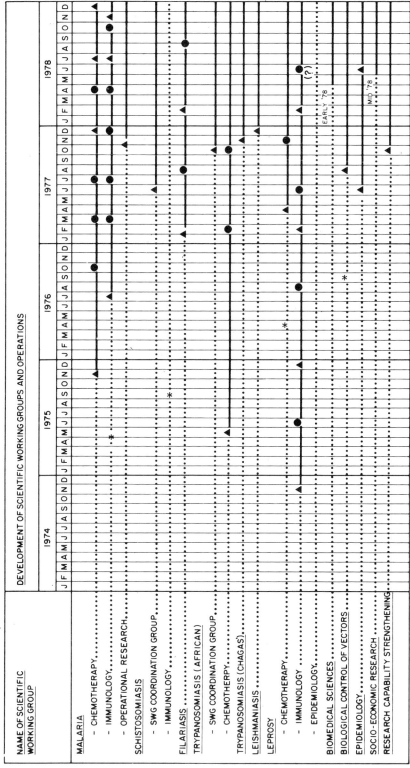

Fig. 1 Chart of Scientific Working Groups.

Leprosy

In 1974, the first SWG was established on the immunology of leprosy; it was code-named IMMLEP. The major objectives of the strategic plan included the development of a vaccine, immunodiagnostic tests, and immunotherapy to boost immunity in lepromatous patients and to reduce the adverse effects of immune reactions in tuberculoid and borderline patients. At the end of its first year of operation, IMMLEP had recorded significant achievements including an improved method of purification of bacilli from infected armadillos, development and field-testing of three different soluble antigens and immunochemical analysis of isolated mycobacteria demonstrating 45 definable components.

Progress made by the IMMLEP SWG during the second year includes:

(a) increased supply of *Mycobacterium leprae* to the Programme (approximately doubled);

(b) improvement of methods for purification of bacilli from infected host tissues. The modified methods are more gentle and at the same time have increased the recovery of bacilli;

(c) an antigen reference system using crossed immune electrophoresis has been established for *M.leprae*;

(d) double-blind studies have been carried out in two non-endemic areas with two different *M.leprae*—derived skin-test antigens. A proportion of the subjects (about 10%), especially subjects showing strong responses to tuberculin, were found to respond to both antigen preparations. Thus, further purifications are at present being undertaken to determine whether one can obtain more specific skin tests;

(e) mycobacterial strains showing close antigenic similarities to *M.leprae* have been identified;

(f) induction of cell-mediated immunity reactions with killed *M.leprae* preparations had been achieved in guinea-pigs and mice;

(g) induction of resistance to *M.leprae* infection in mice with killed *M.leprae* has been established.

With regard to vaccine development, research on experimental animals continues, plans have commenced for studies in man, with especial reference to safety precautions. Work is progressing on the improvement of recently developed skin tests but IMMLEP has also taken note of the observation by Abe and his colleagues (1976), that *M.leprae* specific antibodies can be identified by a fluorescent antibody technique. IMMLEP is therefore planning to evaluate the potential usefulness of serological tests.

Another SWG on leprosy is dealing with chemotherapy: THELEP (its acronym) began work a year ago. The THELEP planning committee had identified four areas urgently in need of further research:

(a) assessment by means of surveys in the field of the risk of emergence of dapsone-resistant *M.leprae* in patients treated with dapsone as monotherapy;

(b) evaluation, by means of formal clinical trials, of combinations of already existing drugs in lepromatous leprosy patients of three types:

(i) previously untreated persons;

(ii) those already having relapsed with organisms proved to be dapsone-resistant; and

(iii) those treated with dapsone as monotherapy who have responded but who may be presumed to harbour larger than normal proportions of dapsone-resistant *M.leprae*.

(c) implementation of selected laboratory studies designed to yield information relevant to clinical trials and to field surveys for dapsone resistance;

(d) development of new drugs, both by screening existing compounds for activity against *M.leprae* and by undertaking novel syntheses in selected drug areas.

At its first meeting, THELEP refined the draft of a Standard Protocol for Chemotherapy Trials in Lepromatous Leprosy. Field trials on drug combinations are being set up in South-East Asia and Africa.

Malaria

Similarly for malaria two SWGs are currently operating, one on chemotherapy and the other on immunology. A third SWG on applied research had its first meeting in December 1977.

The SWG on Chemotherapy of Malaria met in November 1975 and established a research programme. The Group has developed a programme of which the primary goal is to provide improved and new tools for the control of malaria, including research on the mechanism of action of antimalarial drugs, the improvement of drugs in clinical use, the improvement of existing and the development of new drug-screening procedures, the development of new drugs, and clinical studies.

The Programme has developed close working relations with the Antimalaria Drug Development Programme of the Walter Reed Army Institute of Research (WRAIR), industry, academia, government and foundation institutes. In the short and medium range, emphasis is being given to: clinical trials of mefloquine, a drug developed by WRAIR; the formulation of sustained-release systems of highly potent drugs such as 8-aminoquinolines and triazines; comparative trials of existing drugs and their combinations; and the screening of selected compounds for tissue schizontocidal and sporontocidal activity. In the long-range programme, promising candidates (e.g. menoctone-type drugs, related naphthoquinones, diamino-quinazolines and 8-aminoquinolines) are being followed up and investigations are being conducted on parasite-drug interaction, mechanism of drug resistance, lead-directed synthesis of compounds, and other subjects related to the chemotherapy of malaria.

The SWG on the Immunology of Malaria met in July 1976 and established a research programme which is mainly oriented towards research in the areas of malarial antigens; mechanisms of immunity and immune evasion; immunodiagnostic tests; immunopathological phenomena, development of blood stage, sporozoite and gamete vaccines in animal models, and eventually the vaccination against malaria in humans.

Much of applied malaria research has been conducted under the auspices of national malaria control or eradication programmes, the majority of which were assisted by WHO. Specific research programmes related to the epidemiology and control of malaria were already being conducted by the Organization and since 1977 they continue in the framework of the Special Programme.

A research project (MPD–012 TDR–005) is at present being implemented in Bendel State, Nigeria, with the aim of finding practical solutions for malaria control problems in Africa. This project follows intensive epidemiological studies, carried out in Garki, Nigeria, between 1969 and 1976, which provided a wealth of technical information on malaria transmission in Africa and the relative value of intervention methods. In the course of these studies, an epidemiological simulation model was developed and is being used for planning purposes. The present project has the objective of selecting those economically feasible and simple methods of malaria control that would produce the best, and an acceptable, degree of reduction in mortality and morbidity resulting from malaria. These methods are being employed in various ecological situations typical in tropical Africa. The results of the project should assist African countries in developing realistic and feasible strategies of malaria control. The research project is a joint effort of WHO and the Nigerian Government. In 1977 the team set up laboratories, selected study areas in four different ecological strata and collected epidemiological data.

Meanwhile, several Regional Advisory Committees on Medical Research (ACMRs) have indicated particular priority areas of applied malaria research, such as baseline assessment and monitoring of drug sensitivity in *Plasmodium falciparum*, evaluation of community participation in antimalarial activities, chemoprophylaxis in children of malaria-endemic areas, approaches towards malaria control in problem areas, impact of pattern application of insecticides, and strain distribution of *P. falciparum*. Efforts are being made within the framework of the Special Programme to achieve the implementation of these programmes. Work on strain differentiation and on drug-susceptibility testing and monitoring (*in vitro*) in *P. falciparum* is already being implemented in the South-East Asia Region, as is a project on chemoprophylaxis in maleria-endemic areas of Africa.

Other Diseases
Similarly the activities with respect to filariasis, schistosomiasis, Chagas' disease and leishmaniasis are being developed. The SWGs on epidemiology and biological control of vectors have also met and are developing research plans, and the other two trans-disease SWGs on biomedical and socio-economic research will meet shortly.

Research Capability Strengthening

The objective is to increase the capability of the tropical countries to meet their own research needs relative to disease control, particularly with special emphasis on the diseases included in the Programme. The Research Strengthening Group (RSG) has had its first meeting at which it adopted the following terms of reference: to establish comprehensive policy criteria that will govern Special Programme operations in the Programme Area; to plan and develop a network of WHO Collaborating Centres in Tropical Diseases; to plan and develop training activities; and to monitor and evaluate activities in this area of the Programme.

Training
Support to training activities of two types: for group training initiatives and for the training of individuals. Requests for support for both types of activity must originate in the tropical countries themselves (governments of institutions within or outside the Special Programme network), from Regional ACMRs or from Special Programme SWGs.

Requests for support of group training activities may range from formal and *ad hoc* courses to seminars, workshops and scientific meetings.

Ad hoc courses and formal training programmes
The Special Programme will support formal or *ad hoc* courses in tropical countries, preferably at sub-regional or regional levels by:

(a) providing experts to improve the scope and quality of courses;
(b) providing or helping to create technical material;
(c) supporting the attendance of trainees, normally only for those who come from outside the country where the course is being held (for this purpose, the existing WHO Fellowship Programme at the Regional Office level should suffice for undergraduate and early

postgraduate levels of training, particularly attendance at regional courses; other trainees can be supported through Special Programme Research Training Grants or Exchange of Research Workers Grants); and

(d) promoting and funding research projects aimed at improving existing training (training for operational research would be particularly suited to innovative approaches).

The criteria for granting support will be based mainly on the relevance of the objectives and contents to national and sub-regional needs, including career structure and opportunities for research, and on an assessment of the efficacy of the proposed activity. Requests for support, together with adequate background information, will come to the RSG through WHO Regional Offices.

Workshops, seminars and scientific meetings

Criteria for supporting workshops, seminars or scientific meetings are:

(a) their relevance to the Special Programme objectives, and

(b) the inclusion of well-defined activities of direct importance to the Programme.

Individual training

The Special Programme will support the training of individuals by:

(a) providing Research Training Grants to potential research leaders and to teachers from tropical countries, for specific training objectives, e.g. to attain a Ph.D. degree or for work as a post-doctoral trainee on an agreed project carried out at an institution outside his/her own country;

(b) awarding Exchange-of-Research-Workers Grants to established scientists from the tropical countries for specific training outside their countries, including short courses and seminars, or workshops, as well as research discussions;

(c) providing on-the-job training opportunities through the research and development component of the Special Programme (the SWGs). The programme will advertise such opportunities, which will be especially relevant to the training needs of less highly skilled researchers; and

(d) awarding re-entry grants for trainees returning to their home countries. Such grants will be awarded on the basis of a formal proposal and protocol with the objective of allowing the application of the new knowledge acquired, e.g. setting up a technique, starting a new research line, etc.

Institution Strengthening

The Special Programme will assist institutions in tropical countries affected by one or more of the six diseases to assume their appropriate role in research aimed at identifying, analysing and solving local and regional health problems, particularly in relation to the six diseases.

To this end, the Special Programme will strengthen research and training institutions in these countries, so that they can better respond to national as well as Special Programme needs; will support training of persons from the tropical countries, to help meet national manpower needs; and will contribute to a rapid transfer to the affected countries from the industrialized world of the knowledge, technology and skills that are relevant to their health objectives and within the sphere of the Special Programme.

These Special Programme activities will also ensure an increasing involvement of scientists from the tropical countries in the Programme's research and development activities.

Collaboration with national programmes

To maximize its impact in respect to the above-mentioned policy guidelines:

(a) This Programme Area will be implemented in particularly close collaboration with national authorities, so as to facilitate the implementation of decisions taken by governments and institutions in the tropical countries to promote health research, particularly research relevant to the control of the six diseases.

(b) Such national commitment as expressed in terms of research training interest, research career-structure opportunities and importance of research components in health and educational planning, will be considered an important element when deciding on support for activities within this Programme Area.

(c) Only national or regional institutions or the national component of research institutions in tropical countries will be eligible for Special Programme support from this Programme Area. Institutions which include a significant percentage of staff foreign to the country or the region will receive support only if such staff are accomplishing a specific task for which qualified local personnel are not available and if there are definite plans to train local counterparts.

Contribution of institutions and scientists from non-tropical countries

The contribution of institutions and scientists of industrialized countries to increasing the research capability of the tropical countries will be further developed, improved and expanded. Institutions from non-tropical countries involved in tropical diseases research will be asked to train selected research workers from the tropical countries in specific aspects for which training opportunities are not available in the tropical countries; and to collaborate with local institutions to strengthen research activities and training.

When research workers from outside the region are recruited to strengthen national institutions, inter-institutional arrangements will be preferred to WHO staffing of the institution; thus it is hoped to overcome the scarcity of competent scientists able to spend prolonged periods in the tropical countries by organizing various types of linkage agreements. Such agreements between two institutions can include secondment of research staff from the more developed research centre, exchange of research staff. joint research projects and training programmes, etc. The agreements must provide for the involvement of research workers from more developed countries, as an integral part of their professional careers based in their own countries, while at the same time providing training opportunities for research workers from the tropical countries.

Other Features

The Programme has a number of interesting features which can be briefly summarized.

Management Within WHO

There is a full involvement of the relevant technical Divisions of WHO which are responsible for the control of these diseases: Malaria and other Parasitic Diseases; Vector Biology and Control; Prophylactic, Diagnostic and Therapeutic Substances; Leprosy Unit; Unit of Immunology. Others concerned are the Divisions of Communicable Diseases, Co-ordination, Non-Communicable Diseases and the Office of Research Promotion and Development. The Division of Health Manpower is involved in the training component.

It is a global programme with co-ordination at the most appropriate level for each activity, national, regional and global. Thus, the national medical research councils are involved in the identification of institutions and scientists to participate in the Programme in the context of rationally defined priorities, especially on the aspect of training and institutional strengthening.

Technical Co-operation

The Programme involves the worldwide community of scientists in the planning, execution and monitoring of the activities. The research and training are being carried out in the global network of collaborating institutions. For example, the first 17 laboratories involved in IMMLEP spanned Venezuela to Japan in a moving-belt type of operation with the provision of armadillo-derived bacilli, antigenic analysis through to field-testing in an endemic area (Burma) and in a non-endemic population in Europe.

Goal-oriented Research

The objectives of the Programme are sharply focused and as far as possible they are set out as clear time-phased operations. This is not intended to confine the activities in a rigid framework but to facilitate the evaluation of the Programme. With the limited resources available the Programme would make little contribution if attempting to cover the whole field of tropical disease research in an open-ended way. It is for this reason that clear-cut specific objectives are being defined. The Programme includes a mixture of short-term, low-risk projects, such as field research to improve the application of existing tools, and long-term high-risk programmes to find new drugs or vaccines, which could make radical changes in the strategy for controlling these diseases.

Reference

Abe, M., Izumi, S., Saito, T. and Mathur, S. K. (1976). Early serodiagnosis of leprosy by indirect immunofluorescence, *Leprosy, India*, **48,** 3, 272–6.

19. Science Knows no Country: The Contributions of the National Institutes of Health to Tropical Medicine Research

Richard M. Krause

"Science knows no country because knowledge belongs to humanity, and is the torch which illuminates the world."

Louis Pasteur, 1876

In 1876 at the International Congress of Sericulture in Milan, Italy, Louis Pasteur gave the above toast at a banquet. In a sense these remarks embody the theme of this Conference. They are also the philosophical foundations on which the United States National Institutes of Health (NIH) is basing its strategy for future research on tropical diseases. This position has also been embraced by President Carter who in his message to the Thirtieth World Health Assembly in Geneva in May 1977, supporting the WHO Tropical Diseases Research Programme said, "these efforts will bring us closer to our goal: a world in which all people can live free from fear of crippling and debilitating diseases". On 31 October 1977, Dr Peter Bourne, Special Assistant to the President for Health Issues, reiterated the President's position in a speech "US Global Health Strategies in an Age of Interdependence" to the annual meeting of the American Public Health Association; he referred to "the new awareness of global interdependence and a commitment by the President to a new world partnership directed toward meeting the basic human needs of people everywhere".

This Conference has focused primarily on malaria and schistosomiasis, and rightly so. These diseases are among the most serious, widespread and intractable problems in tropical medicine. Surely our future research strategies for malaria and schistosomiasis will be a model for the larger task embracing health in all its aspects.

In these remarks on the contributions of the NIH to the strategies of the future concerning tropical medicine, I limit myself primarily to the research programme of the National Institute of Allergy and Infectious Diseases (NIAID). This Institute is responsible for the bulk of the research at the NIH on the diseases of the WHO Tropical Diseases Research Programme, while it also has responsibility for a broad range of other infectious diseases which are peculiar to tropical countries and the developing world, other components of the NIH are likewise engaged in these areas. Furthermore, what the United States Government does about tropical medicine will not be done by the NIH alone. Although there may seem to be a display of divergent objectives and a cacophony of dissonant voices, there is, fortunately, less thrashing about inside the system than appears to be the case from the outside. Over the years there has emerged a reasonable, although certainly not perfect, delineation of responsibilities. For example, the NIH has primary responsibility for the generation of new medical knowledge; the Center for Disease Control has primary responsibility for implementation of procedures and programmes to monitor, detect and control the occurrence and outbreaks of disease; and the Agency for International Development has responsibility for the development of health resources in the developing world.

So the business of the NIH is the generation of new medical knowledge through biomedical research. Such new knowledge must then be applied by a process now called technology transfer. It is at this very point that a major policy issue arises throughout the health enterprise. That policy issue concerns the distribution of the resources between biomedical research on the one hand, and the application of knowledge to prevent and treat disease on the other, and is being intensely debated in the scientific and medical community both within and without the United States Government. We should not minimize the divergence of views which prevail on this issue, whether within Congress, in the Executive Branch of the Government, or in the Institute of Medicine. It is not surprising, therefore, that this policy debate on the distribution of resources between biomedical research and the application of knowledge colours discussions concerning the future objectives of our policies pertaining to tropical medicine.

But I take comfort in the vigour of this debate: it reflects a genuine concern for the complex issues pertaining to medicine and health. We should recognize, too, that this disagreement is an old argument. Science has lived with it from the very start of our modern age, and in my view, we should not be hampered by the technicalities of the issue. This contribution makes a case for both biomedical research and the application of knowledge in instances where both are clearly necessary; the middle ground should be allowed to sort itself out. When this controversy produces more passion than reason, reassurance may be gained from the wisdom of men of the past who were also caught up in this argument. Benjamin Franklin, in addition to his career as a printer, writer and a representative of the colonies to the Courts of England and France, was also a bit of a scientific tinkerer. We learned as schoolchildren about his experiments to probe the mystery of electricity by flying a kite during a thunderstorm. On yet another occasion, when describing a series of experiments, he was asked at the end of a lecture, what good could there possibly be in such knowledge? Franklin's immediate response was "What is the purpose of a newborn babe?" Faraday was involved in a similar exchange shortly after his discovery of electromagnetic induction. While he was demonstrating this new phenomenon to the Prime Minister, he was asked "What is the possible purpose of your new discovery, Dr Faraday?" To which Faraday quickly replied "Mr Prime Minister, some day you will use it as a source of taxes". Pasteur, too, was drawn into the vortex of the argument over basic research and the application of new knowledge, and spent much time circulating this dipole. But he was content with his belief that "There are science and the applications of science, linked together as the fruit is to the tree that has borne it."

Two points may be made concerning the NIH strategy for the future: the first concerns an inventory to determine the tropical diseases which are currently controlled by existing public health measures and those other diseases which will require additional biomedical research before control is achieved; the second deals with what I have termed the synergistic application of new discoveries of biomedical research to conventional public health measures for the control of tropical diseases. This paper then closes with four specific proposals on NIH initiatives for the future.

In April 1977, when I gave the Annual Geographic Medicine Lecture at Case Western Reserve University School of Medicine, I discussed what in my judgement was the first order of business in overall strategy for an attack on tropical diseases. I suggested that we examine tropical diseases from two points of view. First, identify those diseases for which application of known social, economic and public health measures would provide effective control now; and second, identify those other diseases for which there is little likelihood that in the foreseeable future application of socio-economic and public health measures will have any appreciable beneficial impact. In these latter cases, we must be prepared to devote research manpower and research resources to develop new diagnostic procedures, new therapy and new preventive measures. I recognize, of course, that complex diseases such as those that occur in the tropics do not break out neatly into one category or another; few things are that simple. It is also true that because of social and other environmental factors it may not be possible to apply the same scheme for any single disease on a worldwide basis. It is entirely likely that a tropical disease controllable in one country by currently available means would be impossible to contain in another. We have been told that in China intensive application of public health and sanitation procedures has gone far to eliminate the problems of schistosomiasis. Similarly, schistosomiasis has decreased dramatically in Puerto Rico. But in Egypt, on the other hand, a lifestyle dating back to the time of the Pharaohs, is so ingrained, so keyed to the rise and fall of the Nile and the irrigation of the canals, that one suspects it may be difficult, in our lifetime, to put into effect what we think of as good public health and sanitation practices, or to put into effect a new way of life that would go a long way towards the control of schistosomiasis. For the foreseeable future, it may be that the only alternative is an intensive research programme focused on the development not only of new public health measures, but also of new drugs, new treatment programmes, new molluscicides and perhaps even vaccines.

The overall strategy which I have suggested was in a sense applied to schistosomiasis at the recent Edna McConnell Clark Foundation meeting at Bellagio, Italy, the purpose of which was to discuss the current state of the measures available for the control of schistosomiasis. A review of recent work on this disease revealed several general conclusions: well-designed studies of various methods of control of schistosomiasis have been completed and evaluated; studies on morbidity of schistosomiasis in nearly every case reveal a correlation between the intensity of infection and the extent of disease; and while immunological studies of this disease have uncovered a great deal about immune mechanisms, the possibility of a vaccine remains remote for the present.

These general conclusions lead to several specific points in regard to the future efforts in schistosomiasis control.

(1) In most cases the aim of control programmes should be the sustained reduction of prevalence and intensity to a point at which clinical disease is of low public health importance in relation to other diseases in the area. Parasite eradication is not a goal of schistosomiasis control.

(2) Completed studies of single methods of control that were reviewed indicate that chemotherapy may be the most cost-effective method of reducing prevalence, incidence and intensity of infection at present. Highest priority should be given to operational research involving improved delivery systems of these new drugs.

(3) New methods of chemotherapy delivery systems such as selective chemotherapy or subcurative single-dose therapy may substantially decrease egg contamination of the environment and thereby decrease transmission, cost of control, morbidity and mortality.

(4) Despite the advances in chemotherapy, in many epidemiological situations, control will require the use of secondary methods such as molluscicides, and management of water supplies and sanitation.

The NIH will conduct research on these specific points where there is still insufficient knowledge to implement them, and it does not take lightly the continuing need for applied research on existing control measures. But I must say we have a responsibility to go one step further —a step which takes us right into the importance of biomedical research as a strategy for the future.

The most powerful argument for biomedical research on tropical diseases stems from the unanticipated re-emergence of medical problems for which solutions had earlier been developed. Over and over again in medicine we are faced with the re-emergence of old problems in new guises: an example is the recent and alarming occurrence of antibiotic resistance among pyogenic bacteria such as gonococci, pneumococci and *Haemophilus influenzae B*. Widespread occurrence of plasmid-mediated resistance to antibiotics among pyogenic bacteria has forced us to reassess our research strategies for the disease control which was thought to have been achieved with antibiotics. Indeed in the USA in 1964, because of the emergence of sulphonamide-resistant organisms, we made a deliberate public health decision to embark on meningococcal-vaccine development for the control of meningococcal meningitis. In the face of the subsequent worldwide dissemination of sulphonamide-resistant meningococci, there was no alternative to control epidemic meningitis but the development of a new vaccine, and that vaccine required resources, basic research, brains and new ideas. In 1968 I made a special unsolicited trip to Geneva to urge that WHO give meningococcal Group A vaccine field-trials the highest priority in the meningococcal belt of Africa. Dr Karel Raska, then the Director, Division of Communicable Diseases at WHO, seized the opportunity, and meningococcal Group A vaccine is now a public health measure in Africa. In Zambia the vaccine has been used widely during the past two years in the northern provinces around Ndola.

The re-emergence of malaria as a major disease problem—one more directly related to the focus of this conference—also underscores the continuing need for basic research. Malaria was thought to have been solved: the application of traditional public health measures using more recent tools such as DDT and chloroquine was believed adequate for the control of this disease, throughout the world and for all time. How wrong we were. The emergence of chloroquine-resistant malaria parasites and DDT-resistant mosquitoes has laid bare our complacency. We had overlooked the durability of a species; a durability for survival in changing environments, arising out of adaptability. We lost sight of the underlying evolutionary processes. Even now at the close of Darwin's century, we too often think of biology as a static process, as if each species of all living things were caged in solitary confinement in a Linnaean garden.

So in the face of these adaptations of nature such as drug resistance among microbes, we must reassess our means to control malaria, and plan research strategies for new treatment and control methods. And when we have achieved that, make no mistake about if, it we are not vigilant, the course of evolutionary events will again overtake us. And so our strategy includes the study of the biology of malaria, mosquitoes, schistosomes and snails: it is the course of prudence and vigilance.

Darwin, I suspect, would have anticipated the emergence of DDT-resistant mosquitoes or chloroquine-resistant malaria, understanding as he did the meaning of selective pressure in the survival of the species. It is indeed ironic that at the close of Darwin's century we grasp the molecular mechanisms of evolution, but in the applications of modern medicine to public health we fail to recognize the predictable consequences. The job of the NIH, as I see it, is to remain alert to those predictable consequences.

The second point on NIH strategy for the future concerns the practice of what I call synergism—the reinforcement which occurs between the use of conventional public health practices and the enhancement of those practices through the additional benefits of biomedical research. Indeed, our most immediate past experience with plagues in our own countries reveals the importance of this synergism between the application of conventional public health measures along with the new benefits of medical research. What better example of such synergism than the modern control of tuberculosis. Long before the age of antibiotics, much was done in the control of tuberculosis with the isolation of cases and improvement of nutrition, housing, and so on. But in the 1950s modern chemotherapy broke upon the scene as the culmination of seventy-five years of intensive bacteriological research. Only then was it possible to combine public health practices synergistically with modern chemotherapy and to control tuberculosis beyond what would have seemed possible at the turn of the century. I mention tuberculosis because this remains a disease which is not yet controlled in the developing countries.

Another example: synergism remains an important strategy in the control of yellow fever. When conventional public health practices were coupled with the use of Max Theiler's attenuated vaccine the beneficial effects were synergistic rather than additive. This synergistic approach to yellow fever control can still be used without continuous modification of the vaccine. We have been less fortunate in the synergistic application of stagnant practices to the control of malaria.

The overall strategy for the future will be to apply what we know now and to apply it vigorously. At the same time, the particular strategy of the NIH is to develop new modalities for diagnosis, treatment and prevention through basic and applied research. We will work with our own various government and private agencies in the USA, and with other countries, either formally or informally; in particular, we will work with all countries through the good offices of the World Health Organization. We most especially endorse the Tropical Diseases Research and Training (TDR) Programme of WHO. We have followed its development with interest and have participated when asked in the development of its plans and objectives. Hundreds of American scientists supported by the NIH and other government agencies are currently working on the six diseases identified by WHO as of first importance.

Figure 1 lists 1977 estimated expenditures by United States agencies

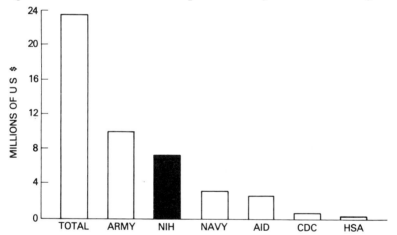

Fig. 1 1977 USA expenditures for the six WHO tropical diseases by agency. AID Agency for International Development; CDC Center for Disease Control; HSA Health Services Administration.

on the six WHO tropical diseases in the TDR programme. The total was approximately $24 million. The NIH spent just over $7 million. Figure 2 shows the 1977 estimated expenditures on each of the six diseases: note that agencies other than the NIH have a major effort in malaria.

Much is said about new initiatives in international health; this new intensity of interest has received widespread notice including an editorial in *Science* last June written by Dr Howard Minners whom we have seconded to WHO to assist in the management of research. But the time has come to act, to take the first steps in the implementation of new

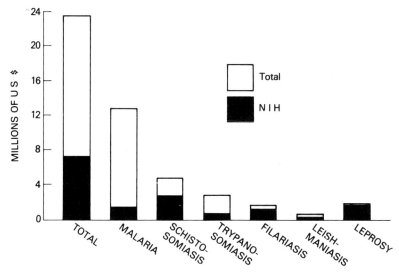

Fig. 2 1977 USA expenditures for the six WHO tropical diseases.

initiatives, and this we at the NIH shall do. I announce these first steps here with the approval of Dr Donald Frederickson, Director of the NIH. A continuation as well as an expansion of our current efforts in tropical medicine will focus on four broad objectives.

(1) The strengthening of tropical medicine in United States universities within the framework of existing biomedical disciplines, e.g. internal medicine, paediatrics, pharmacology, biochemistry, immunology, etc. This will not only enhance the present research effort in our universities, but will also provide long-term career opportunities in the usual medical disciplines for investigators with a specialized interest in tropical medicine.

(2) An extension of current United States research to the developing countries through "linkages" between American investigators and those in the countries where tropical diseases prevail. The WHO TDR programme has called for a network among the research centres in the countries where the diseases exist and in the developing countries. When I attended the Donors and Participants Meeting at WHO a year ago, I emphasized then my preference for the process of linkage between scientific and medical groups in both regions with common goals in biomedical research and development and training.

To facilitate this linkage we shall announce a new research grants programme for international collaboration in infectious diseases research. These grants will require a US investigator to have a defined linkage with a foreign investigator for research done in a truly cooperative way including laboratory and field studies in the overseas environment. Emphasis will given be to the disease entities in the WHO TDR Programme and to those investigators who have identified linkages with colleagues in developing African and Latin American countries, although not to the exclusion of other locations.

(3) Assistance in the establishment or strengthening of centres of excellence in developing countries. The linkages described under objective (2) can be important in reaching this goal. Resources in US public and private sectors as well as the developing countries will be required.

(4) Expanded opportunity for research training in the USA for young medical scientists and health professionals from developing countries. This is particularly true for training related to the tropical diseases, and we have plans in process for an International Tropical Diseases Research Fellowship Program of NIAID. It will be established in co-operation with WHO, and will be administered by the NIH Fogarty International Center. This research fellowship programme will focus especially on the six diseases of the WHO TDR Programme. The objective of this new international fellowship programme is to provide junior or mid-career health professionals and scientists with an opportunity to acquire the special skills which will be applicable to infectious diseases in their own country.

This is a bare outline of the NIH strategies for the future: our business is the generation of new medical knowledge through basic and applied research, and this we shall do on the tropical diseases, in collaboration with colleagues in the United Kingdom and throughout the world. We endorse the objectives of the WHO TDR Programme as a sensible and realistic beginning, recognizing that other diseases are also of major importance in the developing countries. Expansion of our current efforts in tropical medicine will focus on four broad objectives. Included in these are: (a) a new research grant programme to establish research linkages between investigators in the USA and our colleagues in the developing countries; and (b) new research training fellowships for young medical scientists from developing countries to work in the USA. Finally, the control of tropical diseases can have an elusive quality—the re-emergence of malaria is a notable example; we had not anticipated the occurrence or the consequences of chloroquine-resistant malaria parasites or DDT-resistant mosquitoes. In our strategy for the control of tropical diseases, we must recognize that this type of re-emergence is programmed in the genetic machinery of biological evolution. We must therefore remain both vigilant and venturesome: if we are not alert to the sovereign stream of evolution, we shall be swept away by the inevitable consequences of biological adaptability in the microbial world.

20. The Academic Potential

C. E. Gordon Smith

The promotion of health and the control of diseases in large populations require co-operation between a wide range of disciplines—medical, behavioural, agricultural and economic—as well as much greater co-ordination between the disparate organizations which fund them. They also demand greater institutional, inter-institutional and, most of all, international co-operation and integration than the medicine of individuals. While smaller institutions and individual university departments can do excellent work on the basic medical science of tropical diseases, the development, implementation, evaluation and integration of control measures into health services demand the support of broadly based institutions or groups of institutions with a comprehensive approach to preventive medicine and community health.

The main causes of morbidity and mortality (especially in children) in many tropical countries remain gastro-intestinal and respiratory infections aggravated by under-nutrition or malnutrition, and while great expectations for the eventual control of six major diseases are now raised by the World Health Organization Special Programme for Research and Training in Tropical Diseases, governments and foundations who support work on diseases of tropical countries will need to re-examine their priorities lest other disease problems fall into neglect—not least because of the natural tendency of scientists to change or modify their interests in response to the exceptional availability of large grants.

There has been an undoubted and widespread failure, as much in industrialized as in tropical countries, to implement or even test the potential value of research findings in health services. High priority must be given to ensuring that both existing and new knowledge is effectively communicated to those who can utilize it, is appropriately tried and evaluated and, if beneficial and cost-effective, is implemented.

The component subject areas of such a broad attack on the health problems of tropical countries differ greatly in their strengths and states of development—and of course from place to place. They fall into three main categories.

(1) Subjects largely or wholly devoted to communicable diseases important in the tropics (e.g. clinical tropical medicine, medical microbiology, medical helminthology, medical protozoology, medical entomology). Paradoxically these have tended to be stronger in relevant institutions in industrialized than in developing countries. In some of the latter they are weak, especially in the teaching of medical undergraduates; ignorance of the diagnosis and most appropriate treatment of common tropical diseases is by no means confined to doctors in the temperate zones. Everywhere, these subjects are short of medically qualified scientists and mostly they were fairly well stretched in terms of both research and training even before the advent of the WHO Special Programme. An interesting exception is immunology which during the past few years has begun to grow in tropical countries and in relation to tropical diseases, largely due to the efforts of WHO and foundations such as the Wellcome Trust. With the exception of cosmopolitan aspects of microbiology, these specialities have at present only a small number of senior posts worldwide, compared with other scientific and medical disciplines. Thus career prospects, even for present incumbents, are less attractive than in other medical specialities. More recruits of quality (especially medical), and therefore more career posts, are required everywhere, but especially in tropical countries.

(2) Subjects which are strong in industrialized countries but which have not yet developed sufficient interest in tropical medical research. Examples include epidemiology, medical statistics, clinical pharmacology, biochemistry and advanced clinical research in important areas such as gastroenterology and renal disease. The need here is to create more academic nuclei in the tropics and, by collaborative international multidisciplinary projects, to attract the interest of the experts in these fields. This, too, needs additional recruitment and the creation of more career posts especially in the tropics, and if these new disciplines are to make effective contributions to tropical problems, they will need the close collaboration of the basic sciences mentioned earlier—a further demand on their already stretched resources.

(3) Subjects which are weak even in industrialized countries. These include operational research in relation to health services, to the planning and evaluation of disease control programmes, and to the health problems of development programmes, health economics, and health education (particularly its evaluation). In all of these, academic resources are quite inadequate to meet the needs of industrialized countries and hardly exist in tropical countries. We need rapidly to develop a few strong nuclei in broadly based academic centres of international community health, so as to generate an academic base and to train

leaders for the development of satellite nuclei elsewhere. And in all of them we need to be able to attract expertise of high quality from outside the traditional health sector. We need operational researchers and economists from the management and industrial sectors. In health education we need educationalists, experts from the media (especially radio and television) who are capable of developing the subliminal education (probably through entertainment) which will be most likely to influence behaviour for health, especially in largely illiterate communities, and epidemiologists and sociologists capable of evaluating its effects. If the media can be used for political purposes surely they can be used equally effectively for health if similar financial and intellectual resources were harnessed. Without economic and operational analysis, and without the backing of effective health education, few disease control programmes, however scientifically sophisticated, are likely to be successful in large populations. It is much easier to acquire funds for esoteric laboratory research of almost any sort than to get even seed money in these subject areas. Some sources of funding should give urgent attention to the needs of these very neglected disciplines.

To turn now to the specific strengths and weaknesses in industrialized and in tropical countries, the following suggestions are offered as to how some of them may be overcome, and how the essential components could be drawn together to ensure an integrated approach to training and research, and to the effective application of knowledge.

Industrialized Countries

The focal institutions in industrialized countries are the schools of tropical medicine which are small in number and vary greatly in breadth and strength. Most cover only a small range of the required spectrum, but even fairly broad and strong ones such as the London School of Hygiene and Tropical Medicine recognize the pressing need to attract the collaboration of complementary resources in other institutions, and all recognize the need to develop strong and long-lasting co-operation with institutions in the tropics. They realize that they cannot encompass the necessary range of expertise and experience within their own staffs, and that without broad and long-lasting involvement in the real problems of tropical countries, they will lose both credibility and effectiveness. They also realize their importance in enhancing the interest of subjects not yet adequately committed to the tropics and in fostering research and teaching centres in subjects not yet sufficiently developed.

The efforts of these schools are spread over many countries and involving teaching, research, service and advisory activities. Most are on tight budgets with little more than minimally effective staff strengths. Their senior staff members were able to acquire long-term experience and knowledge of tropical countries and their health problems by serving in them during the colonial period. Since then, a number of able younger workers (with some disregard of their longer-term career prospects) have carried out excellent long- or medium-term research in the tropics, mainly funded by foundations. But there is a pressing need to provide many more opportunities for younger workers to spend longer periods of teaching, research and service in tropical countries, in places where they can accomplish good work in a good and co-operative intellectual environment. It is to be hoped that the WHO Special Programme will create additional strong centres of opportunity in tropical countries, supplementing other efforts to create and promote long-term international collaboration. Funds should be made available in particular to encourage two-way visits between tropical and temperate-zone institutions for shorter or longer periods of planned joint research. Such opportunities and links should not, of course, be confined to schools of tropical medicine but should also involve relevant departments in medical schools (e.g. gastro-enterology), elsewhere in universities and in research institutes.

The achievement of all these goals will depend on the availability of able people prepared to devote at least substantial portions of their lives to the understanding and solution of the problems of health and disease in the tropics. These will be recruited only if there are clearly visible career opportunities. Priority must therefore be given by all the organizations concerned to increasing the numbers of career posts. Realistically these must be based on the home countries of the people concerned and, because of the long commitments involved, on institutions in their home countries. A number of industrialized countries, including Britain, have already made provisions for careers for medical and related scientists who wish to research and/or teach in developing countries but, because of the age structure of interested scientists, these posts are filled fairly quickly and will remain filled for many years. There is therefore an urgent need for all industrialized countries which are interested in promoting better health in tropical countries to recognize the need for more career opportunities. In order to offer them encouragement and a structure to relate to, WHO should create a "tropical diseases research service" (or similar body) to which scientists with career posts could be seconded for service in the tropics. The foundations should also move further towards providing career appointments for proven scientists in these fields.

Turning to training, while it is clear that wherever possible scientists and doctors from developing countries ought to receive as much as possible of their training in their own countries or regions, tropical countries vary greatly in their educational development. For this and a variety of other (including political) reasons there is still a need to provide early postgraduate training in industrialized countries, at least in subjects relatively new to medical research in the tropics, and in those insufficiently developed anywhere. This need will continue for some considerable time—especially in teaching the teachers and researchers who will be able to create and mould the future teaching and research resources in the developing countries. A permanent role, for those institutions with sufficient breadth, is in providing a milieu in which the future leaders (teachers, researchers or administrators) in the broad fields of health may gain international understanding and advanced training. The London School of Hygiene and Tropical Medicine has defined this as its long-term objective and already brings together postgraduates with a wide variety of health interests from over 80 countries in any one year.

In their capacities as visiting lecturers, researchers, examiners, advisers and the like, academics from industrialized countries play important roles in establishing contacts and enhancing standards in developing countries. However, there should be more opportunities for them to combine an advisory with a service role, perhaps especially in large-scale development or disease-control programmes. Younger academics in particular can provide complementary expertise and gain valuable experience as members of teams largely composed of indigenous scientists.

Tropical Countries

After much assistance from aid programmes and foundations, the universities and their medical schools in many developing countries are expanding rapidly and successfully, especially where there is economic and political stability. Their greatest strengths are often in the advanced medicine of the individual rather than in the array of subjects so important for resolution of the major health problems of tropical populations, and they often lack facilities (and sometimes the will) for the continuing involvement in field-work so essential if major diseases of large populations are to be controlled.

The man-power training of tropical countries has been concentrated on scientific and medical staff (sometimes unduly on the Ph.D.) without comparable attention to the creation and training of adequate cadres of supporting staff. Scientists cannot be effective without good technician support, and much more attention is urgently needed to the provision of adequate status, careers, salaries and training for technicians if research is to prosper in tropical countries.

If the WHO Special Programme is to achieve lasting benefits the governments of the countries concerned must use it to develop an appropriate research and training system closely integrated with both their universities and their health services and clearly related to a realistic and balanced career structure. Thus could they much improve their prospects of making the best use of existing and new knowledge for improvement of the health of their populations and of greatly reducing the need for overseas training except for potential leaders.

But to achieve and maintain standards in both aspects it will continue to be important for the leaders of research and teaching in tropical countries to understand the problems of other countries and to spend periods working with specialists of international standing in their subject areas. Genuine exchanges of research and teaching staff must become commoner worldwide, and it is to be hoped that many more universities will recruit the best they can attract, regardless of nationality.

Enhancement of International Collaboration

Collaboration depends on people knowing and respecting each other, finding a common interest and wishing to pursue it together. Administrative arrangements can facilitate but not create such relationships. The priority must therefore be to increase the opportunities for people with common, or (better) complementary interests to work together for periods sufficient to develop a lasting relationship. In parallel with the widespread activities funded by aid programmes, foundations and other WHO programmes, the Special Programme, with its network of centres, should greatly increase opportunities for personal contact. If the foundations can judiciously supplement and complement these activities (particularly in fields other than the six diseases) the collaboration so essential for real progress may develop.

Large-scale projects—development or disease-control programmes—offer a very fertile potential source of long-term collaboration. These generally involve indigenous and foreign governments and the international organizations. Development programmes cause large-scale changes in the environment and large population movements, and often profoundly alter the risk of a variety of diseases, e.g. schistosomiasis, malaria, arthropod-borne virus diseases. They therefore require careful prior assessment of the disease risks and careful monitoring as the project proceeds and for at least 10 years afterwards. Such projects, varying in scale, are numerous throughout tropical countries and, because they are planned activities, offer excellent opportunities for broad-based research leading to the design and implementation of health measures and services appropriate to the specific needs of the population concerned. These complex programmes demand a multi-disciplinary team which, ideally, should remain with the project from the preliminary stages until at least 10 years after completion—a period perhaps of 20 years in all. Such teams need to comprise not only health-related experts and officials but also representatives of other relevant disciplines: agriculturalists, agronomists, hydrologists, econo-mists, etc. Such teams should be predominantly indigenous but should be supplemented by experts from outside, wherever possible giving opportunities for younger workers from the industrialized countries to participate. Many project teams exist throughout the developing world but few are as effective as they could be in these various respects. More often than not they succeed or fail because of the ability of their project leader. Every attempt should be made to identify, train and provide careers for people with the relatively rare combination of qualities which make successful leaders for complex field projects.

Conclusions

In conclusion, the priorities for enhancing academic potential for the promotion of health and the control of diseases in the tropics are: firstly, to enhance the potential of those already in relevant disciplines by pro-viding them with satisfactory career opportunities, and with the best possible opportunities (especially in the tropics) for training, research and experience. Secondly, by providing more career opportunities, to increase recruitment of high quality people, especially into relevant subjects relatively new to medicine in the tropics or poorly developed everywhere. Thirdly, to focus the development of research and training on the universities, to encourage interdisciplinary collaboration and to ensure that universities in the tropics extend their relevant activities more widely into the problems of their majority populations. Fourthly, to foster international co-operation and exchange, in research, training and service—particularly in relation to large-scale develop-ment programmes which offer such excellent opportunities for the test-ing, evaluation and implementation of existing and new knowledge. There is, at the moment, a rising tide towards solutions of the health problems of the millions of deprived people in the tropics. If we fail to take full advantage of it, and to ensure that a firm base is laid for long-term action, little that is effective may be achieved, however satisfied we are with our own research—and there will not be another such rising tide in our lifetimes.

21. The Role of the Foundations

John H. Knowles

Any discussion of the role of foundations must take into account certain historical and contemporary facts. The Rockefeller Foundation was established in 1913 to "promote the well-being of mankind throughout the world", in the grandiloquently amorphous but prescient words of its charter. Born in the progressive era of our country, it institutionalized our faith in pluralism and voluntarism, in education and science, and in the rule of reason—articles of faith and values transported to our shores largely from England. (The word "voluntary" dates from 1725 with the founding of Guy's Hospital and is defined in the *Oxford English Dictionary* as "free from state interference or control . . . supported largely by free-will offerings".) It was also a typically pragmatic, American response to two problems: the populist assult on the massive concentration of wealth in the hands of a few; and the honestly humani- tarian, if somewhat guilt-laden desire of the captains of industry— Carnegie and Rockefeller (and later Mellon and Ford)—to return at least part of their good fortune to the people of their country in the form of good works. The secular joined the sacred impulse, for Rockefeller was a devout Baptist and his adviser in all his philanthropies was Frederick T. Gates, a Baptist minister. Gates read Sir William Osler's *Principles and Practice of Medicine* and immediately convinced Rocke- feller that there was nothing more important than health, and the best hope for helping mankind would be found through the eradica- tion of disease and the advancement of medical science. Hookworm was rampant in the south-eastern USA and the Foundation established field-control programmes and helped to build and support local public health units. By 1915, extensive field-control programmes for malaria and yellow fever were initiated. (To this day, the members of the International Health Division of the Rockefeller Foundation are re- membered in the countries where they worked. When in Bahia, Brazil, last year, I was asked about Fred Soper who directed the campaign against the *Anopheles gambiae* mosquito, transported from Africa to

North-east Brazil—the carrier of the lethal, falciparum form of malaria.)

In 1916 the Foundation began its programme of support for the development of schools of public health in the USA—Harvard, Johns Hopkins, Michigan and many others, and abroad, whether in Yugoslavia or in England where the Foundation provided the $2 million for the building of the London School of Tropical Medicine and Hygiene in 1924. In 1921, the Peking Union Medical College was established, bringing Western medicine to China, and functioning to this day.

In 1932, the Foundation began to aid in the establishment of departments of psychiatry in American medical schools and teaching hospitals. The yellow fever vaccine was developed in 1935 by Max Theiler, a Rockefeller Foundation officer working in the laboratories of the Rockefeller Institute (now University) for which he received the Nobel Prize in 1951. In 1937, the field of molecular biology was stimulated in its development when Warren Weaver of the Foundation and Linus Pauling put their heads together. By the 1960s the Arbo-Virus Unit of the International Health Division was established at Yale, and the work on Lassa fever by the Rockefeller staff had attracted attention. In 1967 a field station was established in St Lucia, West Indies, for the study of schistosomiasis.

Meanwhile, a new interest had developed in response to a study requested by the Foundation in the early 1940s. George Harrar, an agricultural scientist, was recruited and sent to Mexico to work in the field on problems of increasing food production for the world's rapidly expanding population. One of his first appointees was Norman Borlaug who received the Nobel Peace Prize in 1970 for his development of high-yielding wheat (albeit water and fertilizer-intensive) in what is now one of the worldwide systems of international agricultural institutes (CIMMYT). High-yielding varieties of rice were developed at the International Rice Research Institute (IRRI) in the Philippines at Los Banos. Most recently, the Foundation has helped to establish the ninth such institute, the International Laboratory for Research on Animal Diseases (ILRAD) in Nairobi, Kenya, where a most important development has already taken place in the first year of its operation—the successful cultivation of trypanosomes *in vitro* by Hirumi.

Because of the Green Revolution, per capita protein consumption kept pace with the doubling of populations in the less developed countries (LDCs) which occurred between 1950 and 1975. But it was recognized by most, and certainly by the Foundation staff, that we were merely buying time, and that the geometric expansion of population had to be reduced lest the Malthusian prediction became true globally, as contrasted with just regionally, as now applies. In the 1960s the Foundation established its interests in population problems, stressing, as always, the building of institutions and the advanced training and education of promising young people. In 1966 we initiated support for the development of centres for the study of reproductive biology, at Harvard, Yale, North Carolina, University of California at San Francisco, and the Salk Institute, where Roger Guillemain, one of our early awardees, has just received the Nobel Prize in Medicine. Support for the training of fellows from the LDCs, and for policy research by indigenous scholars in the LDCs (in conjunction with the Ford Foundation) is an important part of the strategy. Review of global activities in population problems at our Bellagio Study Centre in Italy has been undertaken roughly every three years.

The Rockefeller Foundation does not have infinite resources, and as agricultural and population interests generated enthusiasm and excitement, health interests began to wither away. By 1972, the word "health" was no longer listed on our programme statement, and the work in St Lucia on schistosomiasis was listed at the end of our annual report as an "allied interest". Some work continued in our University Development Programme, initiated under Dean Rusk's presidency in the 1950s, much of it field-work, some fundamental research at the East African Universities, the Universities of Ibadan, Nairobi, del Valle (Columbia), Philippines, Mahidol (Bangkok), and more recently, in Zaire, Bahia, Brazil and Jogjakarta, Indonesia. The International Health Division has been phased out and the Yale Arbo-Virus Unit was cut free. Even foundations reflect and follow their culture and do not always lead, and the lack of interest in health was equalled in the LDCs planning which stressed economic development and not health, and their plans in turn reflected the World Bank—whose Pearson Report in 1969 did not even mention health as a prime variable in economic development nor its indirect effect on the inexorable expansion of population. The steadily growing number of developed countries' agencies for international development followed suit, and the World Health Organization struggled and straggled along.

Meanwhile, the world began to change remarkably and the speed of change and the dire forebodings which accompany it leave us like a Greek chorus groaning at all that transpires. The news of guerrilla warfare and personal violence, hijackings and kidnappings, and ethnic strife in Ireland, Ethiopia, the Middle East, South Africa—coupled with the fact that the world expends $300 billion annually for weapons of destruction, $15 billion in aid, and only $7000 million for health and population problems—is cause for deep concern for the world's future. Environmental pollution and exhaustion of the world's non-renewable resources with particular reference to energy and oil arouses alarm; the gap between north and south, developed and developing countries, is widening; human rights are violated and the possibility, as well as the actual occurrence, of conflict is steadily increasing.

The expansion of production and consumption of the developed countries proceeded at a phenomenal rate between 1950 and 1970, and with it a marked expansion of agencies for international development, of support for the United Nations and its agencies, and the World Bank and regional banks. The Rockefeller Foundation found itself no longer alone in the field, but was now joined by the substantial technical expertise and massive amounts of money of all these agencies. On the domestic scene, the National Institutes of Health (NIH) and the Department of Health, Education and Welfare (HEW), the National Academy of Science (NAS), the National Endowment for the Arts (NEA) and the National Endowment for the Humanities (NEH), to name but a few, are *de facto* foundations.

It is this great complexity that must be grappled with daily at the Rockefeller Foundation, and at the very least I try to simplify, then generalize, and then particularize in the quest to maintain and improve upon the record of the Foundation. The Trustees have just completed a constructive review of the past five years:

Q. Should the Foundation be maintained?
A. Yes.
Q. At the same level of expenditure?
A. Yes, roughly $45 million annually.
Q. How much domestic versus international expenditure?
A. About 33% is spent outside the USA and our interests are increasing in the international sphere.
Q. How much direct (field-work and New York officers) versus indirect (grants and fellowships to others) expenditure?
A. Keep indirect above 60% of our expenditure.
Q. Are we too diffuse, because of the erosion of our assets both by inflation and the slowing of growth and capital expansion in the USA?
A. Yes.
Q. Then what should be phased out?
A. University development in the LDCs, as we simultaneously invite specific grant applications from new-established universities in the LDCs, treating them like our own universities; and the quality of the environment—maintaining those relevant interests within our programmes in agriculture, population, health and international relations.
Q. Can we and should we add anything?
A. Yes, as strong a re-entry into the field of international health as possible, with particular emphasis on the great neglected diseases of mankind, co-ordinating our efforts with other individuals and institutions, public, private, national and international.

Q. What are the fundamental elements of our strategy in all our programmes?

A. To advance knowledge and to be knowledgeable in advance, to
strike at the roots of problems, to build and/or maintain institutions,
to support promising young investigators and their institutions; to
sustain commitments over time, to avoid the fallacies of reduc-
tionism and of dealing in absolutes; to collaborate with others and
by the excellence and quality of our staff and their work, to lead
and demonstrate to those politically constrained national and
international organizations where they might place their billions
without the risks we are still privileged to assume.

Q. What are the most threatening problems, aside from destructive
conflict?

A. Global inflation and massive unemployment of youth, and the
transformation of the ideas of progress and uncontrolled growth—
whether that of populations or of industries. Special Commissions
should be structured to review these problems in the search for
opportunities for the Foundation.

Q. How do things look in the USA?

A. Mixed. There has been a general erosion of confidence in leaders
which began with Vietnam and has run right through Watergate
to the present incumbent of the White House. In the latter instance, the liberals are dispirited and seem to have lost confidence—
over quantity and quality in education, inflation and unemployment, the plight of minorities (now adding a new and rapidly
expanding Hispanic force), over the failure of legislation and money
and good intentions. We seem to be stalled in diastole in the Age of
Anxiety. Perhaps Schopenhauer was correct when he noted the
two basic causes of unhappiness: not having what you want, and
having it. We are all worried about energy and particularly oil.

Q. What is your prognosis?

A. Guarded but hopeful. The glass is half full, not half empty, but the
cup is not running over. There are many opportunities for the
Rockefeller Foundation in this great age of discontinuity, dis-
junction and transformation of some of the greatest and most
energizing ideas of western civilization. What could be more important than to sustain and to try to improve upon our record in
health, agriculture, population and education—these interests,
coupled with strong support for the arts and humanities while we
look for new opportunities *vis-à-vis* minorities, ethnic strife, unemployment of youth.

Q. Well, after those generalizations, now be specific.

A. You invited me here to speak on the role of the foundations in
tropical medicine and I will not repeat what I have written elsewhere which I think is quite specific (Knowles, 1976), nor bore you
with the details of how we accomplished our re-entry, except to say
that (a) foundations themselves resist change and have powerful
constituencies; (b) our resources are finite and expansion in one

area has to be accompanied by contraction in another; and (c) the individual divisional director is the key to our past, present and future, and the quality of that individual has been and always will be the key to our success or failure.

I must decry what seems increasingly to be a combination of insensitivity, the ignorance of chauvinistic super-specialized idiot savants and just plain political laziness—the phenomenon of forgetting the past or beating straw men, or pushing aside past or present efforts in the rush to the new, the exciting. The Rockefeller Foundation, in turning its attention to the creation of an international network of biomedical research groups to study the great neglected diseases of the developing world, is not turning its back on field experiments or traditional public health disciplines, and it is fully aware that while new knowledge and more effective technologies are needed, the old and existing methods and tools of public health are as important as ever and will be for the foreseeable future. It merely says that we believe our history,traditions, strategies and present finite resources can be most fruitfully applied as described below. We understand as much as we can about the interdependent variables of food–nutrition–health–population–economic development in the quality-of-life equation and we hope and expect to learn much more. We believe that all elements can and should be addressed simultaneously and we subscribe to the idea of meeting basic human needs rather than the trickle-down theory—which too often has meant a trickle down into the ruler's pockets or into weapons of destruction.

The following proposal was unanimously approved by our Trustees on 5 December 1977, when Dr Kenneth Warren presented our recommendations.

Great Neglected Diseases
of the Developing World

Proposed Action
Resolved that the sum of Six hundred thousand dollars ($600 000), or as much thereof as may be necessary, be, and it hereby is, appropriated for allocation by the officers for the creation of an international network of biomedical research groups to study the great neglected diseases of the developing world; this sum to be available for allocation during the period ending 30 June 1978.

Classification: Population and Health—Great Neglected Diseases (Health Sciences)

Summary: The sophisticated biomedical research establishment of the industrialized nations has thus far largely ignored many of the diseases that afflict hundreds of millions of people in the developing world. These conditions include schistosomiasis, hookworm, malaria, sleeping sickness, amoebic dysentery and fatal diarrhoea of infants. The Foundation renders valuable service by encouraging outstanding basic and clinical scientists to shift their attention to these great neglected diseases.

It is proposed, therefore, to create a network of high-quality investigators who would constitute a critical mass in this field, attract the brightest students, and conduct research of an excellence now rarely seen in this area. A significant part of the investigators' effort would be spent in applied collaborative research in developing countries. The overall result should be breakthroughs in diagnosis, treatment, and prevention, leading to more rapid and complete control of these widespread infections.

The officers envisage this network as consisting of up to 12 research units, each to be supported at the level of about $150 000 annually for a maximum of eight years. The proposed grant would be allocated for initial support of the first seven centres. The funds would be used largely for the salaries of young professional personnel and for travel to collaborative centres in the developing world.

Relationship to Programme: This proposal relates to the Foundation's traditional and now renewed interest in tropical medicine and to the schistosomiasis programme.

Previous Support: During the period 1972–6, the St Lucia project required the expenditure of $2 382 497; support for schistosomiasis research projects, mainly in immunology, totalled $1 237 700; and there were five grants totalling $116 645 for basic research in onchocerciasis. In addition, in 1974 a grant of $525 000 was made to develop a unit devoted to research on the great neglected diseases of the developing world in the Department of Medicine at Case Western Research University School of Medicine. Since 1971, under the Conquest of Hunger Program, $1 million has been provided for support of an animal-disease research and training laboratory in East Africa, and for co-operative immunological research related to trypanosomiasis and East Coast fever.

Description: During the present century, research in tropical diseases has been supported mainly by crash programmes mounted by the Armed Forces during periods of war (Second World War, the Korean and Vietnam conflicts); during peacetime there has been an almost complete termination of interest and funding. Malaria has been the chief target of such research, and new insecticides and antimalarials have been developed. Unfortunately, both the mosquito and the malarial parasite have become resistant to these agents in many endemic areas. Large-scale epidemics of malaria are occurring again in South-east Asia, Africa, and Latin America. In addition, cholera is spreading through the Middle East, and one of the principal means of controlling it is an inadequate vaccine offering only partial protection for limited periods. Other major diseases—including schistosomiasis, elephantiasis, African sleeping sickness, leprosy, and amoebic dysentery—have received little attention from war-motivated research.

Recently, however, international agencies have become concerned about these neglected problems, which are perceived to be a significant hindrance to both economic development and acceptance of population control. The World Bank is expending $120 million over the next 20 years in stop-gap measures to prevent river-blindness in West Africa by insect control, despite little knowledge of the infection and no adequate drugs and vaccines. The World Health Organization has embarked upon a Special Programme for Research and Training in Tropical Diseases for which it has now received commitments of £12 million, largely from European countries. But WHO must work under several constraints: the necessity to distribute funding politically and geographically, and not necessarily on the basis of scientific excellence; the limitations of the tropical medicine establishment of the industrialized world, which suffers from mediocrity bred by decades of neglect; the lack of an infrastructure to administer a large granting establishment; and the uncertain future of support, which at present comes largely from Scandinavian sources and is being given principally to the USA, the United Kingdom and the developing world.

During the past 40 years, however, tremendous strides have been made in research methodology, instrumentation, and knowledge of biological systems. These techniques, if applied to the worm, protozoan, and bacterial infections of the developing world, should result in a series of breakthroughs of major practical significance. Contrast the World Bank's $120 million for temporary suppression of the insect vectors of river-blindness with the Foundation's investment of about $100 000 which may already have produced a highly effective means of treating this infection in man. Contrast the tens of millions of dollars being invested in partial control of schistosomiasis through dumping toxic snail-killing chemicals into vast bodies of water (e.g. the Nile, Lake Victoria) with the few hundreds of thousands of dollars which have already produced a rapid, cheap radioimmunoassay for the diagnosis of schistosomiasis, as well as new concepts of targeted mass treatment for controlling this great infection of mankind. Thus, a relatively small investment made in the right place can have an enormous impact on these diseases.

Highly competent basic biomedical and clinical investigators are developing an interest in the great neglected diseases of the developing world for both scientific and humanitarian reasons. Only an organization like the Foundation, which commands their confidence, can enable them to make a major commitment in time and energy to this area. The present proposal is aimed at the establishment of a network of research groups in a number of the best medical research institutes in the world, each led by outstanding scientists who will attract cadres of excellent students and young investigators. The rapid establishment of up to 12 of these groups should result in a critical mass of investigators with a high output, both quantitatively and qualitatively. Each of the groups from the developed countries would establish links with medical schools or research laboratories in the developing world. The network units organized in centres of excellence in less-developed countries would function as research and training centres for their own country, their region, and for investigators from the developed world.

Preliminary discussions have indicated a readiness for commitment to this field by the following leading scientists:

(1) *Dr Sheldon Wolff*, Professor and Chairman, Department of Medicine, Tufts, USA. His group work on bacterial diarrhoeas and amoebiasis, with field programmes in Brazil and Guatemala.

(2) *Dr David Weatherall*, Nuffield Professor of Clinical Medicine, University of Oxford, England. His group would work on malaria, with field programmes in the Gambia.

(3) *Dr John David*, Professor of Medicine, Harvard Medical School, USA. His group would work on the immunology of worm infections, with field studies in Kenya.

(4) *Sir Gustav Nossal*, Director, Walter and Eliza Hall Institute, Melbourne, Australia. His group's immunological research would be directed to both worm and protozoan infections, with field studies in Southeast Asia.

(5) *Dr Leslie Webster*, Chairman, Department of Pharmacology, Case Western Reserve University School of Medicine, USA. His group has extensive and sophisticated equipment (e.g. for nuclear magnetic resonance spectroscopy and high-pressure liquid chromatography) that will be applied to developing new and improved drugs against a variety of worm infections.

(6) *Dr Anthony Cerami*, Head of the Laboratory of Medical Biochemistry, Rockefeller University, USA. His group would concentrate on the development of new methods of treatment of protozoan infections, with field studies in Kenya and Brazil.

(7) *Dr Aziz El Kholy*, Director, Biomedical Research Centre for Infectious Diseases, Cairo, Egypt. This centre would be used for research on parasitic infections by outstanding young Egyptian investigators and by visiting research personnel from network and other laboratories.

The formation of these seven units into a research network can be catalyzed at a relatively small cost, ranging from $50 000 to $150 000 per unit per year. As part of this programme, annual meetings of the network would be held each year. Since few of these outstanding investigators have a broad knowledge of these diseases, the first meeting would be a short, intensive course in tropical medicine at the London School, originally built with support from the Foundation. The heads of the participating units would comprise an advisory committee to the programme.

Evaluation: The officers would evaluate the units individually on the basis of site visits, reviews of research work in progress, and scientific publications. In addition, the proposed annual meetings would permit evaluation of each team's research contributions by the other investigators; as well as an evaluation of the total programme. The output of both practical results—such as new methods of diagnosis, treatment, and prevention—and applied operational research would be monitored.

Budget and Sources of Funds: The proposed appropriation of $600 000 would be available for allocation by the officers during the period ending 30 June 1978. The funds would be allocated for initial support of the seven centres listed above. In each centre, core support would be provided from other sources.

The Foundation funds would be used largely for the salaries of outstanding young professional personnel and for travel, living expenses, and research supplies for carrying out research in tropical endemic areas. In certain instances, funds might be provided for technical personnel, special items of equipment, and supplies and animals for laboratory research.

Comment: The proposed new Foundation programme in tropical disease research would add a high level of quality to the recently established WHO Special Programme by stimulating some of the best basic scientists in the developed and less-developed world to turn their attention and expertise to the pressing disease problems of the tropics. New techniques, drugs, and vaccines produced in the sophisticated research laboratories of the industrialized world could be subjected to field testing and evaluation in conjunction with WHO-sponsored projects.

Implications for Future Support: During the next several years, the officers expect to identify up to 12 research units. They plan to recommend support for each of these at the level of about $150 000 per year for a maximum of eight years. It is anticipated that the excellence of the research produced by these units would generate funds from other organizations, and by monitoring the programme annually the Foundation will be able to phase out its funding as the units become self-sufficient.

I think this meeting will be looked upon as a watershed in man's attempts to control and eradicate disease. I do believe this is an historic occasion. I would like also to express my sentiments about coming here and being with friends and colleagues at an intellectual feast in the country of Sir Patrick Manson (and Lt-Col. Robert Knowles, Professor of Zoology in the Calcutta School of Tropical Medicine and Hygiene, for whom monkey malaria is named), and of the transforming experience of visiting the Wellcome Museum and being greeted not by a giant worm or a mosquito, but a model of DNA!

Reference

Knowles, J. H. (1976). American Medicine and World Health, 1976. *Annals of Internal Medicine*, **84**, 483–5.

Discussion: Who Can Do What—Gaps and Overlaps

Sir John Dacie (*Chairman*), opening the final session of the meeting, said that Professor Monekosso had put his finger on the problem in asking "how should we help the Third World to help themselves?". This was certainly essential, and also, by so doing, how could humanity as a whole be helped? This was a point that he felt the meeting should discuss.

In referring to Dr Lucas' programme, he commented on the very wide-ranging activities being undertaken by WHO at the present time, and on their plans for the future. Sir John agreed with Dr Krause that the career problem was fundamental for those entering medical research, and said that he had given the meeting an important summary of the role of the National Institutes of Health in the USA. He had also been impressed by the presentation by Dr Gordon Smith on the role of institutes and universities, and that of Dr Knowles on the new proposals by the Rockefeller Foundation. In view of the many fields of activity covered by speakers during the Symposium, he felt that the forthcoming discussion would be most important.

Dr Williams in reviewing the situation in tropical medicine, said that for many years the subject had been grossly neglected and attempts by him to raise interest in research in such institutions as WHO, the Rocke-feller Foundation and NIH had been unsuccessful. The Wellcome Trust had, however, undertaken to support research in tropical medicine to the extent of some $2 million a year, and it was now very exciting to see the large organizations lending their support once more. During the years of neglect, the Wellcome Trust had instituted the London Harvard Scheme in an attempt to maintain the interest of the USA in tropical medicine.

Dr Williams said that his own view was that foundations ought to be innovators. They were small, and had the opportunity to start projects which should eventually be taken over by the major government agencies. Six diseases had been discussed, and although Dr Williams realized WHO did not intend to confine itself precisely, the Special Programme left an enormous gap of tropical medicine completely untouched. This was one of the gaps that the meeting should consider. Another important function of the foundations which Dr Williams felt was quite clear, was career support. Governments were not finding extra money to support the young men needed in tropical medicine, and the foundations could possibly do so. The third point that he felt foundations should remember, was that they were not rivals. He expressed his delight that the Rockefeller Foundation was again coming into the field, and hoped that they and the Wellcome Trust could work together with a unity of purpose. He felt very optimistic about the future in view of the policies announced at the meeting by both the Rockefeller Foundation and the National Institutes of Health, and congratulated the Royal Society of Medicine on its timing of this symposium.

Sir John Dacie thanked Dr Williams for his remarks, and for his reference to the Royal Society of Medicine, and said that the Royal Society of Medicine Foundation in New York should receive the credit.

Dr Knowles added a small qualification to what had been said: WHO, the Rockefeller Foundation and the NIH had announced grand schemes, but it would take a great deal of sustained effort to bring about the hoped-for results.

He agreed with Dr Williams' remarks concerning those tropical diseases not mentioned in the planned programmes, and about career support. He pointed out the NIH grant more fellowships than any other institution in the USA and said that the Rockefeller Foundation shared their view that it was a prime strategy: whatever else was done, unless the critical mass of young investigators was enlarged through the provision of incentives, it would not be possible to sustain an effort over generations.

Finally, he took the point made about rival institutions and said that there was no real question of rivalry. He saw one of the roles of the Rockefeller Foundation as helping to raise additional funds for NIH and AID, influencing the World Bank and working with WHO to help raise more money from the USA.

Sir John Dacie raised two points for discussion—careers for postgraduates returning to their own countries, and the question of the other diseases which must be tackled.

Professor Monekosso said that the question of career structures in less developed countries was very serious because in many cases no research organization existed. Those concerned were doing all they could to try to stimulate government and politicians to support research. He felt that it would be useful if biomedical research were linked with the universities, since the functions of teaching and research were interrelated and the numbers of people involved were small. A career structure could be started in that way, at least until such time as research organizations were established.

On the question of other diseases, he felt that the pre-selected six were the most crucial in terms of biomedical research, although others needed attention. For many of the diseases it was a matter of operational research and applying what was already known.

Dr Lucas took up the question of the role of the foundations. His own experience over many years of working in a developing country, was that the foundations made a most important contribution to the development of science and particularly to tropical medicine. The Rockefeller Foundation gave considerable support to the medical school in Ibadan for example at one time running six Fellowships, two of which were earmarked for public health. This concentration on an area previously neglected enabled Dr Lucas to leave the Department in 1977, with 16 full-time teachers and 6 trainees in place, even though the Rockefeller support had been phased out. This sustained support over a crucial period had made it possible to find and train environmental science engineers and medical statisticians, of whom the Department now had two. He referred also to their research work on schistosomiasis and recalled that when equipment was needed, an appeal to the Wellcome Trust brought support necessary for field-work to be carried out. Ciba had also given support to some of their activities.

He wished to make it clear that the foundations, at a time when governments had been struggling to provide the minimal essentials, stimulated the research which went beyond the minimum. They managed also to bring pressure to bear in order to provide support for neglected areas such as public health and field research in schistosomiasis.

Professor A. W. Woodruff, considering the provision of personnel for a career structure in research, pointed out an interesting development in the University of Ibadan which he thought important, and in which the research foundation might assist. After qualifying, candidates at Ibadan carried out a period of one year attached to a hospital, working on a research project and ultimately presenting a thesis on the year's research. In this way they became identified with their own country and with its problems. He felt that this system would provide an introduction to research which was much needed, and which might help in the recruitment of a research cadre. He hoped the idea would be taken up by other medical schools and universities, and possibly be supported by some of the foundations.

Dr Karl Maramorosch (*Rutgers University*) commented on the work of Hirumi, who had worked with him for ten years. When Dr Hirumi left for Nairobi the laboratories were not ready, so he constructed a collapsible hood from six pieces of plastic. Using that hood he started work in his hotel room where he tested the 90 media and, four months later, he had the culture of *Trypanosoma brucei*. Dr Maramorosch pointed out that many of the people who visited well equipped laboratories would not have such equipment when they returned to their own countries. It was most important to teach them to invent equipment, as Dr Hirumi had done, or to find alternative methods. If ingenuity and inventiveness could be encouraged in order to make use of the materials available, this might minimize the risk of people who had been trained for a period in say England or the United States, becoming frustrated with the lack of facilities and consequently leaving the bench. At the same time, strong emphasis should be placed on improving the facilities where possible.

Dr C. W. Schwabe (*University of California*) returned to the question of careers, and the need to explore unconventional resources and unconventional approaches. He referred to a project carried out in East Africa some 20 years previously, where all sera had to be sent to South Africa for complement fixation tests and this took a considerable time. Only ten miles away, the Kenya Veterinary Research Laboratory were running about a thousand complement fixation tests a day, with the aid of expert technicians.

Another example of duplication of effort was found by Dr Schwabe in West Bengal, where he recently discovered two parallel rabies diagnostic services under the veterinary services and health service, neither of which, for budgetary reasons, was offering a full range of modern diagnostic facilities for rabies. The obvious solution was to combine the two.

Considerable progress was made in India against smallpox because there were trained vaccinators throughout rural India, who had been trained in the campaign against rinderpest in cattle. In view oth these examples, he felt that interactions between professions could prove mutually beneficial.

Dr Schwabe pointed out that the idea was not new—many committees of WHO had discussed the value of interaction between the larger health establishment and the relatively small veterinary services. He reminded the meeting that veterinary services in many Third World countries are more organized in rural areas than are the health services, and suggested that attempts should be made to avoid duplication of effort, establish co-operative activities and a link with related programmes in agriculture.

There were many possibilities, he felt, for unconventional approaches. Although the veterinary profession was small, it had certain attributes and experience in preventive medicine in different populations. His final point was that it was not enough to know the most modern and satisfactory procedure, it was also necessary to know the cheapest reasonably satisfactory procedure available.

Dr Warren said that the Edna McConnell Clark Foundation had contributed greatly to the whole field, although it had entered only four years previously and had concentrated on one area, schistosomiasis.

He commented that the approach of the Rockefeller Foundation meant that the individuals or groups to whom they gave grants could work on any of the great neglected diseases they chose, and do so in their own way, the only proviso being that it was work on a great (i.e. affecting many people) and neglected (i.e. little work had been done on it) disease.

With regard to careers, he pointed out that the grants would be given not to the established investigators leading a group, but to young research workers. The aim was to encourage bright young people into a career in the field. Their policy with regard to training was not to bring workers from the Third World to the West, but to send workers from the West to the developing countries to work with young people there and to learn how to cope with research under those conditions.

Dr Hitchings said that his contribution would be essentially pessimistic. He wondered how significant was the omission of the pharmaceutical industry in calculations for the future. The industry was cramped both economically and by regulations, which in turn exacerbated the economic pressures. This was, he felt, misguided, since it was evident that the industry had done much for society, and its ability to create and innovate was being compromised.

Commenting on malaria, he said that resistance problems had been appreciated, but were largely ignored. Even now the best prophylactic drug was reserved for therapy and the best therapeutic drug was used for prophylaxis. The pessimism he had spoken of came largely from the view that whatever advances were made, they would be obstructed by bureaucrats and administrators.

Dr Krause disagreed with the idea that it had been generally appreciated that antibiotic resistance would occur. Although it may have been known by a few people, the medical profession and medical planners had thought that infectious diseases were cured, leaving such problems as cardiac disease and cancer. This idea caused many people to leave the field; the general opinion was that antibiotics would take care of the problem, and this resulted in complacency. Clearly it was known that antibiotic resistance could occur, but it was not *widely* appreciated that this would become epidemiologically important. When meningococcal meningitis resistant to sulphonamides appeared, there was no-one in the USA capable of modern research on the meningococcus and a whole new group of microbiologists had to be recruited.

Dr Ormerod said that it had been most encouraging to hear considerable support being given to causes for which they had campaigned over many years, but introduced a note of caution. He had certain misgivings about the proposed programmes and their effects on the ecology of tropical countries. The World Bank figures indicated an enormous increase in poverty in the Third World over both the past and the coming decades; this would lead to increased child mortality, decreased lifespan and an increase in the already large proportion of the population who are severely malnourished. Although some claimed that these were economic and political problems he did not believe that, and felt instead that they were ecological problems, dependent upon the different climate and terrain of tropical countries. The health programmes exacerbated the ecological fragility of tropical countries. He was not suggesting that the programmes should be cut, but he did feel that their effects should be monitored, and there was no monitoring of such effects on the ecology of Third World countries today.

Dr Lucas said that this statement was incorrect. The World Bank was third co-sponsor of the Special Programme and the monitoring of the effects of the health programmes was of special interest to them. In addition he pointed out that a part of the programme would support a study-group considering socio-economic questions.

Dr A. P. Hall (*Hospital for Tropical Diseases, London*) pointed out that a drug which had not been mentioned was mefloquine, a very powerful single-dose antimalarial drug developed by the US Army in an $8 million per year programme begun in 1963. He felt that Dr Hitchings was being over-pessimistic in his views.

He also suggested that in order to reduce the price of quinine, WHO might consider the cultivation of cinchona trees on a large scale.

Dr S. J. Kingma (*Christinm Medical Commission, Geneva*) thought that a greater effort should be made to make current technology available in Third World countries, in particular those techniques which villagers could use such as oral re-hydration in infantile diarrhoea, some therapeutic methods for malaria, and water technology.

Dr John R. David (*Harvard Medical School*) spoke of the enthusiasm they had encountered in a district near Nairobi during the course of a school study there. Fifty-eight of the 60 patients arrived for the study. At its conclusion they asked if their parents could come, why the study was limited to the school and what else they could do. He felt sure that this enthusiasm and desire to help could also be found elsewhere.

Sir Kenneth Stuart (*Commonwealth Secretariat*) said that the Commonwealth Secretariat were emphasizing the establishment of centres of excellence in the developing world, and wherever possible these centres would be located in universities. His one concern was that such centres and people of excellence should fit in with the planning and executive capacities of the people they sought to serve. The critical area was where science became contiguous with people, and unless special efforts were made to facilitate the transfer of information across this barrier, the activities of foundations and special programmes would not achieve the maximum possible benefit. He felt that the foundations and those responsible for special programmes should look specifically at this interface and assist nations who needed to maintain categories of staff and levels of activity that they did not traditionally support. He wondered what plans had been made to establish this final common pathway through which the achievements of foundations and special programmes would have to be channelled.

Dr Lucas said that WHO was aware of the problem, but pointed out that it was the Ministries of Health of the 150 member states of the World Health Assembly who had demanded an intensification of research, and who had set up the Special Programme. WHO were hoping to be able to feed the research results to the countries concerned through dialogues with national governments. They suggested that each government in an affected area should review its mechanism for identifying research needs in the context of national health priorities, and set up a mechanism for co-ordinating the research within its own territory, linked on an international basis, to contiguous areas and to the global programmes. If this proved possible, the strengthening of institutions, training of personnel and conduct of research would be in the context of priorities identified by the national governments, and so capable of being applied by them.

Professor Monekosso added that as Dr Williams had said earlier, one of the needs of these programmes is for decentralization, so that the activities took place at grass roots level rather than at WHO centres.

Closing Remarks

Richard M. Krause

Perhaps I should do no more than express a note of thanks to those who organized the meeting of which this book is a record. Two years ago Sir John Stallworthy made a masterly summary of the Anglo-American Conference on Sexually Transmitted Diseases which I cannot duplicate, but I do feel that there are some thoughts which need to be drawn together.

First of all, we were given a hieroglyph by Dr Mahmoud which represented schistosomiasis in Ancient Egypt. There is another, that all physicians use; the Rx is a direct derivative of an ancient hieroglyph. I use four hieroglyphs which embrace the theme of this volume, Dx (diagnosis), Rx (treatment), Px (prevention) and Cx (control). In papers 3 and 4 Dr Joseph and Dr Williams emphasized the importance of keeping our minds on these four hieroglyphs for a programme on tropical medicine.

In preparing these Closing Remarks I have been searching for a persistent theme and what I detected was not so much a theme as a mood—a mood of impatience—if we only had the answers to the issues of diagnosis, treatment, prevention and control now and not some time in the distant future. I applaud this mood of impatience because it stems from our common humanity and our desire as physicians to do the best we can for our patients. However, we must not impede progress with impatience. We must think matters through and time is required to verify, explain and exploit new knowledge. We must not move so quickly to implement new knowledge that unknown deleterious consequences outweigh potential benefits. We should have a healthy scepticism balanced by a brisk optimism.

Each of the technical papers gave a brilliant display of human ingenuity. It was Victor Hugo who said that there is no greater power in the world than the idea whose time has come. Surely this is so for tropical medicine. We can all perceive the opportunities that will flow from Dr Trager's experimental design to grow malaria, advances in physiology, immunology, pharmacology and, finally, prevention, treatment and control. Surely Dr Hitchings and Dr Gillies will exploit this *in vitro* system for biochemistry on the one hand and entomological dissection on the other.

Turning to schistosomiasis, Dr Chernin gave us the first model of the conference—warmth, water and poverty with a dash of snails and faeces, setting the stage for the lively discussion which followed.

I could not summarize here the discussions by Dr Smithers and Dr Butterworth on the immunology of schistosomiasis, or by Dr Cohen on malaria, but I would like to discuss the subject of immunology. I am not as pessimistic as some about the possible benefits of immunology in schistosomiasis and malaria control because I do have two points on the issue of immunology and schistosomiasis. I cannot believe that there is no immunity to schistosomiasis. It may be more complex than the immunity for the common bacterial infections or the immunity for influenza as we perceive it, but here I would remind you that immunity is often more complex that it seems. Immunity has two aspects. For a bacterial infection as simple as pneumococcal pneumonia it has, first of all, the immunity of *prevention*. There is also the other immunity responsible for the recovery processes that often occur in chronic infectious states of pyogenic infections. The immunity of prevention has a rather simple requirement for several micrograms of antibody per ml; the immunity of recovery from otitis media due to the streptococcus and the pneumococcus is much more complex.

I think that there is an analogy here of which we must not lose sight. Nine years ago when we started a programme on the gonococcus, I was told by workers in the field that there was no immunity to the gonococcus, even the textbooks said so. Of course there is immunity to gonococcus; it is a matter of dissecting it out and discovering what it is.

I applaud the comments of several contributors on the importance of the need for immunochemistry. We must persuade the immunobiologists to think in biochemical terms; to purify, obtain and put into a bottle the biological substances of significance that are isolated from the parasites.

If we are to direct our attention to the immunology of malaria and schistosomiasis, we shall need new generations of workers to study the antigens of significance and to use them in the immunological systems that will dissect out the mechanisms of immunity.

On the issue of a possible vaccine, I take heart from the new immunology. So far in vaccine development we have been concerned almost entirely with only one parameter—interference with the immune system at one point—vaccine in, antibody out. However, we are now dissecting out the nature of the immune system as an organ system, which in the future we may well manipulate just as we now manipulate the cardiovascular system for the treatment of heart failure, not only at one but at several points in the system. As a result, to continue the analogy, we now treat heart failure with digitalis to improve the pump; with diuretics to improve the output of fluid by the kidney. Similarly, there may be whole new avenues for manipulation of the immune systems which will be discovered through the new immunology.

Finally, in the treatment and control of these tropical diseases Dr Mahmoud told us of new opportunities for the use of new drugs by the application of epidemiological principles, and Dr Wright introduced many of us for the first time to the arcane world of mollusc biology. He recognized the importance of exploring the void in the role of snails as hosts for schistosomiasis, and that is certainly an exciting corner of comparative biology and biochemistry that should be examined.

We concluded with thoughtful guidance on the control of schistosomiasis and malaria. Dr Stauffer Lehman particularly discussed the interrelationships between disease control and economic development. He raised one important point, that we must start the health planners talking with those who shape development. That is, perhaps, an important role for the foundations to play. Finally, there has been much thoughtful and exciting discussion on future aims, and how we might achieve them.

Subject Index

A

ABH 154
ABO system 154
Adenosine
  deaminase 88
  kinase 88, 92
Ades crucians 105
Ades quadrimaculatus 100, 105, 210
Anaplasma 77
Anopheles 27, 65, 101, 103
  albimanus 102, 104, 107
  biological control 103–107
  DDT resistant 29–34, 37, 250, 253
  freeborni 103
  gambiae 101, 102, 103, 105, 213
  genetic control 37, 101–103
4—aminoquinilines 210
Aotus trivirgatus 50, 56, 77, 94
Ascaris 139

B

Babesia 77
Bacillus
  sphaericus 104
  thuringiensis 104
Bancroftian filariasis 214
Biomphalaria glabrata 194
Biomphalaria pfeifferi 118
Birth control 42
Bulinus africanus 198, 199, 200
Bulinus bavagi 199
Bulinus beccarii 199
Bulinus camerunensis 201
Bulinus cernicus 199
Bulinus forskali 199, 200, 201
Bulinus obtusispira 199
Bulinus senegalensis 199
Bulinus tropicus 199
Bulinus truncatus rohlfsi 118, 198, 199–202

C

Chloroquine 29, 52, 92
Chomismate 81
Coelomomyces 104
Co-enzyme A 79, 93

Co-enzyme Q 93
Colonial Research Service 17
Colonialism 14–18
  medical advances during 16
Culex 103
  control with *Hydra* 103
Cyclops 104

D

DDT 27–30, 36–37, 210
DNA synthesis 86, 90, 91
Diamino diphenyl sulphone 92
Diarrhoea
  childhood 9
Dieldrin 28, 29, 37, 101
Dihydrafolate 80, 84, 90, 91
Dihydropteroate 81, 82
2, 3—diphosphoglycerate 93

E

Effector mechanisms 157–164, 164–165
Eimeria 82
Environmental approaches
  to tropical infections 209–214
Eosinophils 159, 160, 161, 164, 165
  ECF-A 165
Epidemiology 209–214
Erythrocytes
  DNA 89
  duck 89, 90
  human 80
    for *P.falciparum* culture 51–52
  mouse 92
  nucleotides of 88
Escherichia coli 81,82

F

Family planning 40, 41
Fasciola hepatica 196
Fc receptor
  lymphocytes 159, 169
Filariasis 8, 16
Folates 79, 80
  biosynthesis 82, 89, 90
Forssman antigen 154

G

Glycolipids 154, 155
Granulocyte 162, 163
—mediated damage 163

H

Haematuria 173
Haemoglobin S 53
HCH 28, 29, 37
Health Services 225–226
  personnel training 226–227
Helisoma 194
Helminth
  density 174, 175
Hepatosplenomegaly 174, 181
Histocompatibility locus 154, 155, 158
  D 155
  I 155
  K 155
Host-parasite relationship 190–202
Hycanthone 121, 174, 177, 178, 182
  side effects 177, 178
Hydroxymethylpteridine 82

I

IgE 159
Ig G 156, 158, 159, 160
Immunology
  malaria 36
  vaccine
Insect growth-regulators 101, 107
Institutes 17, 18, 21
  Central research Institute at Kasauli
    16
  Haffkine Institute in Bombay 16
  King Institute at Guindy 16
  Medical Research Council Units 17, 18

K

Kala-Azar 16
Kato technique
  of stool examination 176–177
Koch, Robert 99
Kwashiorkor 230

L

Leishmaniasis 8
Leprosy 8, 237–238
Leukocytes 161
  Cytotoxicity 162, 165
Lewis antigens 154

M

Macaca
  fascicularis 70
  mulatta 70
  rhesus 141
Macrophaye
  activation 157, 159
Malaria 10, 16, 27–48, 238–240
  annual incidence 27, 29
  annual mortality 29
    infant 32
  chemotherapy 36, 91, 92, 211
  economic burden 39–41
  eradication 29–41
    cost of 34–35, 39—41
  immunology and 65–73
  life cycle 65–66, 75
  populations at risk 31–33
  vaccine 8, 36, 37, 54, 67–73
  vector control 99–108
    chemical 100–101, 192, 193
  vaccine 72
Malathion 29, 37
Malnutrition 16
  protein-energy 9, 12
Mansoni japonicum 113
Marisa cornuarietis 122, 194
Measles
  vaccination 8–9
Medical research
  third world programmes 228–229
  organization 229–230
Mermithids 105
Merozoites 36, 57, 66
Metarrhizium 104
Metrifonate 174
Metrizamide 161, 162
Mice
  athymic nude 140
Microsporida 103
Microsporidiae 196
Molluscs 190–202, 211, 212, 218
  biological control 193–197
  molluscicides 180–181, 190, 192, 193,
    198
  N-tritylmorphdine 200
  resistance 202
  parasites 195, 196
    microsporidian protozoa 196
    trematodes 195, 196
  predators 193
MNS 154

Monkeys
  douroncouli 69, 70
  rhesus 69, 71
Manolayers 100, 101
Mycobacterium leprae 237–238

N

National Institutes of Health
  Allergy and Infectious Diseases 246
  contribution to tropical medicine re-
    search 245–253
Nematode 105, 106
Niridazole 114, 177, 181, 201
Nosema evrytremae 196

O

Onchocerciasis 16
Oncomelania 122
Orotate 85, 86, 90
  phosphoribosyl transferase 85
Ouchterlong diffusion 136
Oxamniquine 174, 178–179, 182

P

P-aminobenzoic acid 80, 81
Pan American Health Office 40
Pantothenic acid 79
Parenchymal cell
  hepatic 65
Pigeons 81
Plague 16
Plasmodia
  metabolism 79–94
  vitamin requirements 93
Plasmodium berghi 66, 68, 80, 82, 84, 85,
  90, 92, 93
Plasmodium chabaudi 82, 84, 87, 91, 92
Plasmodium coatenyi 62
Plasmodium cynomolgi 71, 87
Plasmodium falciparum 29, 70, 80, 93, 239–
  240
  cultivation of 49–60
    additional strains 50
    large scale 54–60
  gametoocytes 53–54, 66
  morphology 57, 58
Plasmodium gallinaceum 80, 85, 90
Plasmodium knowlesi 68, 69, 70, 71, 80, 84
  85, 86, 90, 93

Plasmodium lophurae 58, 79, 84, 85, 86, 87,
  90
Plasmodium malariae 60
Plasmodium vinckei 84, 86
Plasmodium vivax 60, 68
Population
  control 42
  world
    increase 42
Praziquantel 121, 174, 180
Primaquine 80
Prontosil 80
Propoxur 37
Pteroate
  synthesis 82
Purine
  biosynthesis 87, 88
Pyrimethamine 86, 90, 91, 92
Pyrimidine
  biosynthosis 85, 86
Pyrethoids 100, 107
  biomesrethrin 100
  permethrin 100
  S-bioallethrin 100

R

Rabies 16
Research foundations
  role of 263–266

S

Sanitary engineers 119
Schistosoma
  Schistosomulum 157, 158, 159, 164, 165
    cellular effect mechanisms 158
    granulocyte mediated damage to 163
    leukocyte cytotoxocoty to 162
Schistosoma
  bovis 123, 199
  haematobium 115, 118, 122, 140, 176,
    177, 179, 180, 192, 197, 198, 199,
    200, 201, 202, 214, 219
  intercalatum 199, 201, 202
  japonicum 115, 121, 140, 141, 180, 214,
    219
  mansoni 115, 118, 122, 140, 141, 177,
    178, 180
  mattheei 123
  mekongi 219
  nasalis 123
  spindale 123

Schistosomiasis 8, 10, 16, 113–204, 210, 213
  cell biology and 153–166
  cercariae 157, 175, 196
  chemotherapy 173–183, 197, 218
    hycanthone 178, 182
    metrifonate 179–180
    newei agents 177–180
    niridazole 177, 181, 201
    oxamniquine 178–179, 182, 185
    praziquantel 180
    selective 181
  dynamics of infection 174–175
  egg 136, 137, 141, 165
    antigens 137, 140
    counting 175, 176–177, 178, 179, 180, 181, 182
    culture 143
    granuloma formation 137, 138, 139, 140
    morphology 201
    production 197
    proteins 201
  environmental approaches 217–219
  immunology and 134–144
    immunodiagnosis 136–138
    immunopathology 138–140
  life cycle 175
  Macaca rhesus 141, 143
  membrane 143
  molluscs 190–202
  prevalence of infection 116–117
  protective immunity 140–144
  St Lucia project 173, 182-183, 218
  tegument 142
Schizonts 57, 65
S-isobutyl adenosine 53
Snails *see* Molluscs
Sporozoites 36, 65–68, 87
  antibodies to 67
    CSP 67–68
    exoerythrocytic 65, 66
Sulphadiazine 92
Sulphanilamide 80, 81, 82
  sites of action 91

T

Tartar emetic 173

T-cell 157
  cytotoxocity 155, 157–158
  mediator 159
Thymidine kinase 84
Thymidylate 83, 90
  synthetase 91
Toxoplasma 82
Trematode 195–196
Trophozoites 57
Tropical medicine
  history of 14–20
Trypanosoma brucei 62
Trypanosomiasis 8, 16, 193

U

U.N.I.C.E.F. 40
Unikaryon pyriformis 196
United Nations Environment Programme 37

V

Vaccination programmes
  measles 8–9

W

World Health Organization 19, 22, 28, 30, 31, 33, 229, 231, 233–244, 257
  Executive Board 35
  Expert Committee on Bilharziasis 117
  Expert Committee on Malaria 34, 38, 41
    in Parasitic Disease 8, 116, 233, 251
    in Tropical Diseases 23, 251, 254, 260
  Programme in Expanded Immunization 9
  Research strengthening group 240–243
  Scientific working groups 234–238
  Special Programme for Research and Training
  strategies for the future 233–244

Y

Yaws 22
Yellow fever 16